Handbook of Pediatric Surgery

CW00571538

Chandrasen K. Sinha • Mark Davenport (Eds.)

Handbook of
Pediatric Surgery

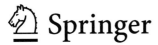 Springer

Chandrasen K. Sinha, MBBS (Honours)
MS MCh(Paediatric Surgery) FRCSEd
FRCSI FRCS(Paeds)
Department of Paediatric Surgery
Kings College Hospital
London
UK

Mark Davenport, ChM FRCS(Eng)
FRCPS(Glas) FRCS(Paeds)
Department of Paediatric Surgery
Kings College Hospital
London
UK

ISBN: 978-1-84882-131-6   e-ISBN: 978-1-84882-132-3
DOI: 10.1007/978-1-84882-132-3
Springer Dordrecht Heidelberg London New York

Library of Congress Control Number: 2010920242

© Springer-Verlag London Limited 2010
No part of this work may be reproduced, stored in a retrieval system, or transmitted in any form or by any means, electronic, mechanical, photocopying, microfilming, recording or otherwise, without written permission from the Publisher, with the exception of any material supplied specifically for the purpose of being entered and executed on a computer system, for exclusive use by the purchaser of the work.

Product liability: The publishers cannot guarantee the accuracy of any information about dosage and application contained in this book. In every individual case the user must check such information by consulting the relevant literature.

Printed on acid-free paper

Springer is part of Springer Science+Business Media (www.springer.com)

A good surgeon is a doctor who can operate and knows when not to operate!

Theodore Kocker (1841–1917)

It is usually a bad sign if the anesthetist is asking you if you are losing a lot of blood during a case – especially when you're not!

Michael Hoffman

It is usually a bad sign if there are three or more anesthetists are in the operating room at the same time and none of them is reading the newspaper!

Michael Hoffman

If an operation is difficult you are not doing it properly.
(This philosophy of perfection characterized the brilliant surgical career of Robert E. Gross, spanning 40 years from 1927 to 1967, at Harvard Medical School, Children's Hospital and Peter Bent Brigham Hospital.)

Be not the first to whom the new is tried, nor the last to lay the old aside

When technology is the master, the result is disaster.

Human mind works best like parachute – works best when open!

Chinese proverb

Hippocratic Oath

It was developed and written in Greek in the 4th century BC. It has been widely quoted by all graduates. It contains fundamental doctrine (do no harm, do not induce abortion or practice euthanasia), which is still pertinent today despite the gap of over two millennia.

I swear by Apollo, the healer, Asclepius, Hygieia, and Panacea, and I take to witness all the gods, all the goddesses, to keep according to my ability and my judgment, the following Oath and agreement:

To consider dear to me, as my parents, him who taught me this art; to live in common with him and, if necessary, to share my goods with him; To look upon his children as my own brothers, to teach them this art.

I will prescribe regimens for the good of my patients according to my ability and my judgment and never do harm to anyone.

I will not give a lethal drug to anyone if I am asked, nor will I advise such a plan; and similarly I will not give a woman a pessary to cause an abortion.

But I will preserve the purity of my life and my arts.

I will not cut for stone, even for patients in whom the disease is manifest; I will leave this operation to be performed by practitioners, specialists in this art.

In every house where I come I will enter only for the good of my patients, keeping myself far from all intentional ill-doing and all seduction and especially from the pleasures of love with women or with men, be they free or slaves.

All that may come to my knowledge in the exercise of my profession or in daily commerce with men, which ought not to be spread abroad, I will keep secret and will never reveal.

If I keep this oath faithfully, may I enjoy my life and practice my art, respected by all men and in all times; but if I swerve from it or violate it, may the reverse be my lot.

Preface

Pediatric surgery was a late starter, breaking off from general surgery only in the last 50 years or so. The surgeons who practised it were a small, often self-selected group who typically dedicated their surgical lives to the care of infants and children. That generation would often have been available round the clock, for most days of the week, simply because there was no-one else to do the job. When they did get out, to discuss cases and compare notes, it was often across borders to meet like-minded people from overseas or out-of town. Thus, like no other specialty, pediatric surgery is an international specialty, suffering much less from parochial constraints and much more receptive to ideas from the outside.

We hope this book helps all those involved in the surgical care of the child (including general practitioners, general surgeons, accident & emergency doctors, and pediatricians) to arrive at the correct decision and improve the quality of their care. However, any advice regarding further improvement of this book will be most welcomed. This book should also be helpful for trainees (especially pediatric surgery, general surgery, pediatric medicine and MEDICAL STUDENTS) preparing for various examinations.

The overriding aim and guiding principle of this book was to utilize capable surgeons as authors from across the world. They are the acclaimed experts in their field, and we thank them and have tried to capture their knowledge and essence within the constraints of a concise, general textbook.

Chandrasen K. Sinha
Mark Davenport
London, UK

Acknowledgements

We gratefully acknowledge the role of Melissa Morton, Denise Roland and Balasaraswathi Jayakumar (Springer), who were very encouraging and steered us smoothly through this turbulent journey.

CKS dedicates this work to Uma, Leena, Ankit, and Akarsh. MD acknowledges the patience and forbearance of his family and dedicates this work, as always, to Keren and Georgina.

Contents

Part V Principles of Pediatric Urology

Part VI Surgery of the Liver, Pancreas and Bile Ducts

Contributors

Meena Agrawal
Paediatric Surgery Department,
Children's Hospital at University
Hospital Lewisham, London, UK
Evelina Children's Hospital,
Guy's and St Thomas' Hospital NHS
Foundation Trust, London, UK

Ravindra Bhat
Child Health Department,
Kings College Hospital, London, UK

Tariq Burki
Paediatric Surgery Department,
Bristol Children's Hospital, Bristol, UK

Robert Carachi
Surgical Paediatrics Department,
University of Glasgow,
Royal Hospital for Sick Children,
Glasgow, UK

Lorna Cook
Department of Paediatric Surgery,
Kings College Hospital, London, UK

Arnold G. Coran
Section of Pediatric Surgery,
C.S. Mott Children's Hospital,
University of Michigan Health System,
Ann Arbor, MI, USA

Denis A. Cozzi
Pediatric Surgery Unit,
Sapienza University of Rome
and Policlinico Umberto I,
Rome, Italy

Joseph I. Curry
Paediatric Surgery Department,
Great Ormond Street Children's Hospital,
London, UK

Mark Davenport
Paediatric Surgery Department,
Kings College Hospital, London, UK

Emmanuel M.L. Endeley
Paediatric A&E,
Buckinghamshire Hospitals – Wycombe
and Mandeville Hospitals,
Mandeville, UK

Ciro Esposito
Pediatrics Department,
"Federico II" University of Naples,
Naples, Italy

Ross M. Fisher
Department of Paediatric Surgery,
The Children's Hospital,
Leicester Royal Infirmary,
Leicester, UK

Ajay N. Gangopadhyay
Department of Pediatric Surgery,
Institute of Medical Sciences, BHU,
Varanasi, India

Milan Gopal
Paediatric Surgery Department,
Royal Victoria Infirmary,
Newcastle Upon Tyne, UK

Dinesh K. Gupta
Paediatric Surgery Department,
Institute of Medical Sciences,
Varanasi, India

Devendra K. Gupta
Department of Pediatric Surgery,
All India Institute of Medical Sciences,
New Delhi, India

Girish Gupte
Liver Unit,
Birmingham Children's Hospital,
Birmingham, UK

Nadeem Haider
Paediatric Surgery Department,
Leeds General Infirmary, Leeds, UK

Rupert Hinds
Department of Paediatrics,
Monash Medical Centre, Melbourne,
Australia

John M. Hutson
Department of Paediatrics,
University of Melbourne,
Melbourne, Australia
Urology Department,
Royal Children's Hospital,
Melbourne, Australia

Saidul Islam
Paediatric Surgery Department,
Great Ormond Street
Hospital for Children,
London, UK

Eric B. Jelin
Department of Surgery, Division of Pediatric
Surgery/Fetal Treatment Center,
University of California at San Francisco,
San Francisco, CA, USA

Masih A. Kader
Paediatric Surgery Department,
University Hospital Lewisham,
London, UK

Jonathan S. Karpelowsky
Paediatric Surgery,
University of Cape Town,
Red Cross War Memorial
Children's Hospital,
Cape Town, South Africa

Dorothy Iwagba Kufeji
Department of Paediatric Surgery,
Evelina Children's Hospital,
St Thomas' Hospital, London, UK

Vijai Kumar
Paediatric Surgery Department,
Institute of Medical Sciences,
Banaras Hindu University,
Varanasi, UP, India

Pablo Laje
Department of Pediatric Surgery,
The Children's Hospital of Philadelphia,
Philadelphia, PA, USA

Hanmin Lee
Department of Surgery,
Division of Pediatric
Surgery/Fetal Treatment Center,
University of California at San Francisco,
San Francisco, CA, USA

Marc A. Levitt
Colorectal Centre, Cincinnati Children's
Hospital, USA

Erica Makin
Paediatric Surgery Department,
King's College Hospital,
London, UK

Marcelo Martinez-Ferro
Department of Pediatric Surgery,
Fundación Hospitalaria de Niños,
Buenos Aires, Argentina

Prema A. Menon
Pediatric Surgery Department, Post
Graduate Institute of Medical Education
and Research, Chandigarh, India

Alastair J.W. Millar
Department of Paediatric Surgery, Red Cross
War Memorial Children's Hospital, Health
Sciences Faculty, University of Cape
Town, Cape Town, South Africa

Vibhash C. Mishra
Urology Department,
Wexham Park Hospital, Slough, UK

Devesh Misra
Paediatric Surgery Department,
Royal London Hospital,
London, UK

Bharat More
Paediatric Urology Department,
Great Ormond Street Hospital,
London, UK

Hanif G. Motiwala
Urology Department,
Wexham Park Hospital,
Slough, UK

Vadivelam Murthy
Department of Neonatology,
Kings College Hospital,
London, UK

Imran Mushtaq
Paediatric Urology,
Great Ormond Street Hospital,
Great Ormond Street, London, UK

Guy Nicholls
Paediatric Surgery Department, Bristol
Children's Hospital, Bristol, UK

George Ninan
Paediatric Surgery Department,
Leicester Royal Infirmary, Leicester, UK

Anindya Niyogi
Paediatric Surgery Department,
Chelsea and Westminster Hospital,
London, UK

Ike L. Njere
Department of Paediatric Surgery,
University Hospital Lewisham,
London, UK

Shawqui Nour
Paediatric Surgery Department,
University Hospitals of
Leicester NHS Trust,
Leicester Royal Infirmary,
Leicester, UK

Anand Pandey
Department of Paediatric Surgery,
Chhatrapati Shahuji Maharaj
Medical University,
Lucknow, UP, India

Christopher J. Parsons
Paediatric Surgery Department,
King's College Hospital, London, UK

Ramnik V. Patel
Department of Paediatric Surgery,
Sheffield Children's Hospital,
London, UK

Shailesh B. Patel
Department of Paediatric Surgery,
King's College Hospital, London, UK

Nitin Patwardhan
Paediatric Surgery Department,
Bristol Children's Hospital, Bristol, UK

Alberto Peña
Department of Pediatric Surgery,
Cincinnati Children's Hospital,
University of Cincinnati,
Cincinnati, OH, USA

Abid Q. Qazi
Paediatric Surgery Department,
Sheffield Children's Hospital,
Sheffield, UK

Ashok Rajimwale
Paediatric Surgery Department, Leicester
Royal Infirmary, Leicester, UK

Katragadda L.N. Rao
Pediatric Surgery,
Post Graduate Institute of Medical
Education and Research,
Advanced Pediatrics Centre,
Chandigarh, India

Steven S. Rothenberg
Pediatric Surgery Department,
Rocky Mountain Hospital for Children,
Denver, CO, USA

V. Scott
Paediatric Surgery Department,
Leicester Royal Infirmary,
Leicester, UK

S.P. Sharma
Department of Pediatric Surgery,
Institute of Medical Sciences,
Banaras Hindu University,
Varanasi, UP, India

Chandrasen K. Sinha
Paediatric Surgery Department,
King's College Hospital,
London, UK

Lewis Spitz
Emeritus Nuffield Professor
of Paediatric Surgery,
Institute of Child Health,
London, UK

Roly Squire
Paediatric Surgery Department,
Leeds Teaching Hospitals,
St James' University Hospital,
Leeds, UK

Shamshad H.S. Syed
Paediatric Surgery Department,
Chelsea and Westminster Hospital,
London, UK

Giorgia Totonelli
Pediatric Surgery Unit,
Sapienza University of Rome,
Rome, Italy

Juan A. Tovar
Department of Pediatric Surgery,
Hospital Universitario La Paz,
Madrid, Spain

Vijai D. Upadhyaya
Department of Surgery,
MGM Medical College,
Indore, India

Benno Ure
Department of Pediatric Surgery,
Medical School Hannover,
Hannover, Germany

Jenny Walker
Paediatric Surgery Department,
Sheffield Children's Hospital,
Sheffield, UK

Harry C. Ward
Pacdiatric Surgery Department,
Barts and the London NHS Trust,
Royal London Hospital,
London, UK

Jean W.L. Wong
Paediatric Surgery Department,
University Hospital Lewisham,
London, UK

Mark Woodward
Paediatric Surgery Department,
Bristol Children's Hospital,
Bristol, UK

Atsuyuki Yamataka
Pediatric Surgery and Urogenital Surgery,
Juntendo University School of Medicine,
Bunkyo-ku, Tokyo, Japan

Suzanne M. Yoder
Pediatric Surgery Department,
The Rocky Mountain
Hospital for Children,
Denver, CO, USA

Part I

Milestones in Pediatric Surgery

Mark Davenport

Circumcision has been illustrated among the petroglyphs of the ancient Egyptians and is recorded as a mark of the covenant between God and Abraham in Genesis (Ch.17 verse 10) (Fig. 1.1.1).

Classical physicians such as Hippocrates (460–370 BC) have described surgical intervention, including specific treatment for long-bone fractures. The Roman physician Aulus Celsus, in his book "De Medicina" (~30 AD), has described relatively complex surgery for cleft palate and tonsillectomy as part of a wider manual for surgical and medical therapies.

Western medicine declined with the fall of the Western Roman empire, but the medical flame was kept alive in the Arab world by Kitab at Tasrif (also known as Albucasis), in Cordoba, Spain, who published an encyclopedia of medicine, in which the subjects were cleft palate, hydrocephalus, and hypospadias. A version of this widely known text was illustrated by Serafeddin Subuncuoglu, a Turkish physician, in 1465 and circulated widely as an atlas throughout the Middle East and Ottoman empire.

The first detailed textbook dedicated to children's conditions is credited to the Swiss surgeon Felix Wurtz, who published it in 1563.

The medical separation between the young and old was first made clear in the 19th century by the establishment of the great children's hospitals across the world, with the first being in Paris (Hopital des infant Malades) in 1802, followed some years later by London (Great Ormond Street) in 1852, and Boston (Boston Children's Hospital) in North America in 1882.

Some of the first widely-read publications dealing specifically with children's ailments and congenital malformations also appeared in this century. For instance, "A Practical Treatise of Children" by Coley was published in 1846 in London. "The Surgical Diseases of Children" by John Cooper Forester from Guys Hospital, London, published in 1860, described both ether and chloroform anesthesia and the surgical treatment of imperforate anus.

Special and separate care of infants probably began in Paris during the 1870s with the introduction of incubators, the concept of sterilization of feeding bottles, and others.

M. Davenport
Paediatric Surgery Department, Kings College Hospital, London, UK

C. K. Sinha and M. Davenport (eds.), *Handbook of Pediatric Surgery*,
DOI: 10.1007/978-1-84882-132-3_1.1, © Springer-Verlag London Limited 2010

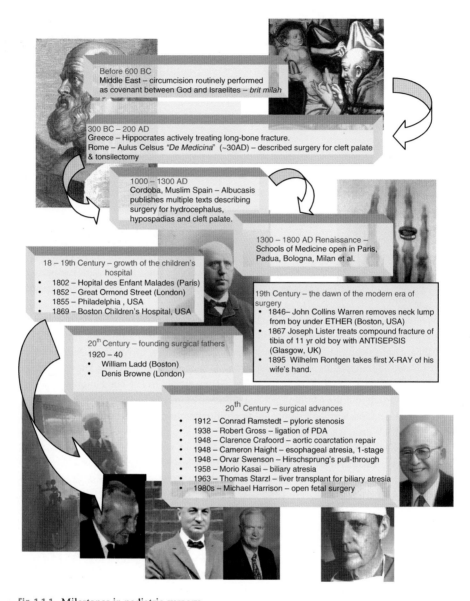

Before 600 BC
Middle East – circumcision routinely performed as covenant between God and Israelites – *brit milah*

300 BC – 200 AD
Greece – Hippocrates actively treating long-bone fracture.
Rome – Aulus Celsus *"De Medicina"* (~30AD) – described surgery for cleft palate & tonsilectomy

1000 – 1300 AD
Cordoba, Muslim Spain – Albucasis publishes multiple texts describing surgery for hydrocephalus, hypospadias and cleft palate.

1300 – 1800 AD Renaissance –
Schools of Medicine open in Paris, Padua, Bologna, Milan et al.

18 – 19th Century – growth of the children's hospital
- 1802 – Hopital des Enfant Malades (Paris)
- 1852 – Great Ormond Street (London)
- 1855 – Philadelphia , USA
- 1869 – Boston Children's Hospital, USA

19th Century – the dawn of the modern era of surgery
- 1846– John Collins Warren removes neck lump from boy under ETHER (Boston, USA)
- 1867 Joseph Lister treats compound fracture of tibia of 11 yr old boy with ANTISEPSIS (Glasgow, UK)
- 1895 Wilhelm Rontgen takes first X-RAY of his wife's hand.

20th Century – founding surgical fathers
1920 – 40
- William Ladd (Boston)
- Denis Browne (London)

20th Century – surgical advances
- 1912 – Conrad Ramstedt – pyloric stenosis
- 1938 – Robert Gross – ligation of PDA
- 1948 – Clarence Crafoord – aortic coarctation repair
- 1948 – Cameron Haight – esophageal atresia, 1-stage
- 1948 – Orvar Swenson – Hirschsprung's pull-through
- 1958 – Morio Kasai – biliary atresia
- 1963 – Thomas Starzl – liver transplant for biliary atresia
- 1980s – Michael Harrison – open fetal surgery

Fig. 1.1.1 Milestones in pediatric surgery

Towards the end of this century, continental Europe appeared to be the area where most of the advances were emerging from and most of the radical physicians were located. Harald Hirschsprung appeared omnipresent describing not only the disease to bear his name but also the pathology and features of pyloric stenosis and enema reduction of intussusception.

The first half of the twentieth century, while devastated by world war and leaving most continental European cities desolate bequeathed something like modern-day surgical practice. This was founded on effective safe anesthesia with basic monitoring of vital signs and the ability to change physiology with intravenous blood and fluids; with operations carried out by trained competent specialist surgeons, experienced in visceral operations, or problems of soft-tissue and bone reconstruction. Life-threatening post-operative bacterial infection no longer stalked the wards, limited by antisepsis and treated with antibiotic.

In the interwar period the "founding fathers" of, at least Western, children's surgery practiced. In the USA, William Ladd and his successor Robert Gross were, for the first time, pediatric surgeons rather than interested bystanders. The influential "Abdominal Surgery of Infancy and Childhood" written by Robert Gross was first published in 1941. In England, Denis-Browne (Great Ormond Street 1928–1957), an Australian by birth was the first surgeon to concentrate solely on children, although he clearly did not believe in specialization-publishing innovative techniques in all sorts of fields. He became the first president of the British Association of Pediatric Surgeons in 1953 – the first real international organization devoted to pediatric surgery. Their equivalents in Europe included Pepe Boix-Ochea in Barcelona, Theodor Ehrenpreis in Stockholm, David Vervat in Rotterdam, Fritz Rehbein in Bremen, Bernard Duhamel in Paris, Mattai Sulumma in Helsinki, and farther afield Chakraborty and Raman Nair in India, Douglas Stephens in Australia, and Osamu Wakabayashi and Keijiro Suruga in Japan.

Part II

Principles of Surgical Science

Fluids, Electrolytes, and Dehydration

2.1

Mark Davenport and S. H. S. Syed

Appreciation of basic physiology is the key to safe preoperative resusciation enabling *appropriate* surgery. *Administration* of *appropriate* postoperative fluid regimens ensures *optimal* outcome.

2.1.1
Normal Fluid Physiology

Most of us are made up predominantly of water.

- ~60% of body weight (BW) i.e. *total body water ~42 L in 70 kg man.*

This is divisible into two compartments:
  (a) *Intracellular* (~40% BW) – high K^+, high [proteins]$^-$. Regulated by active Na^+/K^+ pump at cell membrane.
  (b) *Extracellular* (~20% BW) – high Na^+, high Cl^-

- *Plasma* – Intravascular osmotic pressure maintained by albumin, and regulated by capillary membrane (i.e., Starling's Law – oncotic pressure and pore size).
- *Lymph*
- *Connective tissue, bone water, CSF*, etc .
- *Interstitial* (~5%)

N.B. transcellular compartment – includes the mythical *third-space* (<2%).
  (*NB circulating blood volume* ($\equiv 65$ *mL/kg*) *is made up of not only plasma but red cell mass as well.*)

M. Davenport (✉)
Paediatric Surgery Department, Kings College Hospital, London, UK

C. K. Sinha and M. Davenport (eds.), *Handbook of Pediatric Surgery*,
DOI: 10.1007/978-1-84882-132-3_2.1, © Springer-Verlag London Limited 2010

2.1.2
Age-Related Changes

- ↑ Total body water (80% in neonate vs. 60% in adult)
- ↑ ECF → ICF (almost parity in newborn vs. 3:1 in adult)
- ↑ Surface area/body mass ratio

2.1.3
Normal Fluid and Electrolyte Requirements

In general, normal neonatal fluid prescription depends on (a) body weight and (b) day of life (Tables 2.1.1 and 2.1.2).

Basic prescription is 100 mL/Kg/day (up to 10 kg). *(Beyond neonatal period.)*

Table 2.1.1   Estimated fluid requirements in childhood

	Day of life	ml/kg/day
Premature infant	1st	60–150
	2nd	70–150
	3rd	90–180
	>3rd	Up to 200
Term infant	1st	60–80
	2nd	80–100
	3rd	100–140
	>3rd	Up to 160
Child >4 weeks of age, ≤10 kg	*100*	
Child 10–20 kg	1 L + 50 mL/kg/day for each kg over 10	
Child >20 kg	1.5 L + 20 mL/kg/day for each kg over 20	

Table 2.1.2   Sample fluid requirements (by body weight)

Body weight	Calories required (kcal/day)	Maintenance (mL/day)	Maintenance (mL/h)
3	300	300	12
5	500	500	20
10	1,000	1,000	40
20	1,500	1,500	60
45	2,000	2,000	80
70	2,500	2,500	100

2.1.4
Insensible Fluid Loss

This is an obligate fluid loss, largely from radiation and evaporation related to body surface area and the work of breathing.

$$\sim 300 \text{ mL/m}^2/\text{day}$$

$$\text{Body surface area (m}^2) = \sqrt{\frac{weight(kg) \times height(m)}{3,600}}$$

2.1.5
Postoperative Fluid Regimens

The composition (if not the volume) of postoperative maintenance fluid prescription has recently come under scrutiny (at least in the UK), and is changing from one using predominantly low or no saline solutions (e.g., 5% dextrose, 4% dextrose/0.18% saline, described wrongly as "hypotonic") to using high saline solutions (i.e., 0.9% saline, described as "isotonic"), on the basis that the former regimens lead to hyponatremia, whereas use of the latter seldom leads to hypernatremia (although it gives far more than normal daily requirement of Na Cl – Table 2.1.3).

Further, because of the metabolic response to surgery (see Chap. 2.2), there is "inappropriate" secretion of ADH, and many units will prescribe only two-thirds of the calculated maintenance volume in the first 24–48 h.

Finally, consider ongoing losses from drains, NG tubes, stomas, and fistulas (Table 2.1.4). In principle, replace *Like with Like.* In most cases, this is a ml. for ml. replacement with an isotonic (0.9%) saline solution (±20 mmol of K^+/L).

Table 2.1.3 Sample electrolyte requirements (by body weight)

	Na (mmol/kg)	K (mmol/kg)
Neonate (preterm)	4–6	2–3
Neonate (term) – 10 kg	3	2
10–20 kg	1–2	1–2
20–Adult	1–2	1

Table 2.1.4 Electrolyte content of gastrointestinal secretions

Secretion	Na^+ (mmol/L)	K^+ (mmol/L)	Cl^- (mmol/L)	HCO_3^- (mmol/L)
Saliva	44	20	40	–
Gastric	20–120[a]	10	100	–
Bile	140	5	100	40
Pancreas	140	5	70	70–110
Small intestine	110–120	5–10	90–130	20–40

[a]Depends on pH and therefore reciprocal with H^+

Table 2.1.5 illustrates composition of commonly available intravenous fluids.

_____

2.1.6
Dehydration

> **Dehydration** may be thought of as contraction in predominantly the **ECF**
> **compartment** because of the relative loss of fluids and sodium.
> Is referred to in terms of **% body weight loss**

One principal cause of dehydration is excess intestinal losses due to diarrheal illness, and it is a cause of death in >1.5 million children/year. It is important that a pediatric surgeon has a basic working knowledge of diarrheal illness, as it is so common both in the community (and therefore on the ward).

Infective Causes

- Viruses
  - Rotavirus
  - Calcivirus (incl Norovirus)
  - Astrovirus
  - Adenovirus
- Bacteria
  - *Campylobacter spp*
  - *Salmonella spp*
  - *E. coli*
  - *Clostridium difficle*
  - *Shigella spp*
- Protozoa
  - *Giardia lamblia*
  - *Crypotosporidium*
  - *Entamoeba histolytica*

Surgical Causes

- Intestinal obstruction
- Appendicitis
- Intussusception
- Fistula losses (also stomas)

Table 2.1.5 Intravenous and oral rehydration solutions

	Osmolarity (mOsm/L)	Glucose (mmol/L)	Na (mmol/L)	Cl	K	HCO$_3$	Notes
Intravenous solutions (crystalloid)							
Lactated Ringer's[1]	273	–	130	110	4	25	Lactate Ca^{2+}
Hartmann's[2]	278	–	131	111	5	29	Lactate, Ca^{2+}
0.9% NaCl "normal saline"	308	–	154	154	–	–	
Dextrose (5%)	252	300	–	–	–	–	5 g/L=170 kcal/L
D5+0.45% NaCl	454	300	77	77	–	–	
D4+0.18% NaCl	284	240	30	30	–	–	Not available in UK
Intravenous solutions (Colloids)							
Haemaccel®	293	–	145	145	5	–	Gelatin (35 g)
Gelofusine®	308	–	154	125	<0.4	–	Gelatin (40 g)
Hetastarch	310	–	154	154	–	–	Starch (60 g)
Pentastarch	326	–	154	154	–	–	Starch (100 g)
Albumin (4.5%)	300	–	<160	136	<2	–	
Oral rehydration solutions							
WHO–ORS	330	110	90	80	20	30	
Pedialyte®	270	140	45	35	20	30	
Dioralyte®		90	60	60	20		Common in UK
Electrolade®		111	50	40	20		

(N.B. CHO=3.4 kcal/g, compared with fat 9 kcal/g)

[1]Sydney Ringer (1836–1910) – British physiologist and physician at University College, London.

[2]Alexis Hartmann (1898–1964) – American pediatrician, modified original Ringer solution by the addition of lactate to treat acidosis in children.

2.1.7
Management

In general, the treatment aims to restore normal fluid and electrolyte balance safely without precipitating complications (e.g., hypernatremic convulsions). The key is to recognize the degree of dehydration (expressed in terms of % body weight loss – i.e., 5% of a 20-kg child implies a deficit of 1,000 mLs. of fluid) (Table 2.1.6) and then the type as defined by the plasma sodium level (Table 2.1.7).

Aim for rehydration within 12–24 h, *unless* hypernatremia is documented (Na >150 mmol/L), where the period should be lengthened to ~36–48 h. In general, oral rehydration solutions (Tables 2.1.5 and 2.1.6) should be used whenever possible (may be defined as presence of a functioning GI tract). Intravenous resuscitation may well be required for more severe episodes of dehydration, particularly where there is a shock-like state and fall in CBV.

Table 2.1.6 WHO classification of dehydration

	No dehydration	Mild – moderate	Severe
Adult	*<3%*	*3–9%*	*>9%*
Child	*5%*	*10%*	*15%*
Mental status	Alert	Restless, listless	Lethargic, comatose
Thirst	Normal	Thirsty	Unable to drink
CVS	Normal pulse/BP	Tachycardia, CRT >2 s	Tachy/brady, CRT >>2 s
Respiratory	Normal	Rate	Inc rate and volume
Extremities	Normal	Cool	Cold, mottled
Mucous membranes	Moist	Dry	Dry
Skin fold	Immediate recoil	Delayed (>2 s)	>2 s
Urine output	Normal	Diminished	Absent
Management of nonsurgical dehydration			
	Encourage normal diet and fluids	*ORS –* 30–80 mL/h Consider via NG tube if failing.	*IV initially* e.g., 20 mL/kg NaCl (0.9%)
		REASSESS	
CRT capillary refill time			
ORS – oral rehydration solution (see Table 2.1.5)			

Table 2.1.7 Types of dehydration

Isotonic	130–150 mmol/L
Hypotonic	<130 mmol/L
Hypertonic	>150 mmol/L

2.1.8
Specific Electrolyte Problems

2.1.8.1
Potassium

(*Normal 3.5–5.5 mmol/L – ↑ variability in neonates*)
Hyperkalemia 5.5 mmol/L – NB-beware factitious result due to hemolysis

- Surgical Causes
  — Dehydration, renal failure, transfusion, tumor lysis syndrome, rhabdomyolysis.
- Signs
  — ECG: tall "tented" T waves, ↑ PR interval ↑QRS complex duration
- *Treatment*
- Calcium resonium (oral or rectal) – cation exchange resin
- Calcium gluconate (100 mg/kg, IV if >7 mmol/L) – myocardial membrane stabilization
- Dextrose/Insulin IV
- Salbutamol (IV or inhaled)

2.1.8.2
Hypokalemia

- Surgical Causes
  — Fistula, dehydration. Aldosterone-secreting tumors.
- Signs
  — ECG: (less obvious changes) flat T waves, U waves, AV conduction defects.
- *Treatment*
  (a) Slow ↑K+replacement (do not exceed KCl 0.51 mmol/kg/h IV, unless on ECG monitor)

2.1.8.3
Calcium

(Normal total 2.0–2.5 mmol/L ≡ 8.5–10.2 mg/dL)
(Normal ionized 1.0–1.25 mmol/L ≡ 4–5 mg/dL)
   Most is stored and relatively fixed in bone. Serum calcium is made up of different components (bound to albumin (~40%) and complexed with bicarbonate (<10%) and free ions (~50%)). Ionized calcium is the active part and is <1% of total. Calcium balance is regulated by parathormone and acid/base balance.

2.1.8.4
Hypocalcemia (always check magnesium levels additionally)

Usually neonates

- Surgical causes
    - Chronic renal failure (e.g., PUV), postthyroidectomy, pancreatitis, malabsorption, Di George syndrome, and CHARGE syndrome.
- Signs – tetany, i.e., muscle irritability.
    - Chvostek[3] – twitching of facial muscles by tapping facial (VII) nerve.
    - Trousseau[4] – inflation of BP cuff causes carpal spasm (*main d'accoucheur* – hand of the obstetrician/deliverer)
- *Treatment*
    - Calcium (10%) gluconate (IV)
    - Calcium supplements (oral)
    - Vitamin D metabolites

   Hypercalcemia
Usually children

- Surgical causes
    - MEN (types I, II), Chronic renal failure, parathyroid tumors, hyperthyroidism, rhabdomyosarcoma, neuroblastoma, metastatic disease.
- Signs
    - *"Stones, Bones, Psychic groans, Abdominal moans"*, i.e., renal calculi, osteoporosis, bone cysts, psychiatric manifestations, weakness, confusions, pancreatitis, peptic ulcers.
- *Treatment*
    - Saline rehydration (with furosemide diuresis)
    - Calcitonin
    - Bisphosphonates, etc.

---

[3]Frantisek Chvostek (1835–1884), Austrian physician.
[4]Armand Trousseau (1801–1867) – French physician.

2.1.9
Acid–Base Imbalance

2.1.9.1
Concepts

Definition –	Acid – H^+ donor	Base – H^+ acceptor
	Cation is a +ve ion	Anion is a –ve ion

$$pH = -log_{10}[H^+]$$

- Neutral pH at 37°C = 6.8
- Normal blood pH = 7.4 ($\equiv H^+ = 40$ nmol/L) (range 7.2–7.6)
- Normal intracellular pH = 7.0 ($H^+ = 100$ nmol/L)

Anion gap – "difference" between summated anions and cations – there is always more of the latter owing to unmeasured anions (e.g., [protein⁻]). An elevated anion gap is usually due to an increase in [lactate⁻], [butyrate⁻] and others.

Normal is up to 30 mmol/L (but depends on what is being measured),

Key Equations

Henderson[5] equation

$$[H^+] + [HCO_3^-] \leftrightarrow [H_2CO_3] \leftrightarrow [CO_2] + [H_2O]$$

Henderson–Hasslebalch[6] equation

$$pH = pK + log \frac{[HCO_3^-]}{[CO_2]}$$

2.1.10
Base Excess (or Deficit)

Definition – "the quantity of base (acid) required to return the plasma in vitro to a normal pH under standard conditions."

Normal body equilibration is maintained by a series of buffer systems.

(a) Chemical – bicarbonate, phosphate, protein
(b) Respiratory – elimination of CO_2
(c) Renal – elimination or retention of bicarbonate

---

[5]Lawrence J. Hendersen (1878–1942) American biochemist.
[6]Karl A. Hasslebalch (1874–1962) Danish chemist.

2.1.11
Abnormal Acid–Base States

Metabolic Acidosis $\uparrow [H^+] \downarrow [HCO_3^-] \downarrow [BE]$

Multiplicity of causes, but can be subdivided on the basis of change in anion gap. Thus, the subdivisions are:

- Normal anion gap
  - Loss of base
    — Renal loss of bicarbonate in renal tubular acidosis.
    — Fistula loss of bicarbonate (pancreatic)
- Increased anion gap
  — Tissue hypoxia – anerobic metabolism $\uparrow [lactate^-] + \uparrow [H^+]$
  — Ketoacidosis – diabetic

2.1.11.1
Treatment

(a) Correct the underlying problem
(b) Sodium bicarbonate (4.2% IV) infused over 30 min.
(c) Ensure ventilation adequate to excrete excess CO_2

N.B. give half calculated dose – repeat blood gas

Metabolic Alkalosis $\downarrow [H^+] \uparrow [HCO_3^-] \uparrow [BE]$

This is much less common in pediatric practice. Causes include

- Loss of acid
  — Vomiting of HCl – e.g., pyloric stenosis
  — Loss of acid stools – chronic diarrhea
- Loss of chloride
  — Chronic use of diuretics
- Renal perfusion impairment with changes in renin/aldosterone axis.
  — Dehydration, cirrhosis
- Hypokalemia – causes $\uparrow$hydrogen ion exchange in kidney
- Contraction alkalosis – as the body fluids are "alkali," dehydration causes a fall in total body water and $\uparrow$concentration of electrolytes, hence $\uparrow$pH.

2.1.11.2 Treatment

(a) Treat the underlying cause
(b) Often simple correction of fluid and saline deficit will allow restoration of homeostasis.

Base deficit $(mmol/L) \times$ body weight $(kg) \times 0.3 = mmol/L$ of HCO_3 required for full correction

Further Readings

1. Holliday MA, Ray PE, Friedman AL (2007) Fluid therapy for children: facts, fashions and questions. Arch Dis Child 92:546–50
2. Word Health Organisation (2005) The treatment of diarrhoea: a manual for physicians and other senior health workers. Geneva, Switzerland, 4th revision

Metabolic Response to Injury and Sepsis

2.2

Mark Davenport

2.2.1
Metabolic Response to Injury

There is a programmed set of neuro-hormonal responses in response to "injury" which results in profound metabolic change.

The early period can be divided into:

- "Ebb" (↓ metabolic rate) phase
- "Flow" (↑ metabolic rate) phase

This period is characterized by Na and water retention together with oliguria with intense catabolism to provide substrate (glucose). There is then a later *anabolic recovery and healing phase* characterized by diuresis of excess sodium and water.

2.2.2
Early (Ebb and Flow)

1. ADH release (from hypothalamus)
   (a) ↑ Absorption of water (at distal convoluted tubule)
   (b) Oliguria (concentrated)
2. Renin – angiotensin – aldosterone release (from adrenal cortex)
   (a) ↑ Na^+ ↓K^+ reabsorption
3. Adrenaline/noradrenaline release (from adrenal medulla)
   (a) ↑ Glucose, ↑glycogenolysis
   (b) ↑ Protein breakdown
   (c) ↑ Lipolysis

M. Davenport
Paediatric Surgery Department, Kings College Hospital, London, UK

C. K. Sinha and M. Davenport (eds.), *Handbook of Pediatric Surgery*,
DOI: 10.1007/978-1-84882-132-3_2.2, © Springer-Verlag London Limited 2010

4. Glucocorticoids (via ACTH)
   (a) ↑ Glucose, ↑ protein breakdown, ↑ lipolysis, ↑glycogenolysis
   (b) ↑ Acute phase proteins (from liver[via IL-6 release]), e.g., C-reactive protein, fibrinogen, haptoglobin, etc.

2.2.3
Late

(1) ↑ Insulin release (although still ↑ glucose)
(2) ↑ Growth hormone, 17-ketosteroids, etc.

2.2.4
Tissue Response to Injury

The local tissue response to injury is orchestrated by release of cytokines from monocytes, macrophages, and T cells. This can have both local (paracrine) and systemic effects and can be divided into two basic groups.

- *Pro-inflammtory cytokines*
  — TNF-α (↑ temperature, tachycardia); IL-1β; IL-2; IL-6 (regulates liver production of acute phase proteins); IL-8 and interferon-γ
- *Anti-inflammatory cytokines*
  — IL-1ra, IL-4, IL-10, IL-12, IL-13, TGF-β

2.2.5
Systemic Inflammatory Response syndrome (SIRS)

SIRS can be diagnosed (in adults/older children when two or more of the following are present:

- Heart rate >90 beats per minute
- Temperature <36 or >38°C (>38.5°C in children)
- Tachypnea (>20 bpm or, on blood gas, a $PaCO_2$ <4.3 kPa (32 mmHg))
- White blood cell count (<4 or $>12 \times 10^9$/L)

Various modifications have been made with reference to pediatric age groups (Table 2.2.1).

Table 2.2.1 Pediatric definitions of SRS (modified from Goldstein et al.)

Age	Heart rate		Respiratory rate (bpm)	WBC ($\times 10^9$/L)	BP (systolic)
	Brady	Tachy			
0–1 week	<100	>180	>50	>34	<65
1 week to 1 month	<100	>180	>40	>19 <5	<75
1 month to 1 year	<90	>180	>34	>17 <5	<100
2–5 years	–	>140	>22	>15 <6	<94
6–12 years	–	>130	>18	>13 <4	<104
13–18 years	–	>110	>14	>11 <4	<117

2.2.6
Multiple Organ Dysfunction Syndrome (MODS)

Definition – "altered organ function (>2 systems) in acute illness such that intervention is needed."

Possibly caused by ↓ intestinal mucosal permeability to Gram –ve organisms, ↑ circulating endotoxin and ↓ liver function.

Again in pediatric practice various criteria have been submitted (e.g., liver "failure" is a bilirubin >68 μmol/L).

2.2.7
Differences with Age

There are differences in neonates although much less study has been performed. In principle, the above sequence holds, although first-day neonates may have higher endogenous opioids blunting this response to injury.

Further Reading

1. Pierro A (2002) Metabolism and nutrition in the surgical neonate. J Pediatr Surg 37:811–822
2. Goldstein B et al (2005) International pediatric consensus conference: definitions for sepsis and organ dysfunction in children. Pediatr Crit Care Med 6:2-8

Shock

2.3

Mark Davenport

> Shock may be thought of as contraction in predominantly the *intravascular compartment* due to blood loss, etc.
> It is referred to in terms of *% loss of circulating blood volume*.

Definition – *"failure to supply the metabolic needs of the tissues,"* and can be divided therefore into four groups.

- *Hypovolemic*, e.g., blood loss, dehydration, and fluid loss
- *Cardiogenic*, e.g., infarction, pump failure
- *Distributive*, i.e., inappropriate expansion of vascular bed, ↓ systemic resistance
  - Anaphylactic – histamine release → vasodilation
  - Septic – endotoxin release → vasodilation "warm shock"
  - Neurogenic – spinal injury, leads to ↓ sympathetic vascular tone
- *Obstructive*, e.g., tension pneumothorax, pericardial tamponade

2.3.1
Degree of Shock

The degree of hypovolemic (only) shock can be estimated from an array of clinical signs and correlated with features of known blood loss (Tables 2.3.1 and 2.3.2). Any clinical features imply that at least 15% of CBV (in adults) will have been lost. A child's physiological compensation is much better and at least 25% loss of CBV is required to produce even minimal signs of shock. Underestimation is much more likely than overestimation in children (Table 2.3.3).

M. Davenport
Paediatric Surgery Department, Kings College Hospital, London, UK

C. K. Sinha and M. Davenport (eds.), *Handbook of Pediatric Surgery*,
DOI: 10.1007/978-1-84882-132-3_2.3, © Springer-Verlag London Limited 2010

Table 2.3.1 Modified ATLS® classification (adults)

	I	II	III	IV
	<15%	15–30%	30–40%	>40%
Estimate	750 mL	1,000 mL	2,000 mL	
Heart rate	<100	>100	>120	>140
Blood pressure	N	N	↓	↓↓
Respiratory rate	14–20	20–30	30–40	>40
Mental state	Slight anxiety	Anxious	Confused	Lethargic, comatose if >50%

Table 2.3.2 Modified ATLS® classification (pediatric)

	<25%	25–45%	>45%
Heart rate	N or ↑	↑↑	↓
Blood pressure	N	N or ↓	↓↓
Skin	Cool, clammy	+ Cyanosis ↓CRT	Cold ↓↓CRT
Mental state	Anxious	↓ Conscious level, ↓ Response to pain	Comatose

CRT - capillary refill time

Table 2.3.3 Circulating blood volume (CBV)

	Blood volume (mL/kg)
Neonate	90
Child	80
Adult	65–70

2.3.2
Differences with Age

- Improved compensation with onset of shock
- Tachycardia – often normal in young children
- Hypotension – late sign
- ↑ Surface area/body weight ratio – ↑ insensible losses ↑ heat loss

2.3.3
Management

2.3.3.1
Principles

Restoration of normal circulating blood volume is usually the aim; however, there are caveats to this. In uncontrolled hemorrhagic shock (UCHS), where bleeding may have stopped due to ↓BP, then rapid infusion to normal pressures leads to ↑bleeding ("popping the clot"), renewed failure to control hemorrhage and a poorer outcome than hypotensive resuscitation. *Stopping bleeding* is therefore seen to be the primary aim, before massive resuscitation.

- *"Scoop and run"* – if journey to surgical center is <1 h; then following establishment of airway and breathing → immediate transport (with IV resuscitation along the way). If >1 h, then establish IV line and fluids first.
- *"Permissive hypotension"* – if UCHS consider small aliquots of fluid based on
- Loss of radial pulse
- Mental awareness
- Systolic <80 mmHg (adults)
- Empirical observation suggests that volume of crystalloid required is 3:1 the estimated deficit in CBV.

     (Example: 20% loss in CBV in 10 kg child – assumes 160 mLs blood lost which needs ~480 mLs of saline to compensate.)

Safe practice (neither under nor over) requires bolus administration and then review vital signs and status. The goal is a well-perfused child with warm peripheries (e.g., CRT <2 s), improved mental status (may start complaining and be more aware of pain), and improved vital organ function (e.g., renal – aim for urine output 1–2 mL/kg/h).

Transfusion of blood may be needed (typically for Class III/IV shock): urgently (uncross-matched O negative if >40% loss of CBV); emergently (crossmatched, type-specific) or electively (following fluid resuscitation and hemodilution – aim for Hb >8 g/dL).

2.3.3.2
Colloids vs. Crystalloids

This is a controversial area with proponents of colloids suggesting that they remain in the intravascular space for longer while the latter diffuse across all the ECF and therefore have only short-term effects and exacerbate edema.

2.3.3.2.1
Long-Standing Debate

- *SAFE trial* (Saline vs. Albumin Fluid Evaluation, $n = 7,000$) trial. Randomized albumin vs. isotonic crystalloid in ill adults (multiple causes).
No overall difference in outcome (RR for death with colloid use $= 0.99$).
Two subgroups
    Traumatically injured – more likely to die with colloids
    Severe sepsis – less likely to die with colloids

2.3.3.3
Massive Transfusion

Defined as transfusion of patient's circulating blood volume in <24 h
    (e.g., *5 kg infant (90 mL/kg)* $\equiv 450 mL$)

Potential issues

- $\downarrow Ca^{2+}$ – citrate tends to bind ionized $Ca2^+$ (give calcium gluconate)
- $\uparrow K^+$ – leakage from red cells
- Hypothermia – unless deliberately warmed
- Depletion of 2,3 DPG stores in red cells – shifts O_2 dissociation curve
- Dilutional coagulopathy

> **Typical first bolus – 20 mL/kg IV**
> **0.9% saline (or Ringer's lactate, etc.)**
> **May be repeated (×2)**

Further Reading

1. Alam HB, Rhee P (2007) New developments in fluid resuscitation. Surg Clin North Am 87: 55–72
2. Tien H, Nascimento B Jr, Callum J, Rizoli S (2007) An approach to transfusion and hemorrhage in trauma: current perspectives on restrictive transfusion strategies. Can J Surg 50: 202–209
3. Finfer S, Bellomo R, Boyce N, French J, Myburgh J, Norton R; SAFE Study Investigators (2004) A comparison of albumin and saline for fluid resuscitation in the intensive care unit. N Engl J Med 350:2247–2256

Parenteral Nutrition

2.4

Chandrasen K. Sinha, Shamshed H. S. Syed, and Rupert Hinds

Parental nutrition is indicated when enteral feeding is either not possible or not sufficient to meet the demand.

Parenteral nutrition (PN) is required in the maintenance of fluid and electrolyte homeostasis and nutritional status as well as encouraging growth in infants and children, who cannot tolerate enteral feeding. However, whenever possible, enteral feeding should be given in order to attempt to minimize the complications of PN and promote gut adaptation.

- Extremely premature infants cannot initially tolerate large quantities of enteral feed and require the commencement of PN early after birth.
- Young infants require PN, if enteral feeding is not possible for more than 4–5 days.

The choice of route of administration is dependent on the likely duration of PN. Although peripheral PN is sometimes the only choice in children with a relatively short-term need, ideally percutaneous peripheral central access should be sought. In children with longer-term needs, definitive central access is preferred.

Intestinal failure occurs when the body is unable to sustain its energy and fluid requirements without support due to loss of functional small bowel.

2.4.1
Indications – Short Term

- Failure to establish adequate enteral nutrition
- Functional immaturity (prematurity)

C.K.Sinha (✉)
Paediatric Surgery Department, Kings College Hospital, London, UK

C. K. Sinha and M. Davenport (eds.), *Handbook of Pediatric Surgery*,
DOI: 10.1007/978-1-84882-132-3_2.4, © Springer-Verlag London Limited 2010

- NEC (prevention and treatment)
- Septicemia/multiorgan failure, where enteral feeding is not possible
- Postoperative period (e.g., prolonged ileus)
- Severe burns
- Multiple trauma
- Severe acute pancreatitis
- Acute exacerbation of ulcerative colitis/Crohn's disease
- Inflamed mucosa – following chemotherapy/radiotherapy

2.4.2
Long Term

- *Short bowel syndrome* – after extensive bowel loss (e.g., bowel atresia, volvulus, long-segment Hirschsprung's disease, gastroschisis, and IBD particularly Crohn's)
- *Motility disorders* – chronic intestinal pseudo-obstruction (CIPO)
- *Diseases of intestinal mucosa* (e.g., microvillous atrophy, intestinal epithelial dysplasia, or tufting enteropathy)

2.4.3
Multidisciplinary Team

- The support team should ideally include pediatrician, specialist nutrition nurse, dietician, pharmacist, pediatric surgeon, social worker, psychologist, and microbiologist.
- The role of the support team is appropriate/accurate prescription, safe administration, good care of lines and infusion sites, and cost-effectiveness.

2.4.4
Composition of PN Solution

Estimate resting energy expenditure based on age/weight/height and allow calculation of extra-energy requirement for infection, trauma, or postoperative stress, etc.

Measurement of metabolic rate whilst not always possible in the clinical setting is the best method of accurately calculating nutritional requirements. Various equipments are available, which allow the measurement of indirect calorimetry in children during or immediately after surgery (or stress) to establish the resting energy expenditure (Table 2.4.1).

Table 2.4.1 Approximate parenteral energy needs across the pediatric age range

Age (years)	Kcal/kg/day
Preterm	110–120
0–1	90–100
1–7	75–90
7–12	60–75
12–18	30–60

2.4.5
Constituents of PN

1. *Carbohydrate* (60–75% of non-nitrogen calories) – administered as glucose. Excess is associated with liver steatosis and in the critically ill child, hyperglycemia may increase mortality.

   Premature infants may require a maximum of 12 g/kg/day.
   Term infants tolerate up to 18 g/kg/day.

2. *Protein* – are supplied as a synthetic amino-acid (AA) mixture with its energy value excluded from total calorie requirement. Parenteral AA is less than enteral because the intestine uses a significant proportion of what is normally consumed by mouth.

   Premature infants may require up to 4 g/kg/day.
   Term infants – 3 g/kg/day.
   Older children – 1.5–2 g/kg/day.

3. *Fat* – lipid emulsions provide a low-osmolarity, low-volume noncarbohydrate source of calories, as well as essential fatty acids (EFA). They make up about 25–40% of total calories. Omission for more than a few days in preterm infant may lead to EFA deficiency. Children receiving lipid emulsions should have triglyceride monitoring, with reduction considered in lipid excess. Levels should be checked particularly when the amount of lipid is increased. In children on long-term or home PN, consideration should be given to using alternate day lipids.

   Premature infants may require up to 3 g/kg/day.
   Older children generally need between 2 and 3 g/kg/day.

4. *Other constituents. Electrolytes* are added on a mmol/kg basis and include sodium, potassium, phosphate, calcium, and magnesium. Urinary sodium may provide additional evidence of sodium depletion in addition to serum electrolytes. *Trace elements* (e.g., zinc and selenium) may need to be monitored.

5. Vitamins.
   - Fat-soluble vitamins – A, D, E, K
   - Water-soluble vitamins – B1, B2, B6, B12, C

Table 2.4.2 Recommended parenteral intake of water and lipid-soluble vitamins in children and infants

	Infant (dose/kg body weight/day)	Children (dose/day)
Vitamin A (µg)	150–300	150
Vitamin D (µg)	0.8 (32 IU)	10 (400 IU)
Vitamin E (mg)	2.8–3.5	7
Vitamin K (µg)	10	200
Ascorbic acid (mg)	15–25	80
Thiamine (mg)	0.35–0.5	1.2
Riboflavin (mg)	0.15–0.2	1.4
Pyridoxine (mg)	0.15–0.2	1.0
Niacin (mg)	4.0–6.8	17
B12 (µg)	0.3	1
Pantothenic acid (mg)	1.0–2.0	5
Biotin (µg)	5.0–8.0	20
Folic acid (µg)	56	140

Recommended dosages of vitamins based on ESPGHAN guidelines are displayed in Table 2.4.2.

2.4.6
Modification of PN

- *Calories for catabolism* – it was once thought that postoperative recovery or acute illness increased the need for calories; this is controversial and may not be correct. It is important however to consider the disease process, whether the patient has a temperature and their ventilatory status as this may have impact on the amount of energy, nitrogen, or total fluid requirements. It is important not to overfeed as this may result in subsequent metabolic disturbance.
- *Cholestasis* – starting enteral feeds early promotes gall bladder contraction and bile flow, which may help to prevent bacterial translocation and encourage gut adaptation. Cycling of PN, and particularly the lipid component, may protect the liver and improve preexisting cholestasis.
- Total fluid requirement will be higher, if there is poor absorption and/or high stoma (e.g., jejunostomy) loss.

Nutritional monitoring is required to guide the prescriber as to whether additional electrolyte, trace element, or vitamin support is needed. Frequency of monitoring depends very much on the stability of the patient.

- Electrolytes monitoring 1 or 2 per week
- Trace elements 1/monthly

2.4.7
Concomitant Medications

- *Ursodeoxycholic acid* should be used to prevent or treat PN-associated liver disease (PNALD) (at least 30 mg/kg/day in 2–3 divided doses).
- *Cholecystokinin* has been used with questionable success to improve cholestasis.
- Rotational antibiotics – to try and "decontaminate" the gut, prevent bacterial overgrowth, and avoid bacterial translocation. Although lacking a strong evidence base, probiotics, such as lactobacillus GG have been widely used.

2.4.8
Complications of PN

PN-related complications can be divided into three groups:

- *Mechanical* – injury to adjoining structures (blood vessels, pleura, nerve) leading to hemothorax, pneumothorax, chylothorax, hemopericardium; air embolism; central vein thrombosis; malposition/blockage/dislodgement of catheter, and pulmonary embolism
- *Metabolic* – liver dysfunction; hypo/hyperglycemia; fluid deficiency; fluid overload; electrolyte/other constituents imbalance
- *Infectious* – from local phlebitis to systemic sepsis

The mechanical complications can be minimized by the skills and experience of the operator. The infectious and metabolic complications can be minimized by careful and infrequent use of the line and regular monitoring of PN.

2.4.9
Parenteral Nutrition Associated Liver Disease (PNALD)

PN commonly causes a transient increase in liver enzyme levels, which return to normal after PN is stopped. Prolonged PN may cause cholestasis, steatosis, and gall stones, and if left unchecked progressive liver disease and death.

Possible contributors to PNALD are excessive calorie administration, toxic effects of PN constituents, and nutritional deficiencies, prematurity, sepsis, bowel dysmotility, and short-bowel syndrome.

The likelihood of developing PNALD can be decreased by minimizing excess calories, prescribing it in a cyclical pattern, providing a balanced PN solution, starting enteral feed as soon as possible, and avoiding sepsis.

The lipid component of PN is increasingly being recognized as a major contributor to PNALD. Strategies to diminish this include using lipid sparingly even if this means a reduction in calories in the face of evolving or worsening PNALD. This may be achieved by cycling the PN, and by reducing its frequency to 2–3 times per week in children who remain dependent on PN. Newer lipid solutions which have mixed fat sources, including fish oil are now becoming more widely used and they appear to be hepato-protective.

2.4.10
Suspected Line Infection

Possible strategies are:

1. Blood culture and sensitivity (c/s) should be taken centrally and peripherally before starting antibiotics.
2. Broad-spectrum IV antibiotics through the central line.
   (a) Change according to culture and sensitivity (if +ve – 10–14 days).
   (b) After stopping antibiotic, culture should be repeated after 48 h.
   (c) If the child is systemically unwell, stop PN and start crystalloid solution.
3. If the patient is symptomatic even after 72 h of antibiotics – repeat c/s. Consider using antibiotic locks or the addition of antifungal cover.
4. Line removal should be considered – if patient shocked/persistent infection.
5. If line removed – it is advisable to wait at least 48 h before putting in new line.

Further Reading

1. Goulet O, Ruemmele F, Lacaille F, Colomb V (2004) Irreversible intestinal failure. J Pediatr Gastroenterol Nutr 38:250–269
2. Kauffman SS (2002) Prevention of parenteral nutrition-associated liver disease in children. Pediatr Transplant 6:37–42
3. Koletzko B, Goulet O, Hunt J et al (2005) Guidelines on paediatric parenteral nutrition of the European Society of Paediatric Gastroenterology, Hepatology and Nutrition (ESPGHAN) and the European Society for Clinical Nutrition and Metabolism (ESPEN), Supported by the European Society of Paediatric Research (ESPR). J Pediatr Gastroenterol Nutr 41(Suppl 2): S1–S87

Hematology for Surgeons

2.5

Mark Davenport

2.5.1
Coagulation Tests

2.5.1.1
Normal Process

Damaged and exposed endothelium allows:

1. Platelet adherence to collagen, aggregation, and activation (via surface glycoprotein and vWF) with release of *thomboxane A2*, *V*, and *vWF*.
2. Formation of "prothrombinase complex" (via *VII* and exposed *tF*) to produce initial *thrombin*.
3. Amplification and activation of *XI*, *IX*, *and VIII* to activate *V* and produce more thrombin ("thrombin burst").
4. Thrombin polymerizes *fibrinogen* to form insoluble *fibrin.*

Inhibition of coagulation

1. Thrombin also activates *protein C and S*, which cleaves V and VIII to inactive components.
2. *Thrombin* binds to *antithrombin* – preventing its action.
3. Fibrinolysis, by action of *plasmin* (activated by tPA) on fibrin into smaller soluble fragments (fibrin degradation products, of which D-dimers are one part) (Table 2.5.1).

vWF – Von Willibrand factor.[1]
tPA – tissue plasminogen activator
tF – tissue factor

---

[1]Erik Adolf von Willibrand (1870–1949) Finnish physician: described familial bleeding disorder in 1926.

Mark. Davenport
Paediatric Surgery Department, Kings College Hospital, London, UK

C. K. Sinha and M. Davenport (eds.), *Handbook of Pediatric Surgery*, 35
DOI: 10.1007/978-1-84882-132-3_2.5, © Springer-Verlag London Limited 2010

Most coagulation screens would include *Prothrombin time (PT)*, *activated partial thromboplastin time (APTT)*, *thrombin time (TT)*, and *fibrinogen level*, together with a *platelet count* (and function tests later if all the parameters are normal).

Table 2.5.1   Possible causes for abnormal coagulation tests

	Factors		Possible cause if isolated
PT	II, V, VII, X	Increase	Liver disease, Vit K deficiency, use of warfarin.
APTT	VIII, IX, XI, XII	Increase	Hemophilia, Von Willebrand disease, use of heparin.
TT	Reflects fibrinogen to fibrin time		Hypofibrinogenaemia

Vitamin K (fat-soluble) dependent – factors II, VII, IX, and X

2.5.2
Blood Transfusion (UK-Specific)

The practice of transfusion of whole blood into patients began with Jean-Baptiste Denis's[2] account of a successful (surprisingly) transfusion of sheep blood into a 15-year-old boy in 1667. This was followed by James Blundell[3] who successfully transfused donated blood from a husband into his postpartum wife in 1818. The key discovery of ABO blood groups was made by Karl Landsteiner[4] in 1901, and later the Rhesus antigen in 1937.

- ABO system

Two RBC antigens (A and B), with four possible combinations *(AB, A, B, O)*. Plasma always contains contrary (IgM) antibody (i.e., Group A will have anti-B antibody).
    Marked racial variation – e.g., Norwegian (predominantly Gp A, 42%), Chinese (↑ Gp B, AB, 34%, invariably Rh(D) +ve)

---

[2]Jean-Baptiste Denis (1640–1704) – French court physician to Louis XIV: gave boy 9 ozs of lamb's blood.
[3]James Blundell (1791–1878) – English obstetrician: transfused blood from husband to postpartum wife in 1829.
[4]Karl Landsteiner (1868–1943) – Austrian Nobel prize winner, who discovered both major blood group antigen systems and had time to discover the polio virus!

Table 2.5.2   Group frequency in UK population

	Rhesus +ve (%)	Rhesus –ve (%)
O	37	7
A	35	7
B	8	2
AB	3	1

- Rhesus (D) system

Rh antigen present in 83% of population. If not present then anti-D (IgG) antibody not normally present (unless previously exposed, usually mother from previous Rh (D) +ve fetus) (Table 2.5.2)

- Minor groups

e.g., Lewis (Le), Kell (K)

- Urgent Need for Blood Transfusion

  Type and Screen (takes about 45 mins) – ABO group and screen for alloantibodies (IAT)
  Crossmatched blood
  Uncrossmatched blood – i.e., donor O +ve or O –ve (contains no antibodies). Latter preferred for children

One Unit – Single Donation

- Whole blood ~500 mL stored in citrate phosphate dextrose (CPD)
  - Life ~35 days
- Packed red cells ~350 mL

  (In adults 1 unit should increase Hb by 1 g/dL – administered over 4 h)

2.5.2.1
Platelets

No need for crossmatching

- 1 unit (~50 mL)

2.5.2.2
Fresh Frozen Plasma

Should be ABO compatible – no need for crossmatching

- 1 unit (150–250 mL), usually single donor

2.5.2.3
Cryoprecipitate

No need for crossmatching
  Fibrinogen and factors VII and VIII

- 1 unit (~20 mL)

2.5.2.4
Transfusion Reactions

1. *Hemolytic reaction (ABO incompatibility)* – invariably arises from clerical error.
    (a) Rare – causes rapid-onset chest pain, headache, vomiting with signs of shock, rigors, and hemoglobinuria
    (b) Stop transfusion, resuscitation
    (c) Initiate diuresis – beware acute renal failure
2. *Allergic reactions (IgE mediated to most blood components).*
    (a) Common – skin reactions due to histamine release. Occasionally very severe $\rightarrow$ anaphylaxis (bronchospasm, $\downarrow$ BP)
    (b) Stop transfusion
    (c) Hydrocortisone (IV – 100 mg adult dose)
    (d) Chlorpheniramine (IV – 10 mg adult dose)
    (e) Adrenaline (IV 1 mL of 1 in 10,000 adult dose)
3. *Febrile reaction (nonhemolytic) (anti-leucocyte antibodies)* – usually with history of past transfusions, onset after few hours of pyrexia and tachycardia. As part of histamine release. Severe reactions may cause anaphylaxis.
    (a) Stop transfusion
    (b) Parcetamol
    (a) Hydrocortisone/chlorpheniramine (if severe)
4. *Delayed extravascular hemolysis (recipient antibody-mediated, e.g., Duffy, Kell)* – unexpected fall in Hb at 7–10 days, $\uparrow$ jaundice, +ve Coombs' test.

Coombs' Test[9]

1. Direct Antiglobulin Test (DAT) – detects preformed IgG antibodies (usually) on the red cell. +ve DAT can be
    (a) Immune-mediated (e.g., transfusion reactions, Rhesus disease, drug-induced hemolytic anemia)
2. Indirect Antiglobulin test (IAT) – detects preformed IgG and IgM antibodies in serum. Is used as a screening test for transfused blood, and during pregnancy. A +ve IAT can be caused by
    (b) Minor blood group incompatibility (Rh, Lewis, Kell, etc.)

[9]Robin Coombs (1921–2006) – British immunologist.

2.5.2.5
Transmissible Hazards of Blood Transfusion

- Hepatitis B (1 in 250,000 in USA)
- Hepatitis C (1 in 13,000 in USA)
- HIV (1 in 2 million in USA)
- Variant Creutzfeldt-Jakob[5,6] disease, (vCJD) (no known cases but export of blood products from UK banned since 1999).

2.5.3
Sickle Cell Disease

2.5.3.1
Incidence

- >200,000 new cases worldwide

Sickle cell disease (SCD) includes a number of hemoglobinopathies causing chronic hemolytic anemia and painful episodes associated with the sickle cell gene (valine substitution for glutamic acid at position 6 on β-globin chain).

- Homozygous SCD (Hb SS)
- Compound heterozygotes with Hb C (Hb SC) (milder phenotype)
- Heterozygotes with H β-thalassemia (Hb Sβ)

The abnormal Hb provokes a change in red cell shape (sickle) which tends to cause small vessel occlusion in a wide variety of vascular beds.

2.5.3.2
Sickle Cell Crisis

Not usually seen in first year but may manifest as

1. Dactylitis[7] (i.e., pain/swelling in fingers and toes)
2. Long bone pain (younger children)
3. Abdominal pain (older children and adolescence)
   (a) Difficult to differentiate from surgical pathology (e.g., gallstones, appendicitis, intussusception)
   (b) SCD – ↓ incidence of appendicitis

---

[5]Heinz Gerhard Creutzfeldt (1885–1964) German neuropathologist.
[6]Alfons Maria Jakob (1884–1931) German neurologist.

2.5.3.3
Clinical Features

- Stroke (commonest cause in childhood) (up to 10% of affected children)
- Acute chest syndrome (commonest cause of death)
- Sequestration – causing acute hemolytic anemia and splenomegaly. A similar phenomenon can be seen in the liver in older children
- Orthopedic, e.g., avascular necrosis of hip, oesteomyelitis
- Gallstones – causing cholecystitis and choledocholithiasis
- Priapism[8]

2.5.3.4
Surgery in the Child with SCD

Children with SCD may well require surgical intervention either as a result of their pathology or incidentally. The process, whether elective or emergency, needs to be safe and various areas of best practice are highlighted.

- *Transfusion*
  - Formerly the key component of preparation was to dilute the sickle cells, within a more morphologically normal RBC population (typically aiming for a sickle cell percentage of <30%).
  - Exchange transfusion
  - Latterly, a more tolerant attitude has been adopted whereby the aim has been to aspire to a target hematocrit of >30%.
  - Simple transfusion – for major procedures (e.g., open cholecystectomy)
- *Hypothermia*
  - Use of warming blankets, warmed intra-operative fluids, and temperature monitoring are reasonable standards to avoid peripheral vatemsoconstriction.
- *Tourniquet*
  - Avoid in operations such as hypospadias, hand surgery, and orthopedic procedures.

2.5.3.5
Acute Chest Syndrome

Definition – "the onset of a new lobar infiltration on chest X-ray, excluding atelectasis, accompanied by fever >38.5°C, respiratory distress or chest pain."

---

[7]*Daktylos* (Greek) finger
[8]Priapus – minor Greek fertility god, always denoted with permanently erect penis.

Not uncommon complication (~10%) of invasive surgery (e.g., laparotomy) due to sickling in the pulmonary vasculature. Typically occurs 2–3 days postoperation with ↑ dyspnoea and ↑ temperature. May be limited by aggressive chest physiotherapy and early mobilization.

2.5.3.5.1
Management

1. Oxygenation and ventilatory support
2. Bronchodilators
3. Broad-spectrum antibiotics
4. Transfusion, possible exchange transfusion in severe cases
5. Use of dexamethasone

Further Reading

1. Dick MC (2008) Standards for the management of sickle cell disease in children. Arch Dis Child (Ed Pract) 93:169–176
2. Firth PG (2005) Anaesthesia for peculiar cells–a century of sickle cell disease. Br J Anaesth 95:287–299
3. Stuart MI, Nagel RL (2004) Sickle-cell disease. Lancet 364:1343–60

Postoperative Problems

2.6

Mark Davenport

> Before undergoing a serious surgical operation, put your affairs in order. You never know you may live!
> Victor Hugo (1802–1885)

2.6.1
Postoperative Problems

2.6.2
Analgesia

Relief of pain is a key component of the smooth, uncomplicated postoperative experience – certainly from the patient's perspective!

Assessment of the severity of pain is often led by experience and what is the norm for a particular operation. Nonetheless, no child's response is perfectly predictable and feedback is important. Facial assessment tools (e.g., Wong and Baker) can help in the nonspeaking preschool child. Sometimes it is the accoutrements (e.g., catheter, IV giving set, etc.) of an operation rather than the wound that causes the most distress.

Concept: Multimodal Analgesia

In order to avoid an ↑ in use of opiates, with knock-on effects of nausea, vomiting, and disorientation: use a combination of nonsteroidal anti-inflammatory drugs (Table 2.6.1), together with local anesthetic block (Table 2.6.2)

M. Davenport
Paediatric Surgery Department, Kings College Hospital, London, UK

C. K. Sinha and M. Davenport (eds.), *Handbook of Pediatric Surgery*,
DOI: 10.1007/978-1-84882-132-3_2.6, © Springer-Verlag London Limited 2010

Table 2.6.1 Common postoperative analgesics

	Mechanism of action	Dose	PR	Oral	IV
Paracetamol (acetaminophen)	Inhibition of COX-2 (central)	*20 mg/kg*[a]	Available	125 mg/5 mL 250 mg/5 mL	15 mg/kg (if >1 kg)
Dicofenac Voltarol®	Inhibition of COX-1 (local)	*1 mg/kg* *(50 mg tds)*[b]	12.5 and 25 mg	25 or 50 mg tablets	1 mg/kg
Ibuprofen	Inhibition of COX-1 (local)	*10 mg/kg* *(400 mg tds)*[b]	Available	100 mg/ 5mL	–
Codeine phosphate	opiate	*1 mg/kg*	Available	25 mg/5 mL	C/I

[a]quoted dose ranges varies considerably (10-20 mg/kg). Loading dose of 30 mg/kg recommended.
[b]Adult and >12 years

2.6.3
Local Anesthesia (LA)

Most LAs are tertiary amine bases which require an alkaline tissue pH to equilibrate into ionized and nonionized forms. The latter molecule is able to diffuse across nerve sheath and membrane to enter the axoplasm – its actual site of action. Here they block sodium channels and prevent nerve conduction (Table 2.6.2).

- Selective – unmyelinated C fibers > A fibers (pain > motor)

2.6.3.1
Percentage Solution of LA

- 1% solution implies a concentration of *1 g/100 mL.*

And thus in mg/ml terms should be multiplied by 10.

- 1% lignocaine contains *10 mg/mL.*

Adrenaline (epinephrine) may be added to increase the duration of action, induce vasoconstriction, and allow a higher dose of LA to be used. The usual dose is 1 in 200,000 (i.e., 5 µg/mL). Never use such solutions in proximity to end-arteries (penis, finger, toes).

Side effects

- CNS side effects (usually) include dizziness, circumoral tingling, visual or aural disturbance. Untoward muscle twitching and (rarely) seizures.
- Cardiovascular side effects (rare) – usually with inadvertent IV use, but may include sinus bradycardia and negative inotropism (↓ BP).

Table 2.6.2   Common local anesthetic agents

	Dose	Duration	Notes
Topical			
5% EMLA[®a] also ELA-max[®]	1 tube = 5 g	3 h	Apply under occlusive dressing – 60 mins Avoid <3 months
4% Tetracaine Ametop[®]	1 tube = 1 g	4–6 h	Apply under occlusive dressing – 30 mins Avoid <3 months
TAC[b]	2–5 mL applied directly to wound	1 h	Avoid mucus membranes/burns Use probably superseded by LET
LET[c]	2–5 mL gel or liquid applied directly to wound	1 h	Avoid mucus membranes/burns
Infiltration			
	Upper limit		
Procaine Novocain[®]	7–10 mg/kg		Also vasoconstricts, ↑ allergic reaction
Lignocaine (lidocaine) Xylocaine[®]	3–4 mg/kg *(7 mg/ kg + adrenaline)*	1–2 h	1%, 2%
Prilocaine Citanest[®]	6 mg/kg		
Mepivacaine Carbocaine[®]	5 mg/kg		
Bupivacaine Marcaine[®]	2 mg/kg	3 h	0.25%, Slow onset

[a]Eutectic Mixture of Local Anesthetic (lignocaine and prilocaine)
[b]Tetracaine (0.5%), Adrenaline (1 in 2,000), Cocaine (11.8%) (used mainly in USA, although now declining)
[c]Lignocaine, Epinephrine, Tetracaine (used mainly in USA)

2.6.4
Postoperative Nausea and Vomiting (PONV)

PONV is multifactorial but commonly associated with opiate and inhalational anesthesia use. Physiologically, it is a combination of the effects of chemoreceptor trigger zone (CTZ) on the floor of the IV ventricle and the vomiting center in the medulla. Acetyl choline, 5-HT, and dopamine are all involved in the reflex arc of vomiting.

- ↑ Incidence in 6–16-year old (low in infants) ~40% risk
- ↑ Incidence in ENT (esp. middle ear procedures and tonsillectomy) and ophthalmic (esp. strabismus correction) procedures, laparoscopy

2.6.4.1
Management

Can be thought of as prophylactic or as rescue therapy

- Ondansteron (5-HT$_3$ antagonist, 0.15 mg/kg) and dexamethasone (0.1 mg/kg)
- Dimenhydrinate (not available in UK)
- Cyclizine (antihistamine) – limited evidence for efficacy
- Prochlorperazine and metoclopramide – limited evidence for efficacy

---

2.6.5
Pyrexia[1]

Normal core body temperature $37°C \equiv 98.6°F$
Very common problem, with multiple causes.

2.6.5.1
Immediate (<24 h)

- Underlying reason for surgery (e.g., acute appendicitis)
- Metabolic response to surgery
- Respiratory (basal atelectasis – retention mucus secretions)
  - Treatment – physiotherapy
- Transfusion reactions (see Chap 2.5, 2.4)

2.6.5.2
Early (2–5 Days)

- Respiratory (basal atelectasis, secondary infection)
  - Treatment – physiotherapy, antiobiotic
- IV line colonization – blood culture
  - Treatment – removal (if appropriate), change (if necessary), change antibiotic
- Persisting pathology – inadequate surgery/drainage of collection or abscess

2.6.5.3
Late (>5 Days)

- Wound infection. Culture any discharge.
  - Treatment – drain any subcutaneous collection – open wound – debride wound. Change antibiotic.

[1]*Pyretos* (Greek) – fire. Febrile *febris* (Latin) – fever

- Persisting pathology.
- Anastomotic leakage (esophageal, intestinal, biliary). CXR/US/CT scan.
- Intrabdominal collection/abscess (subphrenic, subhepatic, pelvic, paracolic, interloop). Ultrasound/CT scan.
  - — Treatment – drain collection (if possible). Blood culture. Change antibiotic.
- Urinary tract infection (if catheterized).

2.6.6
Wound Infection

Benchmark ~4% (in pediatric general surgical practice)

Wounds may be defined as: (infection rate %)

1. Clean (e.g., hernia) <2%
2. Clean/contaminated (e.g., appendectomy) 5–10%
3. Contaminated (e.g., resection of bowel for NEC) 10–20%
4. Dirty (e.g., drainage of abscess) >20%

Infection is defined as "discharge of pus," but early signs include increasing pain, erythema, and swelling. This early cellulitic phase can be abbreviated by systemic antibiotics, but typically once pus develops then this has to be drained (by removal of sutures, etc.) and any necrotic tissue removed (debridement). Compared to adults, infection is more often related to duration of surgery and operative events rather than physiology of patient.

2.6.6.1
Organisms

Staphylococci spp (incl. CONS), *Streptococcal spp*, *E. coli*, *Klebsiella spp*, anerobic organisms (e.g., *Bacteroides spp, Clostridial spp*), *Enterobacter spp, Pseudomonas aeruginosa, Candida spp*.

There are many topical therapies which have shown benefit including:

- Iodine-based (e.g., povidone iodine)
- Silver-based (e.g., silver sulfadiazine)
- Alginate-based
- Metronidazole

Empirical (i.e., "best guess") antibiotics

- Flucloxacillin (staphylococcal) for (1) and (2)
- Co-amoxiclav or cefuroxime and metronidazole (broad spectrum including anaerobes) for (3) and (4)

2.6.6.2
Methicillin-Resistant *Staphylococcus aureus* (MRSA)

1. Topical antibacterial agents (iodine- or silver-based)
   If systemically unwell
2. Vancomycin or teicoplanin (both glycopeptides and IV only)
3. Second-line antibiotics include linezolid (an oxazolidinone, oral and IV, requires regular FBC – bone marrow suppression)

2.6.6.3
Necrotizing Fasciitis

Rare, but devastating (20% mortality in children) complication caused by (typically) mixed organisms (e.g., GpA *Steptococcal spp*, *Pseuodomonas aeruginosa*, and anaerobic *spp* such as *Clostridial spp*, *Peptostreptococcus*, *Bacteroides spp*). Rapid spread along deep fascial plane, because of release of toxin, with overlying skin necrosis due to thrombosis.

Can occur primarily – typically scrotal (Fournier's[2] gangrene) or as complication of varicella and in the immunosuppressed.

Suspect if excessive pain (becoming anesthetic later) with surrounding skin erythema becoming mottled and pale. Look for crepitus (gas formation).

Treatment should include high-dose antibiotic (including Penicillin G), wound debridement (early and aggressive), and hyperbaric oxygen (if available).

Further Reading

1. O'Brien CM, Titley G, Whitehurst P (2003) A comparison of cyclizine, ondansetron and placebo as prophylaxis against postoperative nausea and vomiting in children. Anaesthesia 58:707–711
2. Horwitz JR, Chwals WJ, Doski JT, Suescun EA, Cheu HW, Lally KP (1998) Pediatric wound infections. A prospective multicenter study. Ann Surg 227:553–558
3. Davenport M, Doig CM (1993) Wound infection in pediatric surgery: a study in 1094 neonates. J Pediatr Surg 28:26–30

---

[2]Jean Alfred Fournier (1832–1915) French dermatologist described a case in 1883.

Neonatal Physiology and Care

2.7

Vadivelam Murthy, Chandrasen K. Sinha, Ravindra Bhat,
and Mark Davenport

The first few minutes after birth is one of the riskiest periods in life.
The last few minutes are pretty fraught with danger too!!

2.7.1
Transitional Physiology

2.7.1.1
Cardiovascular Adaptation

2.7.1.1.1
Fetal Circulation

Return of oxgenated blood from the placenta, via umbilical vein, left portal vein, and *ductus venosus*[1] to the right atrium (80%, with remaining 20% going through liver sinusoids). Mixing with de-oxygenated blood from SVC, which tends to be streamed to right ventricle and pulmonary artery. Two natural shunt mechanisms avoid futile pulmonary circulation.

1. *Foramen ovale*
2. *Ductus arteriosis*[2]

De-oxygenated blood is returned to placental circulation via the umbilical arteries.

---

[1] Of Arantius (from Julies Caesar Aranzi (1530–1589)) – Italian anatomist in Padua and Bologna.
[2] Of Botali (from Leonardo Botallo (1519–1588)) – Italian surgeon and anatomist.

V. Murthy (✉)
Department of Neonatology, Kings College Hospital, London, UK

C. K. Sinha and M. Davenport (eds.), *Handbook of Pediatric Surgery*,
DOI: 10.1007/978-1-84882-132-3_2.7, © Springer-Verlag London Limited 2010

2.7.1.2
Respiratory Adaptation

There is a reduction in pulmonary fluid production during the later weeks of pregnancy and during normal labor remaining fluid is squeezed out of the lungs. During the first few breaths, the lungs inflate leading to the following changes:

- Establishment of resting functional residual capacity
- ↑ PaO_2 in the alveoli and arterial circulation (causing vasodilatation)
- ↓ Pulmonary vascular resistance
- ↓ Right-to-left shunting (through ductus arteriosus)
- ↑ Pulmonary venous return to the left atrium
- ↑ Left atrial pressure and cessation of right-to-left shunting (through foramen ovale)

After the first breath, there is functional closure of the ductus arteriosis (via ↓ prostaglandinE$_2$) to achieve independence of the two circulations.

2.7.2
Definitions

2.7.2.1
Gestation Age

- <37 weeks – pre-term
- 38–42 weeks – Term
- >42 weeks – post-term

2.7.2.2
Birth Weight

- Low birth weight (LBW) <2,500 g
- Very low birth weight (VLBW) <1,500 g
- Extremely low birth weight (ELBW) <1,000 g
- Small for gestational age (SGA)
  <10th percentile of the expected weight at that gestational age
- Large for gestational age (LGA)
  >90th percentile of the expected weight at that gestational age

2.7.3
General Principles of Management

- In labor room

General assessment of the newborn and securing an airway (suction, bag/mask) should be performed by trained staff. Once respiration is established, the general condition should be assessed. The Apgar[3] score is still an acceptable practical method of systemically assessing a newborn infant. However, a low score does not necessarily signify fetal hypoxia/acidosis and does not predict long-term morbidity (Table 2.7.1).

- Thermoregulation

Infants are covered with vernix and amniotic fluid and can lose heat quickly due to their increased surface area. Simple measures of heat preservation include drying the infant after birth, using warm towels, optimizing room temperature, and early skin-to-skin contact with mum.

- Cord care

Sterile instruments should be used to cut the cord after clamping. The cord should be kept dry and inspected regularly. If there is any suspicion of infection, the infant should be treated with appropriate antibiotics.

- Feeding

Well newborns should be encouraged to bond with the mother soon after birth, by early skin-skin contact with the mum and breast-feeding. High-risk infants should be monitored closely for hypoglycemia and failure to establish breast-feeding may need consideration of alternatives.

Table 2.7.1 Apgar score – performed at 1, 5, and 10 min

Score	Heart rate	Respiration	Color	Muscle tone	Irritability
0	Absent	Absent	Blue/pale	Limp	No response
1	<100	Irregular, slow	Pink torso, blue extremities	Mild flexion	Grimace
2	≥100	Crying, active	Pink	Active	Sneeze

[3]Virginia Apgar (1909–1974) – American pediatrician.

2.7.4
Prematurity

2.7.4.1
Is There a Line

Currently, in the UK, it is considered that there is an achievable survival rate and acceptable quality of life of preterm infants >24 weeks gestation. In contrast, resuscitation of infants <23 weeks is regarded as futile.

2.7.4.2
Respiratory Management

Most preterm infants of <30 weeks, need some form of respiratory support, largely due to respiratory distress syndrome (lack of surfactant), and inadequate respiratory muscle strength (diaphragm and intercostals muscle groups) (Fig. 2.7.1).

1. Surfactant deficiency
   (a) Antenatal maternal steroids
   (b) Endo-tracheal administration of surfactant with in the first hour after birth within first hour postpartum (repeated ×3)
2. Ventilation strategies
   (a) IPPV (Intermittent Positive Pressure Ventilation)
   (b) HFOV (High Frequency Oscillatory Ventilation)
   (c) CPAP (Continuous Positive Airway Pressure)

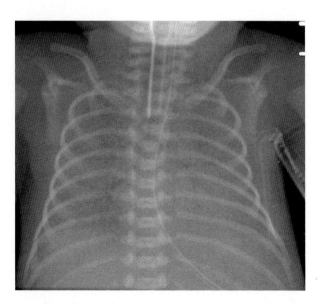

Fig. 2.7.1 Chest X-ray in respiratory distress syndrome (RDS) showing diffuse fine granular opacities with air trapping

2.7.4.3
Hypotension

This is a common problem in extremely preterm infants, due to sepsis, PDA, etc. Most infants will need inotropic support to maintain their mean blood pressure (aim for mean blood pressure above the gestational age of the infant). In most units, invasive blood pressure monitoring is the preferred unless arterial access is an issue.

Commonly used inotropic agents include:

1. Dopamine, dobutamine
2. Adrenaline, noradrenaline, isoprenaline
3. Hydrocortisone

2.7.4.4
Thermoregulation

The preterm are prone to become cold quickly compared to term infants because of

1. Higher ratio of skin surface area to weight
2. ↓ Subcutaneous fat and brown fat
3. ↓ Caloric intake
4. Limited oxygen consumption due to underlying pulmonary problems

Current incubators can maintain warm environments with high humidity (up to 85%) ensuring a thermal range between 36.4 and 37°C.

2.7.4.5
Jaundice

Most preterm infants need treatment for physiological jaundice due to

1. Increased bilirubin production (decreased RBC survival)
2. Defective conjugation due to ↓ hepatic glucuronyl-transferase activity
3. ↓ Hepatic excretion.

As there are no standard and safe limits of billirubin levels in preterm infants that have been universally established, each neonatal unit has adopted its own billirubin level for treatment.

The main principles in management are

1. To exclude haemolytic causes of jaundice
2. Adequate hydration
3. Early phototherapy
4. Exchange transfusion

2.7.4.6
Anemia

Preterm infants are prone to anemia due to decreased production of red blood cells by the immature hematological system.

> *Blood volume in preterm infants and term infants 80–100 mL/kg*

2.7.5
Infections

Preterm infants are prone to infections due to their immature immunological system and underdeveloped skin barrier.

Common Transplacental infections include:

- Toxoplamosis (*T. gondii*) causes choridoretinitis, mental retardation.
- Rubella virus causes deafness,cataract,PDA, mental retardation, microcephaly.
- Cytomegalovirus causes rash, hepatitis, microcephaly, seizures, low birth weight
- Syphilis causes hepato-splenomeagly,anemia, metaphyseal dystrophy

The most common organisms causing neonatal sepsis are:

- First 48 h
  - Group B *Streptoccoci, Escherichia coli*
  - *Listeria monocytogenes*
  - Herpes simplex (HSV-1, HSV-2)
- >48 h
  - *Staphylococcus epidermidis, E. coli, Staphylococcus aureus, Pseudomonas spp.*

2.7.5.1
Clinical Features

Early signs of sepsis in infants include recurrent apneas, temperature instability, hyper/hypoglycemia, and increase in markers of inflammation.

2.7.5.2
Investigations

Blood culture should be performed before the commencement of antibiotics.
C-Reactive protein (CRP), white cell count, platelet count are important in monitoring for infections.

2.7.5.3
Management

Appropriate antibiotics should be started immediately, if there is clinical suspicion of sepsis as deterioration is rapid and outcome is poor in severe sepsis. Fungal infections should be suspected in extreme prematurity and aggressive antifungal treatment should be started if proven. Screen for fungal vegetation in the kidneys, brain, and heart to identify the source.

2.7.6
Neonatal Nutrition (See Chapter 2.4)

See Tables 2.7.2 & 2.7.3

Table 2.7.2   Fluid requirment in Preterm newborn infant

Day	Type of fluid	Volume of fluid (mL/kg/day)
1	10% Dextrose	50–60
2	10% Dextrose	75–90
3	10% Dextrose	100–120
4	10% Dextrose	125–150
>5	10% Dextrose	150–175

N.B. Electrolyte supplementation should be started only after completion of the postnatal extracellular volume contraction and establishment of good urine output

Table 2.7.3 Nutrition requirment for stable Preterm infants

	Units/kg/day	
	VLBW (> 1000 g)	ELBW (<1000 g)
Water (mL)	120–200	160–220
Energy (kcal)	110–130	130–150
Protein (g)	3.4–4.2	3.8–4.4
Fat (g)	1–3	1–3
Carbohydrate (g)	6–12	6–12
Sodium (mmol)	2–4	2–4
Potassium (mmol)	2–3	2–3
Chloride (mmol)	2–3	2–3
Calcium (mmol)	2.5–5.5	2.5–5.5
Phosphorus (mmol)	1.9–4.5	1.9–4.5
Magnesium (mmol)	0.3–0.6	0.3–0.6
Iron (mg)	2–4	2–4
Zinc (µg)	1,000–3,000	1,000–3,000
Copper (µg)	120–150	120–150
Manganese (µg)	0.7–7.5	0.7–7.5
Selenium (µg)	1.3–4.5	1.3–4.5

Further Reading

1. Wood NS, Costeloe K, Gibson AT, et al. (2003) The EPICure study: growth and associated problems in children born at 25 weeks of gestational age or less. Arch Dis Child 88:F492–F500
2. Field DJ, Dorling JS, Manktelow BN, Draper ES (2008) Survival of extremely premature babies in a geographically defined population: prospective cohort study of 1994–9 compared with 2000–5. BMJ 336:1221–1223
3. Tsang RC. Nutrition of the Preterm Infant: Scientific Basis and Practical Guidelines, 2nd edition 2005.

Part III

Fetal and Neonatal Surgery

Fetal Surgery: General Principles

3.1

Eric B. Jelin and Hanmin Lee

Fetal surgery has moved from experimental models to the human condition. But despite dramatic advances in techniques and imaging, fetal surgery, has only been shown to be beneficial in a small subset of patients.

Studies in small and large animals have demonstrated the efficacy and safety of fetal surgery for selected cases of certain life-threatening fetal diseases. The first open surgery on a human fetus was performed for congenital bladder obstruction in 1981 by Dr. Michael Harrison at the University of California, San Francisco (UCSF). Since then, advanced fetal imaging has dramatically improved our understanding of congenital anomalies and has opened the door to new treatments and minimally invasive techniques.

Human fetal surgery is now being performed for diseases such as

- Congenital diaphragmatic hernia
- Mass lesions with hydrops fetalis
- Twin anomalies
- Bladder outlet obstruction
- Congenital high airway obstruction
- Aortic valve stenosis
- Spina bifida

3.1.1
Ethical Concerns

A challenge particular to fetal surgery is that the welfare of both mother and fetus must be considered. The treatment of a fetus with a congenital anomaly confers no direct physical benefit to the mother and subjects her to risk. This is primarily related to the high incidence

E. B. Jelin (✉)
Department of Surgery, Division of Pediatric Surgery/Fetal Treatment Center,
University of California at San Francisco,
San Francisco, CA, USA

C. K. Sinha and M. Davenport (eds.), *Handbook of Pediatric Surgery*,
DOI: 10.1007/978-1-84882-132-3_3.1, © Springer-Verlag London Limited 2010

of preterm labor and its corresponding morbidity, but as with any operation, fetal surgery also carries a risk of infection, bleeding, and damage to adjacent structures. Fetal surgical procedures should only be considered if the in utero anomaly has been shown to have severe irreversible consequences and the procedure is safe and beneficial to the fetus with low risk to the mother.

3.1.2
Accessing the Fetus

The gravid uterus can be accessed by open or minimally invasive (fetoscopic and percu-tanous) techniques. In both approaches, ultrasound assessment for placental position, uterine anomalies, and fetal position are critical for successful intervention, and a skilled sonologist/ultrasonographer is a mandatory member of the operative team.

Open fetal surgery requires:

1. *Maternal* low transverse incision.
2. Exposure and intraoperative ultrasound of the uterus.
3. Analgesia and paralysis of the fetus.
4. Anterior or posterior hysterotomy (depending on placental location) using a uterine stapler with absorbable staples. This makes the hysterotomy, provides hemostasis, and seals membranes.
5. Exposure of appropriate body part of the fetus.
6. Repair of the defect.
7. Return of fetus to uterus – closed with two running layers of absorbable suture and fibrin glue.

Endoscopic techniques for fetal surgery (FETENDO, Figs. 3.1.1 and 3.1.2) have been adapted from laparoscopic surgery. A minimally invasive approach avoids the maternal morbidity incurred with a large open incision and hysterotomy (e.g., postoperative bleed-ing, adhesions, and the inability to deliver vaginally). Percutaneous interventions are usu-ally directed at draining fluid-filled fetal structures or radiofrequency ablation of an anomalous twin. "Real-time" continuous ultrasound guides the placement of percutaneous instruments.

3.1.3
Specific Conditions

3.1.3.1
Congenital Diaphragmatic Hernia

Fetuses with severe congenital diaphragmatic hernia (CDH) and lung hypoplasia continue to have a dismal prognosis. For these selected patients, fetal surgery may improve survival and reduce postnatal morbidity.

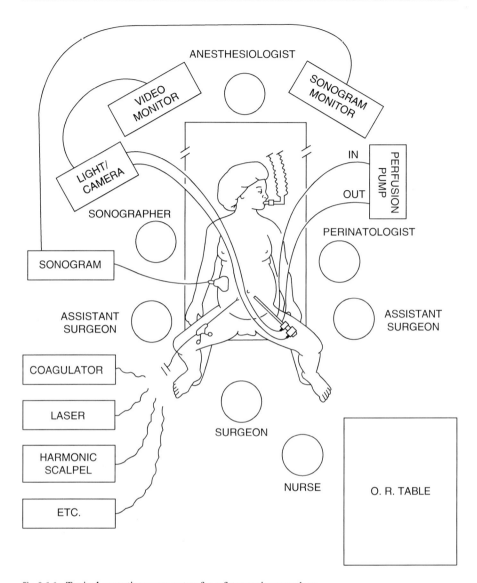

Fig. 3.1.1 Typical operating room setup for a fetoscopic procedure

3.1.3.1.1
Principle

- In utero tracheal occlusion (TO) promotes lung growth and thus improves postnatal lung function.

Using the FETENDO approach, a balloon is inserted into the fetal trachea and inflated at 26–28 weeks' gestation. A randomized control trial comparing *in utero* TO for CDH with

Fig. 3.1.2 Use of FETENDO to place an inflatable balloon in the fetal trachea for CDH

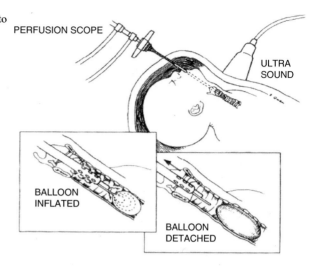

standard postnatal care did not demonstrate improved survival in the TO group (both groups had a 90-day survival of 75%). However, the study had broad inclusion criteria and did not target the sickest subset of patients.

As a result, fetal surgery is now reserved for patients with an estimated survival of <50% based on validated prenatal prognostic indicators. Furthermore, advancements in instrumentation and techniques now permit reversal of TO at 32–34 weeks' gestation, allowing for vaginal delivery and optimal development of surfactant-producing type II pneumocytes. An FDA approved trial is underway at UCSF to perform and then reverse TO in fetuses with severe CDH.

3.1.3.2
Twin Anomalies

3.1.3.2.1
Principle

- Fetoscopic laser ablation of abnormal placental connections

Twin-twin transfusion syndrome (TTTS) – abnormal placental connections cause unequal sharing of blood between fetuses (occurs in up to 15% of monochorionic twin pregnancies). The condition is fatal in >80% of untreated cases and survivors face a risk of brain damage and morbidity.

A 2004 randomized control trial of laser blood vessel ablation showed superiority compared to amnioreduction, the previous therapy of choice, in patients with severe TTTS (≤26 weeks gestation). Survival at 1 month was 76% (laser) *vs.* 56% (amnioreduction group).

Twin reversed arterial perfusion (TRAP) sequence (~1% of monochorionic twins) – characterized by an acardiac and/or anencephalic twin whose blood flow is provided by reversed perfusion through the normal twin's umbilical cord. Fetal demise occurs in approximately 60% of cases and is more likely if the anomalous twin is large, well-vascularized, or both.

Fetal surgery consists of ablation of the blood vessels that supply the acardiac twin, either via fetoscopy with monopolar or bipolary diathermy, YAG laser, or radiofrequency ablation. Survival for the normal twin after radiofrequency ablation has recently been reported at 92%.

3.1.3.3
Fetal Mass Lesions with Hydrops

Large, vascularized mass lesions cause heart failure and hydrops either by impairing venous return or arteriovenous shunting.

3.1.3.3.1
Principle

- Reversal of fetal cardiac failure and hydrops by fetal mass excision

The vast majority of mass lesions are benign and often spontaneously regress; however, some become so large that they cause high-output cardiac failure. The most common are *congenital cystic adenomatoid malformation (CCAM)* and *sacrococcygeal teratoma (SCT)*. Fetal surgery for these lesions involves resection via an open approach (Fig. 3.1.3). A recent review showed improvement in survival of hydropic fetuses with mass lesions from <5% without intervention to 50% with resection.

3.1.3.4
Bladder Outlet Obstruction

Bladder outlet obstruction (e.g., posterior urethral valves (most common), prune belly syndrome, urethral atresia) complicates ~1 in 1,000 live-births.

3.1.3.4.1
Principle

- Relief of urinary obstruction may reduce renal failure and limit pulmonary hypoplasia.

Complete urinary obstruction leads to oligohydramnios, renal failure, and pulmonary hypoplasia. Decompressive fetal surgery has been unable to reverse established renal failure but insertion of a double-J pigtail vesicoamniotic shunt can prevent further deterioration

Fig. 3.1.3 Sacrococcygeal teratoma (**a**) before and (**b**) after fetal resection

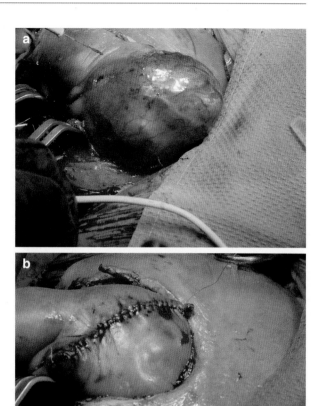

and enhance lung growth. Some centers are investigating the role of fetal cystoscopy to treat fetal bladder outlet obstruction.

3.1.3.5
Myelomeningocele (Spina Bifida)

Neural tube defects (e.g., myelomeningocele (MMC) or spina bifida) occurs in ~1 in 1,000 live-births and is associated with debilitating neurologic injury (e.g., loss of hind limb function, bowel and bladder incontinence, hydrocephalus, and Arnold [1]-Chiari[2] malformation (condition where part of cerebellum herniates through foramen magnum causing hydrocephalus).

---

[1]Julius Arnold (1835–1915) – German pathologist. Malformation recognized and described by both during 1890s.

[2]Hans Chiari (1851–1915) – Austrian pathologist.

3.1.3.5.1
Principle

- *In utero* repair of MMC may preserve peripheral neurologic function and prevent Arnold-Chiari malformation.

The success of prenatal MMC repair in animal models has led to an NIH-funded, multi-center randomized trial to investigate the efficacy of open fetal repair of MMC.

3.1.3.6
Aortic Valve Stenosis

Prenatally diagnosed critical aortic valve stenosis leads to ventricular overload, chronic myocardial wall ischemia, and eventually hypoplastic left heart syndrome. Postnatal therapy involves staged surgical repairs, but mortality is up to 25% after the first operation and survivors face a lifetime of cardiac and neurologic dysfunction.

3.1.3.6.1
Principle

- In utero repair of valve stenosis may preserve ventricular function.

Percutaneous and open fetal aortic valvuloplasty have successfully relieved left ventricular obstruction and minimized left heart damage. The largest series from Children's Hospital Boston (n = 65) reported a technical success rate of >50%. Of the surviving fetuses, however, only one-third developed a functional left ventricle.

3.1.3.7
Congenital High Airway Obstruction Syndrome

Congenital high airway obstruction syndrome (CHAOS) is characterized by a stenosis or mass lesion that blocks the fetal airway. Fetuses with CHAOS that survive until birth face certain neonatal death secondary to airway obstruction.

3.1.3.7.1
Principle

- Correction of airway occlusion while still on placental support.

The EXIT (ex-utero intrapartum treatment) procedure is a specialized mode of surgical delivery developed for fetuses with airway obstruction (Fig. 3.1.4). EXIT maintains the

Fig. 3.1.4 Schematic of an "EXIT" procedure

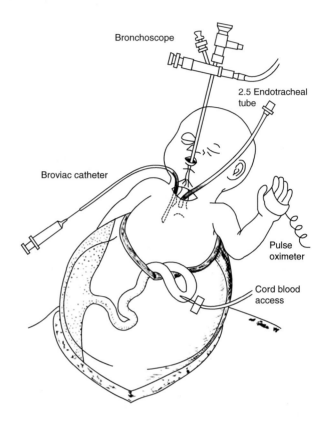

Bronchoscope

2.5 Endotracheal tube

Broviac catheter

Pulse oximeter

Cord blood access

fetus on placental support while an airway is established by orotracheal intubation or tracheostomy. Once oxygenation of the fetus is achieved, the cord is clamped and cut, and the baby is delivered.

The Future of Fetal Surgery

For many fetuses with severe disease, fetal surgery offers the best and sometimes only therapy. The efficacy of fetal intervention is still greatly limited by high rates or preterm labor and preterm birth, but as more is learned about the underlying mechanisms of preterm labor and strategies are developed to combat it, efficacy will increase and applications of fetal surgery will grow. In the near term, minimally invasive techniques will continue to improve and replace open techniques. More distantly, *in utero* gene therapy for metabolic deficiencies, along with stem cell therapy and tissue engineering for organ and tissue deficits promise to be the next frontiers of fetal therapy.

Further Readings

1. Harrison MR (2001) The unborn patient: the art and science of fetal therapy, 3rd edn. W.B. Saunders, Philadelphia, pp. xv, 709 p., [6] p. of plates
2. Harrison MR, Keller RL, Hawgood SB et al (2003) A randomized trial of fetal endoscopic tracheal occlusion for severe fetal congenital diaphragmatic hernia. N Engl J Med 349:1916–1924
3. Senat MV, Deprest J, Boulvain M et al (2004) Endoscopic laser surgery versus serial amnioreduction for severe twin-to-twin transfusion syndrome. N Engl J Med 351:136–144
4. Lee H, Wagner AJ, Sy E et al (2007) Efficacy of radiofrequency ablation for twin-reversed arterial perfusion sequence. Am J Obstet Gynecol 196:459 e1-4
5. Grethel EJ, Wagner AJ, Clifton MS et al (2007) Fetal intervention for mass lesions and hydrops improves outcome: a 15-year experience. J Pediatr Surg 42:117–123
6. Tworetzky W, Wilkins-Haug L, Jennings RW et al (2004) Balloon dilation of severe aortic stenosis in the fetus: potential for prevention of hypoplastic left heart syndrome: candidate selection, technique, and results of successful intervention. Circulation 110:2125–2131

Diaphragmatic Hernia

3.2

Saidul Islam, Chandrasen K. Sinha, and Mark Davenport

A congenital diaphragmatic hernia is a complex anomaly with a significant risk of death, principally due to lung hypoplasia. The aim of postnatal ventilation strategies is to ameliorate this – whereas prenatal intervention seeks to reverse this *in utero*.

3.2.1
Epidemiology

- 1 in 3,000 live-births (1 in 2,000 at ~20 weeks gestation – "hidden mortality")
- M = F
- Predominantly left-sided (80%). Bilateral (<2%)
- Isolated (usually) if live-born
- Late-presenters (~10%) – excellent prognosis

3.2.2
Associations

- Chromosomal defects, e.g., Trisomy 13, 18, 21 (rarely survive)
- *Fryns syndrome* (1–2%) ("coarse" facial features, hypertelorism, cloudy corneas, facial clefts, renal, CVS and genital abnormalities)
- *Pallister-Killian syndrome* (tetrasomy 12p mosaic) ("coarse" facial features, sparse hair, syndactyly)
- *Cantrell syndrome* (formerly a "Pentalogy" of defects including cardiac, sternal defect, exomphalos, and absence of pericardium)
- Cardiac defects, e.g., VSD

M. Davenport (✉)
Paediatric Surgery Department, Kings College Hospital, London, UK

C. K. Sinha and M. Davenport (eds.), *Handbook of Pediatric Surgery*,
DOI: 10.1007/978-1-84882-132-3_3.2, © Springer-Verlag London Limited 2010

3.2.3
Embryology

Key stage – 4–8 weeks of gestation.
The diaphragm is derived from four sources.

- Septum transversum (forming central tendon and some muscle tissue, with innervation by phrenic nerve)
- Pleuroperitoneal membranous folds
- Thoracic body wall mesoderm
- Esophageal mesenchyme

All elements contribute to the muscular rim, and esophageal crura.

Prior to this there is a posterior connection ("canal") between two cavities – the pericardial and the peritoneal. In-growth of the pleuroperitoneal membranes fill and occlude this canal and failure results in the typical postero-lateral CDH (of Bochdalek[1]). There is a left-sided predominance as this canal is larger and closes later than the right. Morgagni[2] hernias occur in the anterior part of the diaphragm either side (usually right) of the xiphisternum. Cantrell defects are typically central and expose the beating heart associated with exomphalos and sternal defects.

The size of the defect varies but complete absence (agenesis) of the hemidiaphragm is not uncommon. A postero-lateral rim almost always is found covered with pleura contiguous with peritoneum. A hernial sac (10–20%) can also be found together with nonrotation and nonfixation of the mid- and hindgut.

3.2.4
Pulmonary Hypoplasia

Classically, it is said that the visceral herniation into the thoracic cavity inhibits ipsilateral lung development. However, recent studies suggest that the lungs have a primary intrinsic defect before being further impaired by secondary visceral herniation ("dual-hit" hypothesis). Consequently, bronchopulmonary generations are permanently reduced in both lungs, resulting in reduced number of alveoli. Impaired development of the pulmonary vasculature is almost invariable, resulting in a hypoplastic pulmonary vascular bed with hypertrophied muscular pulmonary arteries with the tendency to pulmonary hypertension and persistence of the fetal circulation with right-to-left shunting.

---

[1]Vincent Bockdalek (1801–1883) Czech anatomist.
[2]Giovanni Battista Morgagni (1682–1761) Italian anatomist.

3.2.5
Clinical Features

3.2.5.1
Antenatal

The diagnosis is frequently (up to 90% in countries with routine screening) made on ante-natal ultrasound scan. Other features include polyhydramnios, mediastinal displacement, and absence of stomach bubble.

The main benefits of early detection are:

1. Detection of associated anomalies
2. Prognostic indices, e.g., liver position and lung-to-head ratio (LHR). Significant liver herniation and an LHR <1 suggests poor prognosis.
3. Antenatal counseling and in utero transfer to pediatric surgical center

3.2.5.2
Postnatal

Early respiratory distress and cyanosis after birth together with findings of a scaphoid abdomen, tracheal deviation and mediastinal shift are the typical features of CDH.

Diagnosis is confirmed by:

1. CXR – showing herniated intestinal loops and mediastinal shift. If intubated swiftly the loops may remain fluid-filled. The differential of multiple air-filled intrathoracic loops is a macrocystic CCAM (look at the diaphragm outline).
2. US or contrast study – if doubt exists, image diaphragm with US or outline viscera with contrast. Right-sided CDH may cause more confusion as the liver is the typical herni-ated viscus (Figs. 3.2.1 and 3.2.2).

3.2.6
Management

The initial strategy should be to maintain near-normal blood gases but without compromis-ing lung injury (by barotrauma). If cardiorespiratory stability is achieved and maintained on acceptable ventilation modes, then consider definitive surgery.

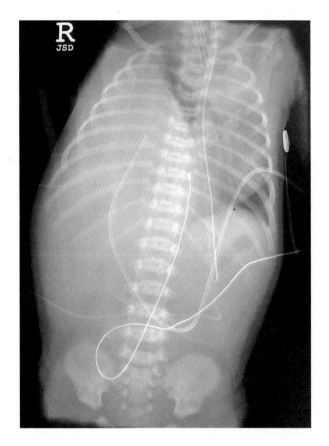

Fig. 3.2.1 Chest X-ray of right congenital diaphragmatic hernia, showing obvious displacement of umbilical vein catheter with liver rotated into right hemithorax

3.2.6.1
Delivery Suite

- Endotracheal intubation and IPPV (not bag/mask as will invariably cause gastric dilatation)
- Naso-gastric tube (to decompress stomach) and venous access

3.2.6.2
In intensive care unit

1. Arterial blood gas – preductal (right radial artery) and postductal (left radial, umbilical artery, etc.) to determine the degree of shunting. (Aim for preductal pO_2 ~60 mmHg , postductal ~40 mmHg).
2. Initial ventilation settings (e.g., rate 30–60 bpm; peak inspiratory pressure (PIP) = 20–30 cmH_2O, positive end-expiratory pressure (PEEP) = 3–5 cmH_2O) to provide adequate tissue oxygenation but avoiding barotrauma at the same time.

Fig. 3.2.2 Postmortem picture of infant who died within 2 h of birth with left diaphragmatic hernia, showing herniation of intestine, left lobe of liver, and spleen. The right lung (also hypoplastic) is barely discernable

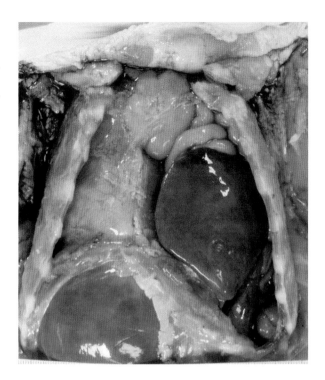

Concept of *"permissive hypercapnia"* or *"gentilation"* is to limit PIP (ideally <25 cmH$_2$O) and FiO$_2$ to produce preductal saturation >90%, while allowing limited rise (e.g., up to 60–65 mmHg) of pCO$_2$.

3. Relative fluid restriction (~50 mL/kg/day)
4. Consider – inotropic agents (e.g., dopamine, dobutamine both 2–20 µg/kg/min) and inhaled nitric oxide (iNO) (1–20 ppm), if signs of significant hypotension or R→L shunting.

3.2.6.3
Second-Line Therapy

1. *High-frequency oscillatory ventilation (HFOV).* Used to deliver a rate of 100–150 bpm, with gas exchange occurring through bulk diffusion.
2. *Extracorporeal membrane oxygenation (ECMO).* Indicated in severe refractory hypoxia although most studies have failed to show real benefit of ECMO in CDH patients. If used, ECMO is indicated if after maximal therapy, the preductal pO$_2$ is <50 mmHg, and pCO$_2$ >50 mmHg, on FiO$_2$=100%. The CDH is usually repaired when the ECMO session is finishing to minimise risk of bleeding etc.

3.2.7
Surgery

The original target in timing of CDH surgery was to get the infant to the operating room as quickly as possible. Nowadays that concept has been discredited and preoperative stabilization has become the norm.

1. Subcostal muscle-cutting incision. Divide umbilical vein and falciform ligament (allows rotation of liver to opposite side).
2. Remove viscera (caution with left-liver and spleen) from thoracic cavity. Any hernial sac (if present ~20%), should be excised.
3. Define anterior and posterior elements of diaphragm (the latter is frequently flattened on posterior abdominal wall). Primary apposition and repair if possible using interrupted, nonabsorbable sutures (e.g., Prolene®) placed around ribs if necessary. Avoid tension and inadequate fascia as this will predispose to recurrence.
4. Placement of viscera within abdominal cavity (in Ladd's position ± appendectomy). If closure too tight consider temporary prosthetic patch/silo.

Alternatives if primary closure is not feasible

- Prosthetic patch (e.g., Gore-Tex®, Permacol® (nonabsorbable), Surgisis® Gold (absorbable))
- Muscle flap (latissimus dorsi or internal oblique)

A right-sided CDH with an intrathoracic liver presents different problems, as the neonatal liver is friable and the hepatic veins and IVC are at risk during dissection and may kink on return to the abdominal cavity. Division of the falciform and rotation around hepatic vein axis aids repair.

3.2.8
Complications and Outcome

There is a reasonable expectation of survival in up to 75% of all live-born infants with isolated CDH. This would be optimistic if the defect was detected antenatally and certainly in the presence of other anomalies.

- *Chronic lung disease* – due to combination of underlying hypoplasia, and barotraumas, may be O_2 dependent for long periods. Bronchopulmonary dysplasia, and restrictive and obstructive lung dysfunction may all be observed in survivors.
- *Recurrence* (10–20%) – associated with prolonged periods of ventilation, prosthetic patches, ECMO, etc. Assess with CXR and, if doubt, CT/MR scan.
- *Gastro-esophageal reflux* (up to 40%) – treat medically initially but may need fundoplication.

- *Chylothorax* (<5%) – due to damage of lymphatics overlying posterior abdominal wall. If significant postoperative hydrothorax presents and needs drainage then send fluid for lymphocyte count, albumen, and lipid content.
- *Deformity of spine/chest wall* (<5%) is multifactorial and due to primary body wall anomalies, ipsilateral lung hypoplasia, and perhaps nature of surgical repair (prosthesis, etc.)
- *Neurodevelopmental impairment* – these are often infants who have struggled for life, with long periods of ventilator dependence, and periods of instability. Hearing loss appears to be particularly common.

Contentious Topics

Fetal Surgery

Effective and reliable discrimination of prognosis at time of antenatal diagnosis has allowed possibility of in utero intervention in selected cases in some institutions. Lung growth in CDH can be increased by tracheal occlusion (as the lungs expel fluid normally). Initial attempts required open hysterotomy and external tracheal clips, which have now been replaced by single-port fetoscopy and intratracheal placement of a detachable balloon (at 24–26 weeks gestation). The balloon is left in situ for 6–8 weeks then removed/punctured to allow the infant a normal delivery.

Minimally Invasive Surgery of CDH

This is an advanced technical procedure but can be done successfully thoracoscopically for Bochdalek hernias, and laparoscopically for Morgagni hernias. The most contentious group for this type of surgery are early presenting neonates as there is no cardiorespiratory advantage (and it may indeed be associated with a detrimental rise in pCO_2); it is an intrinsically longer procedure and the intestinal positioning is left to chance.

Further Reading

1. Lally KP, Lally PA, Van Meurs KP et al (2006) (Congenital Diaphragmatic Hernia Study Group). Treatment evolution in high-risk congenital diaphragmatic hernia: ten years' experience with diaphragmatic agenesis. Ann Surg 244:505–513
2. Harrison MR, Keller RL, Hawgood SB et al. Kitterman JA, Sandberg PL, Farmer DL, Lee H, Filly RA, Farrell JA, Albanese CT (2003) A randomized trial of fetal endoscopic tracheal occlusion for severe fetal congenital diaphragmatic hernia. N Engl J Med 349:1916–1924
3. Nguyen TL, Le AD (2006) Thoracoscopic repair for congenital diaphragmatic hernia: lessons from 45 cases. J Pediatr Surg 41:1713–1715
4. Sinha CK, Islam S, Patel S et al (2009) Congenital diaphragmatic hernia: prognostic indices in the FETO era. J Pediatr Surg 44: 312-316

5. Fryns JP, Moerman F, Goddeeris P, Bossuyt C, Van den Berghe H. A new lethal syndrome with cloudy corneae, diaphragmatic defects and distal limb deformities. Hum Genet 1979; 50: 65–70

6. Cantrell JR, Haller JA, Ravitch MM. A syndrome of congenital defects involving the abdominal wall, sternum, diaphragm, pericardium and heart. *Surg Gynaecol Obstet* 1958; 107: 602–614

Esophageal Atresia

3.3

Chandrasen K. Sinha and Lewis Spitz

The first successful primary repair of an esophageal atresia was performed in 1941 by Cameron Haight in Michigan, USA.
We can probably date this as the birth of modern-day neonatal surgery.

3.3.1
Epidemiology

- ~1 per 3,500 live-births
- M = F
- Isolated (~50%)
- *Associated anomalies* (~50%)

  — These vary in severity and number but two nonrandom associations/syndromes are recognized with EA as a component.

Among the other recognized associations are:

- Congenital heart disease (~30%) including VSD, PDA, and Tetralogy of Fallot[1]
- Anorectal malformation (10–15%)
- GI anomalies (10–15%), e.g., malrotation, duodenal atresia, duplication cyst, pyloric stenosis
- GU anomalies (10–15%), e.g., urethral abnormalities, hydronephrosis, multicystic dysplastic kidney, renal agenesis

---

[1]Etienne-Louis Arthur Fallot (1850–1911) French physician described four key features of this cardiac malformation in 1888.

C. K. Sinha (✉)
Paediatric Surgery Department, Kings College Hospital, London, UK

C. K. Sinha and M. Davenport (eds.), *Handbook of Pediatric Surgery*,
DOI: 10.1007/978-1-84882-132-3_3.3, © Springer-Verlag London Limited 2010

Table 3.3.1   Anatomical classification (after Vogt)

Type	Description	Frequency (%)
I	EA alone	7
II	EA and proximal fistula	1
III	EA and distal fistula	87
IV	EA and proximal and distal fistula	1
V	"H" type fistula. No EA	4

- Tracheo-broncho-pulmonary anomalies, e.g., tracheomalacia, foregut cysts, CCAM, and lung agenesis/hypoplasia
- Skeletal anomalies, e.g., vertebral and rib anomalies, absent radius, phocomelia,[2] sacral agenesis

VACTERL (Previously VATER) Syndrome

This is an acronym coined to describe the main features – Vertebral, Anorectal, Cardiac, Tracheo Esophageal, Renal, and Limb.

CHARGE Syndrome

Again an acronym is used to describe main features – Coloboma, Heart disease, Choanal Atresia, Retarded growth, Genital hypoplasia, Ear (i.e., deafness).

Embryology

1. Twenty-second day – trachea arises from the median ventral diverticulum of the primitive foregut. Rapid growth.
2. Thirty-two days – separation of ventral trachea from the dorsal esophagus.

---

[2]*Phocomelia* (Greek) "*seal*" + (Latin) "limb" - i.e., absent or shortened limbs, typically followed Thalidomide exposure.

3.3.2
Clinical Features: Five anatomical types (table 3.3.1)

3.3.2.1
Prenatal

Maternal US may detect a small or absent stomach accompanied by polyhydramnios. The latter sign is associated with a positive predictive value of ~50%, falling to ~15% in its absence. Other features may also be evident (e.g., skeletal anomalies).

3.3.2.2
Postnatal

Excessive salivation and frothing. Attempting to feed such an infant will lead to choking and distress. The diagnosis should be confirmed by passing a large size (~10 F) NG (or Replogle[3] tube if possible) and taking a CXR. This will show the NG tube at the level of the atresia.

- CXR
  - Air in the stomach suggests distal TEF; absence of air below the diaphragm suggests EA alone.
  - Associated anomalies (e.g., enlarged heart is suggestive of congenital heart disease, hemivertabrae, right-sided aortic arch (~2%)).
- Echocardiogram – define cardiac anatomy, right-sided aortic arch (a left-sided thoracotomy may be an easier approach).

The Type V "H" fistula has a different set of clinical features and typically presents after neonatal discharge with feeding-associated respiratory distress. A number of diagnostic options are available including bronchoscopy/esophagoscopy or a tube esophagogram.

3.3.3
Management

1. The upper pouch should be kept empty by continuous low-pressure suction via a Replogle tube.

---

[3]Robert Replogle – Professor of Cardio-thoracic Surgery, Chicago, IL.

2. Nursed in the horizontal or semiprone position with frequent change in infant's position. In those with lung collapse or pneumonia, the child should be placed with the affected side uppermost and gentle physiotherapy instituted.
3. Incubator humidified air may aid suction of pharyngeal secretions.

3.3.4
Surgery

3.3.4.1
Esophageal Atresia and Distal TEF

Semi-elective operation

1. Posterolateral extrapleural right-sided thoracotomy.
2. Expose and ligate azygous vein. Expose proximal pouch (manipulate Replogle tube) and identify TEF (relation with vagus nerve).
3. Divide TEF close to trachea and then close with nonabsorbable sutures (e.g., Prolene®).
4. Mobilize upper pouch from proximal trachea (excluding a further fistula).
5. Anastomose with a single layer sutures (e.g., 5/0 or 6/0 Prolene® or PDS®).

Most surgeons utilize a trans-anastomotic tube (6–8 Fg) and feed early. A formal gastrostomy and routine postoperative chest drain are less commonly practiced nowadays. Anastomoses considered to be under tension should probably be protected by elective paralysis and the infants ventilated for about 4–5 days with their neck flexed.

3.3.4.2
"Long-Gap" Esophageal Atresia

The ideal management for these cases has yet to emerge and a number of options are available.

Typically, such cases anatomically are defined by *absence of fistula* or prove after division of the distal fistula to have a gap of *>4 vertebral bodies* making primary repair unfeasible. In the past, these infants would probably have had an initial cervical esophagostomy and later esophageal replacement and even now it is a reasonable option where the gap is assessed at >6 vertebral bodies.

Currently, the commonest approach is to perform a delayed primary anastomosis at 2–3 months of life. Thus, Replogle tube drainage is continued and an open gastrostomy performed to initiate enteral feeding. If this regimen protects the lungs effectively, then serial assessment of the gap should be performed (contrast or probe) to document gap shrinkage. When this is felt to be small enough (images should almost overlap) then a thoracotomy is performed (Fig. 3.3.1)

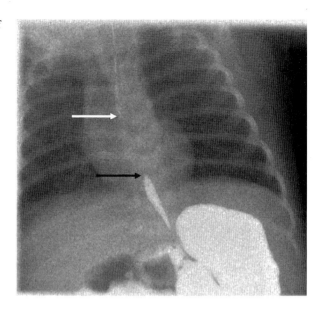

Fig 3.3.1   Contrast study of term infant with Replogle tube in upper pouch (*white arrow*) and contrast in stomach and distal blind-ending esophagus (*black arrow*). Long-gap esophageal atresia (still 3 vertebral bodies)

3.3.4.3
Surgical Complications

1. *Anastomotic leak* (<5%) – major early (<48 h) leaks should be suspected if pneumothorax develops. Most require chest tube drainage and exploration. Later leaks can be managed conservatively (± drain) although may be followed by stricture formation.
2. *Recurrent fistula* (5–10%) – suspected if oral feeding produces coughing and choking. Investigate with contrast esophagram ± bronchoscopy. Requires revision, a catheter passed at bronchoscopy may facilitate indentification.
3. *Stricture* (10–30%) – manifest as early feeding difficulty. Most respond to dilatation (bougie or balloon). Treat reflux but revision occasionally required.
4. *Gastro-esophageal reflux* (~40%) – common, but most amenable to medical therapy. Fundoplication performed in 10–20% of large series.
5. *Tracheomalacia* (~10%) – although of itself a common finding and part of the EA complex it can be a potent cause of "apparent life-threatening events" (ALTE). Investigated by bronchoscopy to show the airway collapse. Treated by aortopexy, tracheopexy, or even tracheostomy.

Preterm Infants with Respiratory Distress Syndrome and an EA/TEF

Dangerous combination as the necessarily high intratracheal pressures are vented through the fistula and can cause acute gastric distension and even perforation. Consider medical means of reducing airways pressure (e.g., high-frequency oscillation) but surgery should be considered early as an emergency with the prime object of ligation of fistula (by a transpleural thoractomy – it is quicker).

Controversies

- *Thoracoscopic repair* is being practiced in some centers with experts skilled in minimally invasive techniques; the first being reported in a 1999 by Thom Lobe[4] et al. in an 8-month-old infant with a Type 1 EA. There is a theoretical avoidance of chest wall deformity, although this should seldom be a real issue now with muscle-sparing thoractomies.
- The *Foker[5] procedure* has been reported for long-gap EA where the two sutured esophageal ends are physically stretched over a period of a week or so to gain length.

3.3.5
Prognostic Classifications

- *Waterston et al. (1962)[6]* classified these patients into three groups based on birth weight, and presence of pneumonia, and other congenital anomalies.
- *Spitz et al. (1994)* simplified this but retained birth weight and presence of major cardiac anomalies.

	Birth weight (kg)	Cardiac anomalies	Prognosis (%)
Group 1	>1.5	Absent	>98[a]
Group 2	<1.5	or Present	59
Group 3	<1.5	Present	22

[a]*Figures derive from original paper in 1994*

Others include *Montreal* (includes ventilator dependence), *Bremen* (includes postoperative complications) and that of *Sinha* et al (where both weight < 1.5 kg and a cardiac anomaly need to be present for bad prognosis) classifications.

3.3.6
Long-Term Outcome

Although for most infants there is effective restitution of normal feeding, allowing normal growth and development, it is probably expedient to defer intake of solids for a while in this group. Swallowing is effective but not normal. Peristalsis is impaired or absent and

---

[4]Thom Lobe – American pediatric surgeon.
[5]John Foker – American pediatric surgeon.
[6]Waterston DJ, Bonham-Carter R, Aberdeen E. Oesophageal atresia: tracheo-esophageal fistula. A study of survival in 218 infants. Lancet 1962; (i) 7234: 819-822.

most children learn to chew well and drink with meals. Typically they also have a higher incidence of respiratory-related issues such as recurrent chest infections, intermittent food-related choking, and a characteristic seal-like bark ("TOF cough" in English!). Such problems tend to subside with age presumably due to airway growth and improved luminal stability.

There may be a long-term malignancy potential during adulthood but the risk remains unquantified.

Further Reading

1. Spitz L, Kiely E, Brereton RJ (1987) Esophageal atresia: five-year experience with 148 cases. J Pediatr Surg 22:103–108
2. Engum SA, Grosfeld JL, West KA et al (1995) Analysis of morbidity and mortality in 227 cases of esophageal atresia and/or tracheoesophageal fistula over two decades. Arch Surg 130:502–509
3. Spitz L, Kiely EM, Morecroft JA, Drake DP (1994) Oesophageal atresia: at-risk groups for the 1990s. J Pediatr Surg 29:723–725
4. Holcomb GW 3rd, Rothenberg SS, Bax KM et al (2005) Thoracoscopic repair of esophageal atresia and tracheoesophageal fistula: a multi-institutional analysis. Ann Surg 242:422–428

Pyloric Stenosis

3.4

Giorgia Totonelli and Denis A. Cozzi

Pyloric stenosis is the commonest cause of surgical vomiting during infancy.

The Danish pediatrician Harald Hirschsprung[1] first described the key features of pyloric stenosis (PS) based on two infants who had died from it in 1888. This was followed by various rarely successful surgical attempts at bypassing or overcoming the gastric outlet obstruction culminating in Conrad Ramsted[2] describing in 1912 two successful cases where only the pyloric musculature was divided.

- 1–3 per 1,000 live-births
- M > F 2:1–5:1
- White > Black > Asian
- Typical postnatal age 3–6 weeks, rare beyond 4 months of age

3.4.1
Pathophysiology

Unknown etiology

1. Genetic component
   (a) Seven percent incidence of PS in children of affected parents (×4 risk if mother affected)

---

[1]Harold Hirschsprung (1830–1916) – Danish pediatrician.
[2]Conrad von Ram(m)stedt (1867–1963) either spelling is correct – German military surgeon, later worked in Munster.

G. Totonelli (✉)
Pediatric Surgery Unit, Sapienza University of Rome, Rome, Italy

C. K. Sinha and M. Davenport (eds.), *Handbook of Pediatric Surgery*,
DOI: 10.1007/978-1-84882-132-3_3.4, © Springer-Verlag London Limited 2010

2. Associated
   (a) Esophageal atresia
   (b) Maternal erythromycin use (via breast milk)
   (c) Young maternal age

PS is characterized by hypertrophy of the circular muscle layer so that the pyloric canal is lengthened and narrowed with pronounced thickening of the whole pylorus.
   There is some evidence that there is:

- ↓ Nonadrenergic noncholinergic nerves with ↑ collagen deposition
- ↓ Interstitial cells of Cajal[3]
- ↓ Expression of neuronal nitric oxide synthase (nNOS)

> Gastric outlet obstruction leads to loss of acid (HCl), Na, Cl, K, and water; i.e., *dehydration, metabolic alkalosis*, and *hypokalemia*. The compensatory response to this is principally renal preservation of Na^+ (initially with loss of further K^+, and then later loss of H^+ as a cation exchange, i.e., "paradoxical aciduria").

3.4.2
Clinical Features

Progressive, nonbilious, projectile vomiting, occasionally containing "coffee grounds" (due to altered blood and gastritis) in a term infant. Symptoms may be atypical in preterm. The key to clinical diagnosis is palpation of the hypertrophied pylorus in the epigastrium or right hypocondrium. Gastric peristalsis may be seen.
   (*Test Feed*: Examine the abdomen from the baby's left while feeding. The "olive" tumor is usually felt around the lateral margin of the right rectus abdominis muscle below the liver edge. A small feed is best since a greatly distended stomach obscures the tumor. In general, it is easier to feel the tumor at the end of the feed, especially if the infant has just vomited.)

3.4.2.1
Investigation

- Urea and electrolytes – ↓ Na^+ ↓ K^+ ↓ Cl^- (↑urea ↑creatinine)
- Blood gas – ↑ pH ↑ HCO_3^-
   (a) HCO_3^- – Mild <25 mmol/L, Moderate 26–35 mmol/L, Severe >35 mmol/L
- *Abdominal US* – noninvasive imaging for accurate diagnosis of PS

---

[3]Santiago Ramon y Cajal (1852–1934) – Spanish pathologist and Nobel laureate.

- Muscle thickness >4 mm
- Pyloric canal length ≥16 mm

3.4.3
Surgery

PS is not a *surgical* emergency – it is a *medical* emergency and initial resuscitation is paramount.

- NG tube.
- IV fluids – stock solution 5% dextrose with 0.45% NaCl (+20 mmol/L of KCl – after confirmation of urine output).
  - ~150 mL/kg/day is reasonable initial rate, modified by serial electrolytes and urine output.

Blood glucose concentrations should be monitored.
Most infants come to surgery within 24 h but long-standing vomiting needs careful preparation over 3–5 days.

3.4.3.1
Ramstedt Pyloromyotomy

1. Incision.
    (a) Classical – vertical, RUQ muscle cutting
    (b) Circumumbilical (described by Bianchi in 1986[4])
2. Evert pylorus out of wound.
3. Longitudinal incision (2–3 cm) along anterior, avascular surface of the pyloric "olive". The back of a scalpel handle is used to split the hypertrophied muscle down to the intact submucosa. Caution with fornix of duodenum (most superficial part).
4. Test mucosal integrity – inflate stomach via NG tube with 60 mL air. Unrecognized perforation will lead to peritonitis, sepsis, and even death.

3.4.3.2
Feeding Regimen

(a) Remove NG tube on completion of surgery.
(b) After 6–8 h, offer 10 mL of sugar water orally, replaced after 3 h by milk, increasing by 10 mL every 3 h until infant takes full feed.
(c) Discharge 24–48 h after surgery.

---

[4]Adrian Bianchi – Maltese pediatric surgeon working in Manchester, UK.

(If known duodenal perforation, continue NG tube aspiration, add 48 h IV antibiotics, and delay oral feeding for ~48 h.)

Complications may include duodenal perforation, incomplete pyloromyotomy, and wound infection. Persistent postoperative vomiting (defined as prolonged vomiting for >7 days), is usually caused by too rapid advancement of postoperative feeding, or of residual pyloric edema. An incomplete pyloromyotomy is possible but unlikely (need for reoperation as <2%). If repyloromyotomy is required, it should be postponed for 2 weeks – most vomiting will actually cease within this period.

Laparoscopic pyloromyotomy, developed in 1990s, using a 5-mm umbilical camera port and two 3 mm working ports. Randomized trials suggest marginal improvements in time to full feeds and discharge with possible ↑ perforation rate.

Further Reading

1. Leclair MD Plattner V, Mirallie E et al (2007) Laparoscopic pyloromyotomy for hypertrophic pyloric stenosis: a prospective, randomized controlled trial. J Pediatr Surg 42:692–698
2. Hall NJ, Pacilli M, Eaton S et al (2009) Recovery after open versus laparoscopic pyloromyotomy for pyloric stenosis: a double-blind multicentre randomised controlled trial. Lancet 31:390–398
3. Cozzi DA, Ceccanti S, Mele E et al (2008) Circumumbilical pyloromyotomy in the era of minimally invasive surgery. J Pediatr Surg 43:1802–1806
4. Allan C (2006) Determinants of good outcome in pyloric stenosis. J Paediatr Child Health 42:86–88
5. Taqi E, Boutros J, Emil S et al (2007) Evaluation of surgical approaches to pyloromyotomy: a single-center experience. J Pediatr Surg 42:865–868

Malrotation

3.5

Ike L. Njere and Mark Davenport

Malrotation is used to describe a spectrum of anomalies of rotation and fixation of the intestines, principally involving the midgut.

3.5.1

- Incidence ~1% (but variable depending on definition, or mode of diagnosis).
- Causes <5% of intestinal obstruction during childhood.
- Most (50–70%) are diagnosed in the neonatal period.
- M=F.

Associated with

- Gastroschisis and exomphalos
- Diaphragmatic hernia
- Duodenal atresia and biliary atresia
- Intussusception (Waugh's syndrome[1])
- Dysmotility (e.g., intestinal neuronal dysplasia) and pseudo-obstruction syndromes

Malrotation occurs when the normal process of rotation is not complete or is erroneous. The commonest variant being failure of the final 90° anticlockwise rotation taking the cecum from the right upper quadrant to the right iliac fossa. Here, it still tries to fix itself

---

[1]Waugh GEA (1920). The morbid consequences of a mobile ascending colon. Br J Surg 7:343.
[2]William E Ladd. see pp. 94.

I. L. Njere (✉)
Department of Paediatric Surgery, University Hospital Lewisham, London, UK

C. K. Sinha and M. Davenport (eds.), *Handbook of Pediatric Surgery*,
DOI: 10.1007/978-1-84882-132-3_3.5, © Springer-Verlag London Limited 2010

to the retroperitoneum, sometimes seen as discrete peritoneal bands running anteriorly to the second part of duodenum (Ladd's[2] bands).

The key pathology is the distance between the two ends of the small bowel mesentery (as marked by DJ flexure and IC valve). When this is diminished, then the risk of volvulus increases – as in the example above.

Embryology

Intestinal positioning occurs between the fifth and twelfth weeks of gestation.

- Stage 1 (5th to 10th week) – midgut herniation into the umbilicus.
- Stage 2 (10th to 11th week) – return of midgut to the abdomen.
- Stage 3 (>11th week) – retroperitoneal fixation of colon and duodenum.

The midgut starts as a straight tube in the early embryo. Its blood supply, the superior mesenteric artery (SMA), with the vitelline duct at its apex, divides the midgut into a cephalad *prearterial* and a caudal *postarterial* segment. Rapid elongation of the midgut causes it to form a loop along the axis of the SMA and then herniate into the umbilicus. The prearterial segment rotates 180° and the postarterial segment rotates 90° (both anticlockwise) along the axis of the SMA. The prearterial segment then reenters the abdomen with an additional 90° anticlockwise rotation. The postarterial segment follows, rotating an additional 180°. The proximal prearterial segment is thus the normal C-loop configuration of the duodenum. The distal duodenum passes beneath the SMA axis and the distal postarterial segment becomes the colon in its "picture frame" position with the transverse colon anterior to the SMA and the caecum in the right iliac fossa (Fig. 3.5.1).

3.5.2
Clinical Features

Malrotation can present at any age though the classic presentation is an infant with bile vomiting (~50%) due to duodenal obstruction (extrinsic due to Ladd's bands or by virtue of the twist of the volvulus). If delayed, then the features are less specific but may include non-bile vomiting, intermittent or acute abdominal pain, diarrhea, constipation, failure to thrive, or passage of altered blood.

Sometimes, chronic midgut volvulus (<10% of cases) may cause mesenteric thickening, with lymphatic obstruction leading to chylous ascites and malabsorption.

On physical examination, the abdomen is soft and nontender to palpation unless volvulus and bowel strangulation has occurred (~25% of all cases) leading to abdominal distension, tenderness, and blood-stained stools.

Fig. 3.5.1   Schematic of normal rotation (**a**) Midline midgut supplied by superior mesenteric artery, initial a/c rotation. (**b**) Prearterial midgut passing behind SMA to reach LUQ and continuation of a/c rotation of postarterial midgut around axis of SMA. (**c**) Final 90° a/c rotation to bring cecum down to RLQ

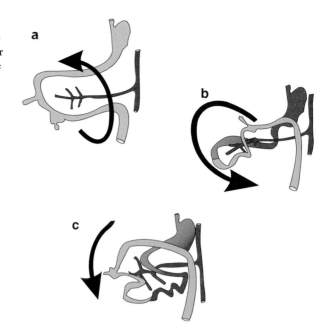

3.5.2.1
Investigations

1. *AXR* is probably "normal" in most cases. But abnormal features may include:
   (a) Malposition of the bowel ("small bowel" to the right and "colon" to the left)
   (b) Lack of distal bowel gas – a "gasless" abdomen or a "double bubble" appearance
   (c) "Whirled" appearance of mid-abdominal bowel
   (d) Thick-walled, tubular loops with thickened folds or thumbprinting (suggesting chronic volvulus)
2. *Upper GI contrast study (Table 3.5.1)*
   (a) Ideally barium, but use nonionic water-soluble contrast if perforation is a possiblilty – investigation of choice (if time permits!)

Lower GI contrast is an alternative to identify position of the cecum, but this is less secure and cecal position may be normal in malrotation (up to 30%) and an unfixed cecum is found normally in ~15% of patients.

3.5.2.2   Ultrasound and CT Scan Identification of Relationship
of Mesenteric Vessels

- The SMA is to the *left* of the SMV (normal).

This relationship can be appreciated on abdominal US and CT scan. If the arrangement is reversed, then malrotation should be suspected. Seems to be operator-dependent and is not widely used.

3.5.3
Management

Consider if volvulus is likely (or even a possibility), *then every minute counts* and the child needs urgent laparotomy for intestinal detorsion. Other elements to be considered while this is being prepared are rapid fluid resuscitation, N-G aspiration, correction of acid/base imbalance, IV broad-spectrum antibiotic regimen, and inotropic agents.

The preoperative preparation can be more leisurely if there is *no* evidence of intestinal ischemia.

3.5.3.1
Surgery: The Ladd's[3] Procedure

There are two preludes to this procedure.

1. Untwist a volvulus – usually this means in an anticlockwise direction – but satisfy yourself that this is completely achieved.
   (a) Assess intestinal damage and prepare for reperfusion syndrome (hypotension, ↑K^+, ↑lactate).
   (b) Resection (if unequivocal necrosis)±anastomosis (if safe). If, equivocal and short bowel is likely then consider leaving "ischemic" gut alone and perform second look laparotomy in 24–36 h.
2. Consider possibility of underlying "windsock" of duodenal stenosis/atresia. Look for duodenal disparity and pass NG tube along into jejunum, if doubt.

The aim is to leave the midgut in a position of complete "non-rotation" with duodenum and small bowel on right, apex of midgut (where a Meckel diverticulum would be) and hence SMA centrally and cecum and large bowel on left. This achieves the widest possible base to the mesentery thus reducing propensity to volvulus.

1. Division of Ladd's bands (lying across the duodenum from abnormal caecum in RUQ).
2. Widen mesenteric base – divide peritoneum overlying central mesenteric vessels.
3. Position bowel – small bowel right and large bowel left.
4. ± Appendectomy.

---

[3]William E. Ladd (1880–1967) – American surgeon working in Boston, MA, regarded as father of American pediatric surgery and pioneer in many areas.

Table 3.5.1 Contrast studies in malrotation

	Normal features	Abnormal features
Overall	"C" shaped duodenum	Redundant duodenum, right-sided jejunal loops
Lateral appearance	Overlapping, posterior position of second and fourth parts	Anterior position of fourth part
Duodeno-jejunal flexure	Left of spinal pedicles; rising to at least level of L1/L2 disk space	Right-sided or centrally placed. Failure of ascent to level of pylorus

Laparoscopic evaluation of a possible malrotation is relatively straightforward if contrast studies are equivocal. Certainly it is the only real investigation, which can evaluate the breadth of the mesenteric base and the mobility of the cecum. Correction of a volvulus though is more problematic and controversial as it can be difficult to appreciate relative position of the intestines.

3.5.4
Outcome and Complications

- Midgut infarction (<5%)
- Recurrence of midgut volvulus post-Ladd's procedure (<2%)
- Adhesional intestinal obstruction (5%)

Further Reading

1. Ladd WE (1936) Surgical diseases of the alimentary tract in infants. N Engl J Med 215:705–708
2. Miller AJW, Rode H, Cywes S (2003) Malrotation and volvulus in infancy and childhood. Semin Pediatr Surg 12:229–236
3. Strouse PJ (2007) Malrotation. Semin Roentgenol 43:7–14
4. Bass KD, Rothenberg SS, Chang JH (1998) Laparoscopic Ladd's procedure in infants with malrotation. J Pediatr Surg 33:279–281

Intestinal Atresia

3.6

Chandrasen K. Sinha, Erica Makin, and Dorothy Iwagba Kufeji

Calder first described two infants with duodenal atresia in 1733. No survivors were reported until the twentieth century, when Vidal (1905) described gastrojejunostomy and Ernest (1914) duodenojejunostomy.

This chapter considers intestinal atresia[1] from the stomach to the colon.

3.6.1
Epidemiology

- 1 in 5,000 F>M (slight) duodenal
- 1 in 3,000 black>white jejunoileal
- 1 in 50,000 colonic

Jejunoileal>duodenal>colonic

Embryology

Primitive gut is divided into *fore-, mid- and hindgut*. Each has its own artery; respectively the *celiac, superior, and inferior mesenteric* arteries, given off the front of the aorta. Endodermal proliferation is maximal between 30 and 60 days and appears sufficient in some parts to almost completely occlude the lumen. Vacuolation, due to endodermal

---

[1]Atresia is derived from the Greek "a" and "tresis" meaning no orifice/perforation.

C. K. Sinha (✉)
Paediatric Surgery Department, King's College Hospital, London, UK

C. K. Sinha and M. Davenport (eds.), *Handbook of Pediatric Surgery*, 95
DOI: 10.1007/978-1-84882-132-3_3.6, © Springer-Verlag London Limited 2010

apoptosis restores the lumen and if this is incomplete it may be responsible for some cases of duodenal atresia (Tandler hypothesis[2]). Differential expression of Sonic Hedgehog (Shh) seems to control key parts of this process.

Rapid jejunoileal growth occurs during the late phase of gestation from about 115 cm (at 24 weeks gestation) to about 250 cm (usual length at term). Rotation of the gut is considered in Chap. 3.5.

3.6.2
Associations

- Pyloric atresia
  - Epidermolysis bullosa
  - HMIA (Hereditary multiple intestinal atresia)
- Duodenal atresia
  - Trisomy 21, Down syndrome[2] – duodenal atresia (up to 30% of unselected series, up to 6% of Down's births)
  - Esophageal atresia
  - Malrotation
  - Cardiac anomalies
  - Vertebral anomalies
- Jejunal ileo colic atresia
  - Abdominal wall defects – especially gastroschisis. Due to localized trauma/ischemia at the entry and exit points
  - Maternal glomerulonephritis
  - Maternal cocaine use
  - Hirchsprung's disease (colon atresia)

3.6.3
Pathology

The cause of most intestinal atresias is unknown, but in utero experimental animal models suggest that atretic segments can be replicated by mesenteric vascular ligation. Less commonly (e.g., HMIA, epidermolyis), disorders in epithelial proliferation and apoptosis could affect luminal continuity.

Julius Tandler - 19th century Austrian embryologist.
[2]John Langdon Haydon Down (1828–1896) – English physician. Published "Observations on an Ethnic Classification of Idiots" in 1866.

3.6.3.1
Classification (After Bland-Sutton[3], Modified by Grosfeld[4]) (Fig. 3.6.1)

Though this was originally described for duodenal atresia it is applicable to all parts of the intestine.

- Type I – Membrane or web
- Type II – Fibrous cord joins two blind ends of bowel
- Type III – Gap between ends with a V-shaped mesenteric defect
  - Subtype (sometimes referred to as Type IIIb), where there is a large defect in the mesentery, significant intestinal loss and distal intestine winds round a single, usually tenuous vascular pedicle ("apple-peel" atresia)
- Type IV – Multiple atresias, often with the appearance of a "string of sausages"

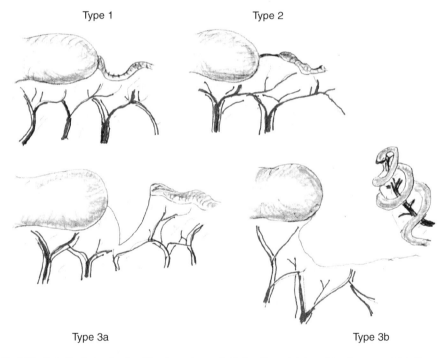

Type 1   Type 2

Type 3a   Type 3b

Fig. 3.6.1 Intestinal atresia classification – (types 1, 2, 3a, 3b, and 4 (combination or multiple))

---

[3]Sir John Bland-Sutton (1855–1936) – English surgeon.
[4]Jay Grosfeld – American surgeon, editor of *Journal of Pediatric Surgery*.

3.6.3.2
Hereditary Multiple Intestinal Atresia (HMIA)

Sporadic or familial condition with multiple atretic segments (from pyloric atresia down, often type 1, and >20). Associated with immunodeficiency and a dilated biliary tree, although many possible surgical solutions exist to retain native bowel, practically, it is almost uniformly fatal. Survivors have often had both small bowel and bone marrow transplants.

3.6.4
Clinical Features

Antenatal US may show polyhydramnios (↑ with the more proximal atresias). A "double bubble," dilated proximal loops or simply "echogenic" bowel may be seen.

Postnatally, infants exhibit bile-vomiting and varying degrees of distension (depending on level of obstruction) together with delay in passage of meconium (not invariable). Stenosis rather than atresia may be tolerated for a period and present later with intermittent vomiting and failure to thrive.

3.6.4.1
Investigations

- *AXR* will show features of obstruction (e.g., dilated bowel loops and absence of distal gas).
  - "Double bubble" and no distal gas – classical feature in duodenal obstruction.
  - More loops will be visible with distal obstructions.
  - Colon atresia – characteristic picture is a single, grossly dilated right-sided loop with a fluid level. This represents the obstructed colon with a competent ileo-cecal valve – a closed loop obstruction.
  - Intrauterine perforation and meconium cyst formation may be suggested by *peritoneal calcification*.
- *Contrast enema* may show a microcolon and is also helpful in ruling out other causes of distal bowel obstruction (e.g., Hirschsprung disease, meconium plug).

Differential diagnosis – meconium ileus ("soap-bubble" sign, no fluid levels), *Hirschsprung's disease* (↑ dilated bowel loops, transistion zone on contrast enema), and *malrotation* (double bubble ± distal gas).

3.6.5
Surgery

Transverse supraumbilical incision

3.6.5.1
Duodenal Atresia (Duodenoduodenostomy)

1. Recognize and treat any associated *malrotation*.
2. Approximate two ends, mobilize to avoid tension (antimesenteric not mesenteric). Recognize possible "wind-sock" Type 1 anomaly if bowel is in continuity.
3. Transverse incision proximal end. Longitudinal incision distal end. Full thickness absorbable sutures. Type 1 membrane may be excised. Caution with area of ampulla.
4. Sometimes because of gross proximal dilatation – consider duodenoplasty and tapering.
5. ± Transanastomotic tube.

3.6.5.2
Jejuno-ileal Atresia (Figs 3.6.2 and 3.6.3)

1. Key observations include *viability* and *length of residual bowel* together with patency of distal lumen. An unrecognized distal atresia or stenosis will inevitably cause proximal anastomotic breakdown.
2. *Bowel Disparity* – main problem in anastomosis if sufficient residual bowel then resect back to more normal caliber. Alternatively, if residual bowel is precious then either imbrication or a tapering enteroplasty can be performed.
3. Strategies to treat short bowel are discussed in chapter 4.11.

3.6.5.3
Colon Atresia

Usually the site of atresia is two-thirds along the transverse colon. Operative options include:

1. *Primary anastomosis* – because of proximal dilatation – resect as right hemicolectomy and ileo-transverse colostomy
2. *Defunctioning colostomy* and *staged anastomosis*

Postoperatively, parenteral nutrition should be started and continued until enteral feeds are established.

Fig. 3.6.2 Jejunal atresia –
type 3a

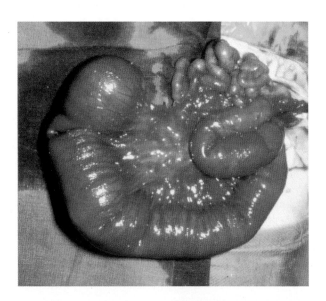

Fig. 3.6.3 Jejunal atresia –
type 3b. "Apple-peel" atresia
complicated by necrosis

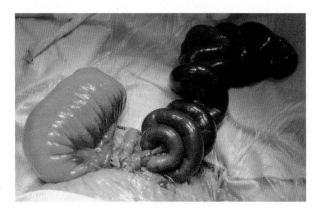

3.6.6
Outcome

Largely dependent on associated anomalies, and length of residual small bowel

Further Reading

1. Alexander F, Babak D, Goske M (2002) Use of intraluminal stents in multiple intestinal atresia. J Pediatr Surg 37:E34
2. Festen S, Brevoord JC, Goldhoorn GA et al (2002) Excellent long-term outcome for survivors of apple peel atresia. J Pediatr Surg 37:61–65

3. Cox SG, Numanoglu A, Millar AJ, Rode H (2005) Colonic atresia: spectrum of presentation and pitfalls in management. A review of 14 cases. Pediatr Surg Int 21:813–818
4. Millar AJ, Rode H, Cywes S (2000) Intestinal atresia and stenosis. In: Ashcraft KW et al (eds) Pediatric surgery. W.B. Saunders, Philadelphia, pp 406–424
5. Dalla Vecchia LK, Grosfeld JL, West KW,. Rescorla FJ et al (1998) Intestinal atresia and stenosis: a 25-year experience with 277 cases. Arch Surg 133:490–497

Necrotizing Enterocolitis

3.7

Lorna Cook and Mark Davenport

First definitive series of necrotizing enterocolitis appeared in 1964 following an outbreak in 21 infants at the Babies Hospital in New York.

3.7.1
Epidemiology

The incidence of necrotizing enterocolitis (NEC) in a neonatal unit varies from 3 to 10% depending on the case-mix of the unit.

- 1–3/1,000 live-births M:F = 2:1 Black > white
- >90% of all cases occur in preterm infants
- Term infants – associated with congenital heart disease or birth asphyxia
- No apparent seasonality or geographic preference
- Reduced incidence in breast vs. formula-fed infants

3.7.2
Pathogenesis

Pathophysiology is unclear but is likely to be multifactorial, with NEC being the common end-point arrived at by different processes. It seems a unique response in the immature, neonatal gut to "stress" (Fig. 3.7.1).

NEC may be focal or diffuse, with the most commonly affected sites being the terminal ileum and colon. Bowel appears distended, edematous, with hemorrhagic fluid in the lumen. Hemorrhage may be visible on the bowel wall mixed with areas of green to black gangrene.

M. Davenport (✉)
Paediatric Surgery Department, Kings College Hospital, London, UK

C. K. Sinha and M. Davenport (eds.), *Handbook of Pediatric Surgery*,
DOI: 10.1007/978-1-84882-132-3_3.7, © Springer-Verlag London Limited 2010

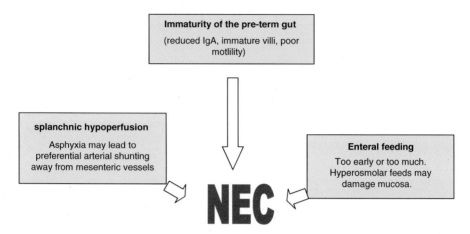

Fig. 3.7.1 Possible causal factors in NEC

Submucosal and subserosal gas-filled cysts may be obvious (N_2 or H_2), from action of gas-forming bacteria.

Histologically it is characterized by mucosal ulceration and transmural coagulative necrosis and gangrene, which may result in perforation. Microthrombi may be seen in mesenteric vessels.

3.7.3
Clinical Features

- Age of onset is most commonly between 7 and 10 days of age and is inversely proportional to gestational age at birth.
- First-week NEC may be predisposed by maternal drug use, perinatal sepsis, and predicted by changes in umbilical artery Doppler characteristics.

Range of nonspecific signs related to sepsis and ischemia (e.g., tachycardia, hypotension, metabolic acidosis, unstable body temperature, increasing O_2 requirement, thrombocytopenia, coagulopathy) together with more specific local signs related to the affected bowel loops (e.g., peritonism, abdominal wall erythema, bile-vomiting, GI bleeding, abdominal mass formation) (Table 3.7.1).

3.7.3.1
Investigations

1. Blood work-up for signs of sepsis and intestinal necrosis
   (a) FBC (esp. platelet count)
   (b) Coagulation screen (INR, fibrinogen, D-dimers)
   (c) Lactate and arterial blood gases

2. Radiology (supine AP±cross-table shoot-though lateral)

   (a) Early signs – nonspecific distension
   (b) Late signs
       – *Pneumatosis* (seen as linear radiolucent bands parallel to the wall of the bowel or "soap-bubble" appearance)
       – *Portal venous gas* (also detectable on US)
       – *Extravisceral free air* is most commonly seen between the liver and the diaphragm and anteriorly outlining falciform ligament ("football sign").
       – *"Ground-glass" appearance* – suggests free fluid.

N.B. Focal intestinal perforation is a poorly defined condition felt to be separate from NEC but may present with pneumoperitoneum without the associated necrosis. Has a good prognosis.

3.7.4
Management

The initial strategy should be supportive and aimed at resting the gut and optimizing the infant's hemodynamic and metabolic condition. This involves:

- Nil by mouth and naso-gastric tube
- Restoration of fluid losses (including third space losses), hematocrit, temperature instability, glucose instability, acid–base imbalance, and appropriate oxygenation, etc.
- Broad-spectrum antibiotics (e.g., penicillin, gentamicin, vancomycin, cefuroxime, metronidazole)
- Analgesia

Table 3.7.1 Bell's staging[1]

	Clinical	Radiology
I – suspected	Irritable, apnea, bile-aspirates, abdo. Distension, +ve fecal occult blood	Intestinal distension
II – definite	GI bleeding ± Abdo. mass	Pneumatosis, "fixed" loops, portal venous gas
III – advanced	Shock, marked GI bleeding	Pneumoperitoneum, severe ascites

Modified subsequently in the 1980s (Kleigman) to divide each type into (A) and (B). More specific but no real change in discrimination

[1]Martin J Bell – American pediatric surgeon working in St. Louis, MO.

Monitoring should be combined with serial radiography to assess onset of complications (e.g., perforation). If improving, then continue for 7–10 days before restarting enteral nutrition.

3.7.4.1
Indications for Surgery

About one-third will require intervention with indications for surgery being:

- Pneumoperitoneum – indicative of perforation
- Failure to progress (after 24 h of full, supportive management)
- Obstructive features – e.g., ↑ distension, ↑ bile-aspirates
- "Fixed-loop" on serial imaging (soft)
- ↑ Abdominal wall erythema – palpable abdominal mass

3.7.5
Surgery

Transverse (usually RUQ) incision

1. Assess site (ileocecal etc.), extent (focal, multifocal), and degree (ischemia, necrosis, perforation). "Pan-intestinal" implies majority of small and large bowel is involved with <25% of viable bowel remaining.

Possible interventions include:

2. *Resection* – focal necrotic areas with either anastomosis (if good condition) or stomas (if not).
3. *Proximal stoma only* – typically if grossly inflamed adherent RIF mass, makes resection dangerous.
4. *"Clip and drop" technique* (for pan-intestinal disease), i.e., rapid resection of obviously dead areas with application of surgical clips to close separate ends. Then after 48 h, second-look laparotomy to fashion stoma and if appropriate re-anastomose distal salvaged segments.

Primary peritoneal drainage (PPD) performed at cot-side under local anesthesia, may be alternative to laparotomy but RCTs have shown no advantage over laparotomy. Some centers use this simply as a temporizing measure for pneumoperitoneum but it can be definitive.

3.7.6
Outcome and Complications

Mortality ranges from 20 to 50% (higher in VLBW and ELBW).

- Recurrence (~5%), usually within a month of initial presentation
- Short-gut syndrome (~25%)
- Strictures (20%) – try to identify after 4 weeks with contrast studies

Prevention Strategies

1. Breast milk (fourfold reduction in NEC incidence vs. formula)
2. Avoidance of indomethacin/ibuprofen/ranitidine and maintenance of gastric acidity – little actual evidence
3. Probiotics (e.g., lactobacillus/bifidobacterium) – inconclusive trials
4. Oral antibiotic (e.g., gentamicin/neomycin) – inconclusive trials
5. Oral/IV immunoglobulin (IgA/IgG) – inconclusive trials
6. Amino-acid supplementation (glutamine) – no trial evidence of benefit

Further Reading

1. Bell MJ Ternberg JL, Feigin RD, Keating JP, Marshall R, Barton L, Brotherton T (1978) Neonatal necrotising enterocolitis. Therapeutic decisions based upon clinical staging. Ann Surg 187:1–7
2. Moss RL, Dimmitt RA, Barnhart DC et al (2006) Laparotomy versus peritoneal drainage for necrotizing enterocolitis and perforation. N Engl J Med 354:2225–2234
3. Rees CM, Eaton S, Kiely EM, Wade AM, McHugh K, Pierro A (2008) Peritoneal drainage or laparotomy for neonatal bowel perforation? A randomized controlled trial. Ann Surg 248:44–51
4. Ron O, Davenport M, Patel S et al (2009) Outcomes of the "clip and drop" technique for multifocal necrotizing enterocolitis. J Pediatr Surg 44:749–754

Meconium Ileus

3.8

Chandrasen K. Sinha, Mark Davenport, and Harry C. Ward

Meconium ileus may define how an infant enters this world, but cystic fibrosis defines its life thereafter.

Definition – Distal ileal intraluminal obstruction due to presence of abnormally viscid meconium. First described in 1905 by Karl Landsteiner.[1]

Meconium[2]

Normal meconium contains bile pigments, desquamated epithelia and is black; CF meconium has ↑↑ albumin, ↓ carbohydrate, ↓(HCO_3^-), and ↓ fluid content resulting in ↑↑viscidity. There is also abnormal intestinal motility and mucin production.

3.8.1
Epidemiology

- ~90% of infants presenting with meconium ileus (MI) will have cystic fibrosis (CF).
- ~15% of CF patients will present with MI.
- MI is the cause of ~20% of neonatal intestinal obstruction.
- M=F.

---

[1]Karl Landsteiner (1968–1943) – Nobel Prize winning (for description of blood groups) Austrian physician, who in spare time also discovered poliovirus.
[2]*Meconium* – (Greek) "poppy juice," i.e., opium – possibly a reference to its tarry appearance or ancient belief that it induced sleep in the fetus.

C. K. Sinha (✉)
Paediatric Surgery Department, King's College Hospital, London, UK

C. K. Sinha and M. Davenport (eds.), *Handbook of Pediatric Surgery*,
DOI: 10.1007/978-1-84882-132-3_3.8, © Springer-Verlag London Limited 2010

Cystic Fibrosis

- Most common (carrier frequency 1 in 25) recessive disease in Caucasians.
- 1 in 3,000 live-births.
- Autosomal recessive disease mutation in the CFTR (CF Transmembrane-conductance Regulator) gene – Ch 7 (q 31.2).
- Commonest mutation is ΔF508 (>1,000 mutations so far identified).
- Chloride channel defect.
  - Respiratory epithelium – viscid secretion and impairment of ciliary mucus clearance. Predisposes to bacterial colonization.
  - Causes ↑ (Cl^-) in sweat.
  - Causes ↓ (Cl^-) GI tract, pancreas, and liver – ↑ viscidity secretions, exocrine gland blockage.
  - Luminal obstruction – vas deferens.

3.8.2
Clinical Features

Antenatal period – hyperechogenic, dilated bowel, or nonvisualization of the gall bladder on US (also seen in Down' syndrome, intestinal atresia, and the normal fetus). Indication for parental genotypes ± amniocentesis.

MI has been classified into two types:

- *Simple MI* – abdominal distension, bile vomiting, and failure to pass meconium. "Doughy," palpable bowel loops on examination
- *Complicated MI*
  - Intrauterine perforation → meconium pseuodocyst
  - Intestinal atresia
  - Local volvulus (usually ileum) → gangrene

3.8.2.1
Investigation

1. *AXR* – dilated loops of bowel with a coarse granular ("soap-bubble") appearance – Neuhauser's sign[3]. Calcification may also be seen in meconium peritonitis.
2. *Contrast enema* – a water-soluble contrast enema will show micro-colon, which may contain small pellets of mucus. The role of contrast enema is often therapeutic but may be diagnostic of either functional or mechanical obstruction.
3. *Postnatal US* – definition of palpable mass (meconium cyst).

---

[3]Edward BD Neuhauser (1908–1987) – Chief radiologist at Boston Children's Hospital.

4. *Confirmation of CF*

  (a) *Sweat test* (pilocarpine iontophoresis) (>1 month postnatal). At least 100 mg of sweat – [Cl⁻] normal <40, diagnostic ≥60 mmol/L).

  (b) *Gene mutation analysis* – common mutations detect >98% of Caucasian CF. Beware in other racial backgrounds.

  (c) *Immunoreactive trypsinogen* – basis for screening. ↑↑ levels in CF.

3.8.3
Management

- Water-soluble contrast enema – in absence of complications.

  (a) Gastrografin® – ~1,900 mOsm/L (i.e., fivefold increase in osmotic pressure than normal). Dilute for effect, but caution with dehydration and IV fluid management.

  (b) Success 60–70% in simple MI with bowel perforation rate ~3% (avoid balloon-tipped catheter, ↑ risk of rectal perforation).

3.8.4
Surgery

Supra-umbilical transverse

1. *Simple MI* – distal ileum is relatively narrow and contains grey, inspissated meconium, further proximally, the mid-ileum is dilated and filled with extremely thick, tenacious, dark green, or tarry meconium. Micro-colon is usually found.

  (a) Ileotomy and passage of catheter (proximal to the inspissated meconium), using *N*-acetylcysteine or normal saline and massage to break up obstruction.

  (b) Options then include – simple closure and return; double-barrelled Mikulicz[4] ileostomy (1953), Bishop-Koop[5] ileostomy (1961), Santulli[6] ileostomy (1957), and a T tube, placed in lieu of a stoma (Fig. 3.8.1).

2. *Complicated MI*

  (a) ± Resection of ischemic bowel (or cyst, atretic segment, etc.) usually with diverting stoma or sometimes primary anastomosis.

---

[4]Jan Mikulicz – Radecki (1850–1905) – Polish surgeon, assisted Billroth in Vienna, and set up famous surgical clinical in Breslau, (then) Germany.
[5]Harry Craden Bishop, C Everett Koop (b 1916) – American pediatric surgeons – latter more famous for becoming Surgeon General in the United States (1982–1989) and first editor of *Journal of Pediatric Surgery*.
[6]Thomas Vincent Santulli (1915–1997) – American pediatric surgeon at Columbia University, New York.

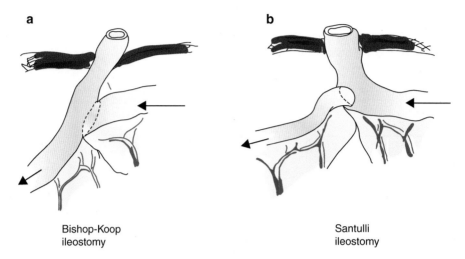

Fig. 3.8.1 Variations in ileostomy for meconium ileus (**a**) Bishop-Koop (**b**) Santulli

3. Postoperative care
   (a) Parenteral nutrition
   (b) *N*-acetylcysteine (10%) enterally (5–10 mLs) if persisting functional obstruction
   (c) Enteral pancreatic enzymes (e.g., Creon®, Pancrease®, etc.)
   (d) Antibiotics
   (e) Involvement of CF team

3.8.5
Outcome

Only 30–40 years ago the diagnosis of CF was regarded as an inevitably leading to death within early childhood. With aggressive respiratory care and improved nutritional awareness most children born today will expect to live into their adult years.

Current average life expectancy ~35 years

3.8.6
Meconium Plug Syndrome (MPS)

Definition – intraluminal colonic obstruction with heterogeoneous etiology
  Associations

- Maternal factors (e.g., eclampsia and diabetes)
- Neonatal factors (e.g., sepsis, prematurity, hypothyroidism, and neonatal intestinal dysmotility)
- Specific (20%)
    — Hirschsprung's disease[7] and CF (debatable).
    — *Small left colon syndrome* – radiological entity with transitional zone at level of splenic flexure, associated with maternal diabetes. ± Histological features of immature ganglion cells.

3.8.6.1
Clinical Features

Neonates present with features of intestinal obstruction, with a differential of meconium ileus and Hirschsprung's disease.

The key investigation is the diagnostic contrast enema followed by a therapeutic water-soluble contrast enema (>95% successful).

Further investigations should include genotype and sweat test ± rectal suction biopsy, to exclude the underlying conditions referred to above.

3.8.7
Distal intestinal obstruction syndrome (DIOS)

Definition – partial or complete obstruction of the ileum or colon, occurring after neonatal period in patients with CF. Formerly known as meconium ileus equivalent.

Colon Strictures and High-Strength Pancreatic Enzymes

In 1994, there was a marked increase in the development of peculiar right colon strictures in otherwise healthy CF children – later termed *fibrosing colonopathy*. This was thought to be due to the recent introduction of high-strength preparations in the market, although it may actually have been due to changes in capsule formulation. It was diagnosed using contrast enema and colonoscopy.

---

[7]Harald Hirschsprung (1830–1916) – Danish pediatrician

- Peak incidence is 6–10 years.
- Affects up to 20% of children and adults with CF at some time.

Etiology – unknown but multifactorial factors include low fluid intake and variable pancreatic enzyme ingestion.

3.8.7.1
Clinical Features

Variable from abdominal pain with cessation of passage of stool to vomiting and features of peritonism. A fictile[8] mass may be present in the RIF. Abdomen tenderness. This makes differentiation from appendicitis and mechanical obstruction due to intussusception, stricture, or adhesive obstruction difficult.

AXR may show a soap-bubble, granular appearance in the right iliac fossa with features of small-bowel obstruction. Consider abdominal US, helical CT scan, and diagnostic contrast enema (even laparoscopy) prior to embarking on therapy.

3.8.7.2
Management

1. Medical
   (a) Oral Gastrografin® (e.g., 50 mls made up to 400 mls solution)/rectal Gastrograffin® (e.g., 100 mls)

Differential Diagnosis of Abdominal Pain in Children with CF

- DIOS – see above.
- Acute appendicitis – tends to present late, possible ↑ incidence of abscess due to concurrent antibiotic use.
    — *Mucocele of appendix* – characteristic of CF, may be asymptomatic.
- Intussusception (older children, not classical age-group).
- Gallbladder – (adolescence and young adults) ↑ incidence of gallstones, typical lesion is micro-gallbladder.
- Ascending colon stricture – see above.
- Small-bowel obstruction.
    — Adhesions (history of meconium ileus)
    — Inguinal hernia – ↑ incidence
- Acute pancreatitis (adolescence and young adults) – needs some residual degree of function. ERCP is indicated for chronic or relapsing pancreatic pain to exclude duct stricture.
- Crohn's[9] disease (adolescence and young adults) – ~17-fold increase in risk.
- Constipation.

---

[8]*Fictile* – (Latin) "clay-like", i.e., capable of being molded.
[9]Burrill Bernard Crohn (1884–1983) – American gastroenterologist

(b) Oral *N*-acetyl-cysteine (e.g., Parvolex®, 30 mls of 20% solution TDS)

(c) Oral poly ethylene glycol (e.g., Movicol® 1 sachet and water TDS)

2. Surgical

The same principles as above can be used. Most can be cleared by intraluminal lavage and manual extraction of luminal content.

Further Reading

1. Escobar MA, Grosfield JL, Burdick JJ et al (2005) Surgical considerations in cystic fibrosis: a 32-year evaluation of outcomes. Surgery 138:560–571
2. Rescorla FJ, Grosfeld JL (1993) Contemporary management of meconium ileus. World J Surg 17:318–325
3. Murshed R, Spitz L. Kiely E et al (1997) Meconium ileus: a ten year review of thirty-six patients. Eur J Pediatr Surg 7:275–277
4. Burge D, Drewett M (2004) Meconium plug obstruction. Pediatr Surg Int 20:108–110
5. Keckler SJ, St Peter SD, Spilde TL et al (2008) Current significance of meconium plug syndrome. J Pediatr Surg 43:896–898

Hirschsprung's Disease

3.9

Tariq Burki, Chandrasen K. Sinha, and Atsuyuki Yamataka

Harold Hirschsprung presented his description of a disease later to bear his name to a pediatric congress in Berlin in 1886. He described two children, who died at 8 and 11 months of age, related to repeated attacks of enterocolitis.

Absence of ganglion cells was documented in 1948 as the cause of Hirschsprung's[1] disease (HD), which subsequently allowed for a rational approach to its diagnosis and surgical management.

3.9.1
Epidemiology

- 1 in 5,000 live-births
- >90% of cases are diagnosed in the neonatal period
- Two distinct clinical types with genetic differences (*vide infra*)
    - *Short segment* (i.e., recto-sigmoid) 75% (M:F 4:1)
    - *Long segment* 25% (M=F)

Associated anomalies variable incidence ~10%

- *Down's syndrome* (~5%)
- Neurocristopathies
    - *Waardenburg–Shah* syndrome – white forelock, bicolored iris, deafness

---

[1]Harald Hirschsprung (1830–1916) – Danish pediatrician, described features of many classical diseases (e.g., pyloric stenosis).

C. K. Sinha (✉)
Paediatric Surgery Department, King's College Hospital, London, UK

C. K. Sinha and M. Davenport (eds.), *Handbook of Pediatric Surgery*,
DOI: 10.1007/978-1-84882-132-3_3.9, © Springer-Verlag London Limited 2010

— *Hypoventilation syndrome* (Ondine's curse[2]) – association with HD termed Haddad syndrome
• Mental retardation syndromes
   — *Smith-Lemli-Optiz* syndrome – mental retardation, polydactly, defect in cholesterol metabolism
   — *Mowat-Wilson syndrome* – mental retardation, characteristic facies
• Development colon anomalies
   — Colon atresia, anorectal atresia
• Miscellaneous
   — *Kaufman-McKusick syndrome* – hydrometrocolpos, hypospadias, polydactyl

(N.B. MEN type 2B (Marfanoid habitus, medullary thyroid cancer, café au lait spots, mucosal neuroma) is associated with *hyperganglionosis* (functionally similar to HD)).

Embryology

Migration of neuroenteric cells from the neural crest to GI tract – aborally.

1. Esophagus fifth week
2. Mid-gut seventh week
3. Distal colon by 12th week

Some studies suggest that ganglion cells are guided to their destination by neural glycoproteins or fibers (e.g., fibronectin, hyaluronic acid).

3.9.2
Anatomy

The normal intestine contains two distinct nerve plexi, between three muscle layers (longitudinal, circular, muscularis mucosae).

1. Submucosal plexus (of Meissner[3])
2. Myenteric or intermuscular plexus (of Auerbach[4])

---

[2]Ondine – water nymph who cursed her unfaithful husband to breathe only while awake. As he fell asleep he died (German mythology).
[3]Georg Meissner (1829 – 1905) – German histologist, also described tactile corpuscles of the skin.
[4]Leopold Auerbach (1828 – 1897) – German neuropathologist.

Each plexi contains a fine meshwork of neurons (ganglion, CD55 +ve) and supporting (glial, CD55 −ve) cells which control motility, absorption, secretion and blood flow. Ganglion cells (nested in groups of four to six cells) receive extrinsic cholinergic and adrenergic signals.

1. Intrinsic neuron stimulation causes muscle relaxation.
    (a) Nitric oxide (NO) is prime mediator
    (b) Other mediators include VIP, Histidine, substance P, Neurokinin A, Enkephalin, Gastrin release peptide, isoleucin, and many others.
2. Extrinsic.
    (a) Cholinergic neurons (contraction)
    (b) Adrenergic neurons (relaxation)
3. Nonadrenergic and noncholinergic (NANC) nervous system – controlled by interstitial cells of Cajal[5] also seem to play an important role in peristalsis.

3.9.3
Etiology

A number of hypotheses have been advanced to explain lack of ganglion cells, including:

1. Failure of migration.
    (a) Distal aganglionosis occurs in chick embryos, when the hind gut is transected.
    (b) Abnormal glycoproteins have been found in the distal aganglionic gut.
2. Hostile environment – loss of neural cell adhesion molecules (NCAM) leads to inability of normal ganglion cells to adhere to smooth muscle cells.
3. Immunologic attack – abnormal immune response mounted by fetus against ganglion cells may lead to destruction of ganglion cells.

3.9.3.1
Pathology

Lack of progression of peristaltic wave into the aganglionic segment of intestine and absent or abnormal internal anal sphincter relaxation is the hallmark of HD.

The gross appearance of intestine varies with age of the child. In the neonatal period the proximal intestine may appear normal but with the passage of time the proximal intestine distends and hypertrophies.

---

[5]Santiago Ramony Cajal (1852–1934) – Spanish pathologist and Nobel laureate.

3.9.3.2
Variable Affected Segment

- Short segment (i.e., recto-sigmoid).
- Long segment – includes total colonic and ileal involvement. Total intestinal aganglionosis is not compatible with life.
- True ultra-short segment disease is believed rare (some believe it to be nonexistent).
- Similarly, segmental disease or "skip" lesions should not be considered in differential diagnosis due to rarity of the condition.

Genetics

- Strong evidence of genetic predisposition.
- The average risk of occurrence in siblings is 3–4% (↑ This risk is further increased in siblings of the individuals with long segment disease involvement).
- Gene mutation
    - *The main gene responsible for increased susceptibility has been diagnosed as RET gene*, which is a proto-oncogene playing a major role in the development of enteric nervous system on Ch 10q11. Associated with Down's syndrome. Dominant mutations in RET gene have been found (50% familial and 15–35% of isolated cases).
    - Seven other candidate genes *have been found to play a role in the pathogenesis of Hirschsprung's disease and these include SOX10, EDNRB* (endothelin receptor type B), *GDNF* (glial cell line neurotrophic factor), *EDN3* (endothelin-3), ECE1, NTN, SIP1.

Mutations in any of these genes may lead to HD. In 50% of familial and 15–35% of isolated cases, dominant mutations in RET gene have been found.

The affected aganglionic bowel looks normal, the ganglionic bowel looks abnormal.

3.9.4
Clinical Features

Two overlapping scenarios

1. Neonatal bowel obstruction
    - Delayed passage of meconium, distension, bile vomiting ± enterocolitis (variable incidence)

(N.B. 95% of neonates will pass meconium within first 24 h of life; almost 100% will pass this within 48 h.)

2. Chronic constipation (not encoparesis)
   - ±Enterocolitis (variable incidence)
   - Failure to thrive

Perforation may complicate HD, and rarely, long-segment HD may present with perinatal proximal (ileal) bowel perforation.

Explosive discharge of fecal matter after rectal examination is a valuable sign and may indicate enterocolitis.

3.9.4.1
Investigations

3. *AXR* – multiple intestinal loops, absence of gas in rectum.
4. *Contrast enema* (Fig. 3.9.1) – ideally before rectal exam. Looking for transitional zone. Delayed films may show contrast retention and are suggestive.
5. *Submucosal rectal biopsy* (suction or occasionally open under GA).
   - 1, 2, and 3 cm above dentate line
   - ± Acetyl cholinesterase staining (90% accurate, less so in neonates and LS HD)
   - ± Immunohistochemistry (e.g., LDH, S100, SDH, etc.)
   - Pathologist-dependent

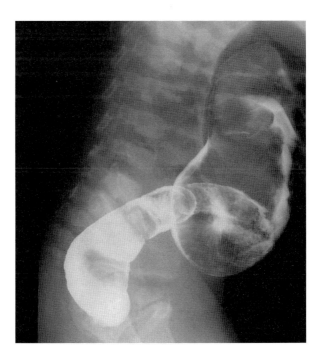

Fig. 3.9.1 Contrast study showing dilated proximal segment and distal narrow segment

6. *Anorectal manometry* – relies on the absence of reflex relaxation of internal anal sphincter in response to rectal dilatation.

   - Not widely available
   - Operator-dependent

3.9.4.2
Differential Diagnosis

- *Mechanical* causes of neonatal bowel obstruction (e.g., ileal and colon atresia, anorectal malformations, meconium ileus, meconium plug syndrome (10% have HD))
- *Functional* hypoperistalsis (e.g., prematurity, sepsis and electrolyte imbalance, small left colon syndrome, and hypothyroidism)

For the older child

- Idiopathic constipation, hypothyroidism, intestinal neuronal dysplasia, hyperganglionosis, etc.

3.9.5
Management

The aim always in HD is to decompress obstructed bowel and may be attempted even before definitive investigation.

If enterocolitis, a potentially lethal complication, is suspected (sepsis, pyrexia, diarrhea, bloody stool) then further active intervention is required including

1. Rectal washout
   (a) 10–20 mL/kg of normal saline is instilled via a rectal tube in small volumes ensuring all fluid inserted is returned. Repeat up to 3× daily.
2. Antibiotics (e.g., vancomycin, metronidazole).
3. ± Colostomy – washouts may not be effective in LS disease.

3.9.6
Surgery

Currently, following diagnostic confirmation most infants can be managed (by parents, at home) with daily rectal washouts until they are considered suitable for a single-stage primary pull-through procedure.

- *Colostomy (indications)*
  — Laparotomy for neonatal intestinal obstruction (in absence of diagnosis)
  — Low birth weight and preterm infants

— Late diagnosis with hugely distended proximal bowel (especially in older children)
— Repeated episodes of enterocolitis (especially in LS disease)

Colostomy (transverse/sigmoid) or ileostomy (LS disease) should be performed in proximal, ganglionic (ideally confirm by frozen section) bowel. Use access to take serial seromuscular or full-thickness biopsies to confirm level of disease in remainder of colon.

3.9.6.1
Pull-Through Procedure

The aim is to resect (largely) the aganglionic segment, bringing the ganglionic bowel through the pelvis and anastomosing it either at the anus or somewhere close. In historical order the commonest are:

1. *Swenson's pull-through[6] (1948)*
   (a) Removal of all aganglionic bowel up to 1 cm from dentate line posteriorly and 2 cm of dentate line anteriorly. Colo-anal anastomosis from outside.
   (b) Potential for pelvic nerve (incontinence) and anterior structure (vas, bladder, vagina) damage.
2. *Duhamel's pull-through[7] (1956)*
   (a) Dissection behind rectum (to minimize pelvic nerve damage) to create tunnel. Ganglionic bowel is brought through ~1 cm above dentate and side-to-side anastomosis created (with GIA or EndoGIA stapler).
   (b) Anterior blind pouch may lead to fecaloma and recurrent obstruction.
3. *Soave's endorectal pull-through[8] (1964)*
   (a) At pelvic reflection, the colon dissection continues in the submucosal plane to ~1 cm from dentate line. Ganglionic bowel is pulled though the rectal muscle sleeve and anastomosed to anal mucosa. Avoids potential for nerve damage.
   (b) Retained aganglionic muscle cuff may cause functional obstruction and constipation or sleeve abscess.
4. *Laparoscopy-assisted transanal pull-through*
   (a) Any of the above can be performed under laparoscopic vision for the pelvic dissection.
5. *Transanal endorectal pull-through*
   (a) Using a circumferential (e.g., Scott) hook retractor, it is possible to dissect entirely from below (submucosa or full-thickness) into the peritioneal cavity, removing the aganglionic bowel and achieving a safe anastomosis.

---

[6]Orvar Swenson (b 1909) – Peripatetic American pediatric surgeon, still going strong at 100-years old.

[7]Bernard Duhamel (1917–1996) – French surgeon, working in Hopital de Saint Denis, Paris.

[8]Franco Soave – Italian pediatric surgeon working in Genoa. As originally described the pull-though bowel was left hanging between the infant's legs and not actually anastomosed.

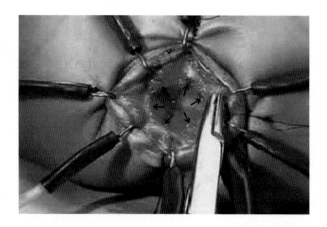

Fig. 3.9.2 The anorectal line (*arrows*) can be identified by hooking the crypts in the dentate line to expose the anal canal with a Scott retractor

(N.B. Dissection starting on the anorectal line as opposed to starting on the dentate line has recently been suggested to improve long-term outcome (Fig. 3.9.2).)

3.9.7
Outcome

- Early complications include enterocolitis, anastomotic leak and stricture, intestinal adhesion obstruction, and perianal excoriation.
- The superiority of one of the above over another has not been shown in long-term follow-up series (although these are few); nonetheless, in general the Duhamel and Soave procedures have a higher rate of constipation, while Swenson's have higher incidence of incontinence. Certainly all the patients need long-term follow-up as they are seldom cured of their pathology.

Further Reading

1. Yamataka A, Kaneyama K, Fujiwara N, Hayashi Y, Lane GJ, Kawashima K, Okazaki T (2009) Rectal mucosal dissection during transanal pull-through for Hirschsprung disease: the anorectal or the dentate line? J Pediatr Surg 44:266–269
2. Minford JL, Ram A, Turnock RR et al (2004) Comparison of functional outcomes of Duhamel and transanal endorectal coloanal anastomosis for Hirschsprung's disease. J Pediatr Surg 39:161–165
3. Conway SJ, Craigie RJ, Cooper LH et al (2007) Early adult outcome of the Duhamel procedure for left-sided Hirschsprung disease – a prospective serial assessment study. J Pediatr Surg 42:1429–1432

Anorectal Malformations

3.10

Chandrasen K. Sinha, Marc A. Levitt, and Alberto Peña

Anorectal malformations (ARMs) are congenital malformations, in which the terminal part of the hindgut is abnormally placed and lies outside (partially or completely) the sphincter mechanism.

3.10.1
Epidemiology

- Incidence ~1 in 5,000
  - More common in Down's syndrome and Cat-eye syndrome.[1]
- Male > female (60:40)
- Second child involvement rare (<1%)

About 5% of babies have no fistula (usually associated with Down's syndrome); the vast majority has a connection between the distal rectum and the genitourinary tract.

Embryology

By 21 days there is a common chamber (*cloaca*[2]) occluded by a membrane, but visible from the outside as an ectodermal pit – the *proctodaeum*. At ~33 days, the posterior hindgut is then separated from the anterior urogenital sinus by mesenchymal ingrowth of the urorectal septum. Cloacal membrane breaks down at ~46 days. The process is regulated by differential expression of the gene Sonic Hedgehog[3] (SHH), and other target genes such as *BMP-4*[4] and the *HOX*[5] genes.

---

[1]Cat-eye syndrome – colobomata and ARM typically due to aneuploidy (e.g., trisomy of Chromosome 22).
[2]*Cloaca* – Latin "sewer."
[3]Sonic Hedgehog *(SHH)* – Blue computer game character popular in 1990s when gene was named.
[4]*BMP4* (bone morphogenetic protein) – part of TGF-β superfamily.
[5]*HOX* – or Homeobox genes. Highly conserved genes responsible for basic patterning in embryo.

M. A. Levitt (✉)
Colorectal Centre, Cincinnati Children's Hospital, USA

C. K. Sinha and M. Davenport (eds.), *Handbook of Pediatric Surgery*,
DOI: 10.1007/978-1-84882-132-3_3.10, © Springer-Verlag London Limited 2010

3.10.2
Classification

See Table 3.10.1

3.10.2.1
Associated Anomalies

VACTERL – Vertebral, anorectal, cardiac, tracheoesophageal, renal, limb anomalies

- Vertebral anomalies – e.g., hemivertebra, scoliosis, spinal dysraphrism (usually tethered cords (~25% of cases)). Tethered cord is the intervertebral fixation of the filum terminale that may cause sensory, motor, orthopedic, cutaneous, bladder and bowel symptoms.
- Cardiac anomalies (~20%), e.g., VSD, tetralogy of Fallot.[6]
- Renal (genitourinary) anomalies (~60%). Marked variation with type so up to 80% of cloacas with a lesser incidence in high ARM and low ARM. Hydrocolpos (50%) and duplicated Mullerian structures (35%) also related to cloacal anomalies.

Table 3.10.1 Anatomical classification of ARM

Males	Females
Rectoperineal fistula	
Rectobulbar urethral fistula[a]	Rectoperineal fistula, Rectovestibular fistula[a]
Rectoprostatic urethral fistula	Imperforate anus without fistula
Rectobladder neck fistula	Persistent cloaca
Imperforate anus without fistula Rectal atresia	Rectal atresia

[a]Common

3.10.3
Clinical Features

Clinical examination is the most important part of management and it makes the diagnosis in 90% of the cases (Figs. 3.10.1 and 3.10.2).

- High anomalies – flat perineum, passage of meconium *per urethra*, short sacrum, and little sphincter muscle contraction.
- Bifid scrotum or a sphincter located close to the scrotum is often associated with prostatic fistula.
- In female babies, a careful examination will tell about the position of the opening (vestibular, perineal, vaginal, or cloacal).

[6]Ettiene Louise Arthur Fallot (1850–1911) – French physician working in Marseille, described details of two cases in 1888, although many previous reports.

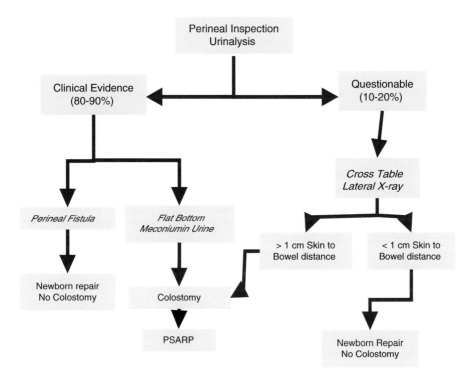

Fig. 3.10.1   Algorithm for male infant

- Cloaca is diagnosed by a single perineal opening.
- Low anomalies are suggested by an opening in the perineum and a "bucket-handle" defect.

3.10.4
Management

- *AXR* – A cross-table lateral film (after 12–24 h) is useful in localizing the distance of rectal gas from perineum, if physical examination is unable to detect a rectal fistula.
  - Sacral ratio (Fig. 3.10.3) – Normal=0.74 (0.7–0.8). Lower values (<0.4) are prognostic for low potential for continence.
- *US*–Useful in detecting associated renal anomalies, vertebral anomalies, and hydrocolpos (in cloaca). Echocardiogram should be done to rule out associated cardiac anomalies.

Initial management includes nasogastric tube, nil by mouth, intravenous fluid, antibiotic prophylaxis, and watchful waiting (for about 24 h) while proper assessments/investigations are done.

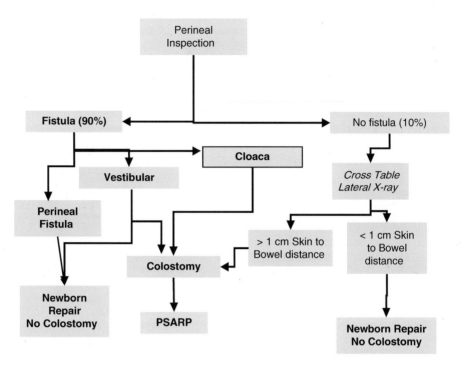

Fig. 3.10.2 Algorithm for female infant

- Babies with a high anomaly are usually treated with initial colostomy, followed by definitive surgery and then colostomy closure.

Defunctioning divided colostomy in the fixed (most proximal) part of sigmoid colon

1. Separate two ends of colon, bridged by skin and separated by an adequate distance so the stoma appliances does not cover the mucous fistula.
2. The distal loop should be washed out to remove any fecal matter. The proximal stoma should be well projecting above the surface of skin, everted and placed at a distance from the mucous fistula, which will prevent spillover and fecal impaction of the distal colon and rectum.
3. Make distal limb smaller to allow insertion of catheter for washouts and imaging, but prevent prolapse of the stoma.

Blind exploration of rectum without a properly done distal high-pressure colostogram must be avoided, as it will lead to damage of the sphincter, bladder neck, ureter, vas deference, seminal vesicles, and urethra.

Definitive surgery can be done around 6–12 weeks.

Fig. 3.10.3 Sacral ratio

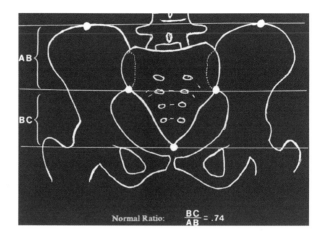

Normal Ratio: $\dfrac{BC}{AB} = .74$

3.10.4.1
Posterior Sagittal Anorectoplasty (PSARP) (Male) [Fig 3.10.4 (a,b)]

1. Identify sphincter position – anal dimple is usually surrounded by an area of discolored skin and indicates sphincter. An appropriate muscle stimulator (e.g., Pena model Radionics Inc.) is crucial in identifying the center of this mechanism as the point to which contractions seem to be directed.
2. Urethral catheterization (for about a week). If catheter comes out, avoid recatheterization to avoid trauma to urethral repair.
3. Midline skin incision – with progressive division of soft tissue, also strictly in the midline. Sometimes, rectum may be too high to reach from below, and a combined abdominal approach will be needed (can be done laparoscopically).
4. Identify rectum, open posterior wall between stay sutures and identify fistula *(bladder neck → bulbar urethra)* from inside. Mobilization of rectum away from fistula and common wall. Safe closure.
5. Consider tapering rectum.
6. Reconstruct muscle complex around mobilized rectum.
7. Anocutaneous anastomosis.

- *Special situations*
    - *Bladder neck fistula*. Problem is usually length of mobilized rectum. Can be corrected by tubularization of flap from dilated end.

3.10.4.2
Posterior Sagittal Anorectoplasty (PSARP) (Female) [Fig 3.10.4 (c,d)]

1. As above, identify "true" sphincter position with stimulator. Anterior perineal orifices are notoriously missed in the newborn period.

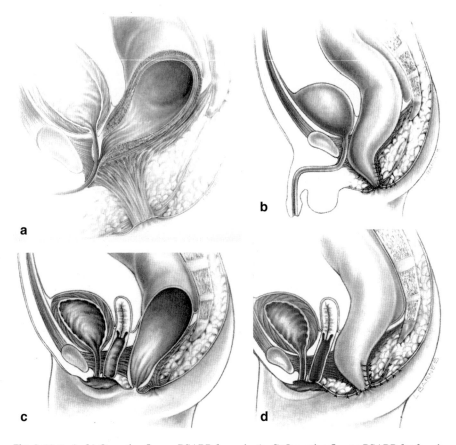

Fig. 3.10.4 (**a, b**) Operative figures PSARP for male. (**c, d**) Operative figures PSARP for female

2. Midline saggital incision.
3. *Anovestibular fistula* – circumferential stay sutures. Mobilize from vaginal vault. Relocate within muscle complex.
4. Reformation of anterior perineal body.
5. Anocutaneous anastomosis.

- *Special situations*
    - *Rectovaginal fistula* – common wall requires careful vaginal reconstruction.
    - *Cloaca with hydrocolpos* – *a* vaginostomy should be performed at the time of the colostomy

Table 3.10.2   Outcome in ARM

Type	Fecal continence (%)	Constipation (%)
Female		
Rectoperineal	100	55
Rectovestibular	95	55
Rectovaginal	70	30
Cloaca	55	30
Male		
Rectoperineal	100	55
Rectobulbar	85	55
Rectoprostatic	60	40
Rectobladder neck	20	15

Definitive surgery *(Mini PSARP)* without colostomy can be done in newborn during 24–48 h after birth if

- Perineal fistula is present.
- Rectum is within 1 cm from skin (on cross-table lateral film).
- Vestibular fistula (if an experienced surgeon is available).

But this can be delayed for 1–3 months if needed, based on the baby's clinical condition. Other operations (i.e., Y–V plasty, cut-back, dilatation) have a higher risk of wound dehiscence, sphincter injury, and suboptimal cosmetic results.

3.10.5
Outcome

- The higher the ARM anomaly, the lower the achieved continence.
- Sacral anomaly – ↓ achieved continence.
- Lower malformations tend to suffer more from constipation (Table 3.10.2).

Further Reading

1. Levitt MA, Peña A (2007) Anorectal malformations. Orphanet J Rare Dis 26(2):33
2. Peña A, Grasshoff S, Levitt M (2007) Reoperations in anorectal malformations. J Pediat Surg 42:318–325
3. Levitt MA, Peña A (2005) Outcomes from the correction of anorectal malformations. Curr Opin Pediatr 17:394–401
4. Rintala RJ, Pakarinen MP (2008) Imperforate anus: long- and short-term outcome. Semin Pediatr Surg 17:79–89

Abdominal Wall Defects

3.11

Chandrasen K. Sinha and Mark Davenport

There are two distinct types of major anterior abdominal wall defect with distinct behavior and outcome.

Gastroschisis[1]	Exomphalos[2] (omphalocele)
1 in 2,000 live-births	1 in 5,000 live-births (↑↑ fetal diagnosis)
↑ Incidence in Western world (reasons not known)	Static incidence
Cocaine/recreational drug use	
Associated with teenage mothers	
No real associations	Associated anomalies
Intestinal atresia – complication	Chromosome anomalies (e.g., trisomies 13, 18, 21)
	Beckwith–Wiedemann syndrome (↑ somatic growth, islet cell hyperplasia (hypoglycemia), macroglossia, and ↑ risk of neoplasia (e.g., Wilms', hepatoblastoma))

Upper midline syndrome (also called *Pentology of Cantrell*) – it consists of exomphalos, anterior diaphragmatic hernia, sternal cleft, ectopia cordis, and cardiac anomaly.

Lower midline syndrome – vesico-intestinal fistula, anorectal malformation, bladder/cloacal exstrophy, meningomyelocele sacral anomalies, and colonic atresia.

---

[1]*Gastroschisis* – (Greek) – "Belly cleft."
[2]*Exomphalos* – *Omphalos* (Greek) – navel or umbilicus.

C. K. Sinha (✉)
Paediatric Surgery Department, King's College Hospital, London, UK

C. K. Sinha and M. Davenport (eds.), *Handbook of Pediatric Surgery*,
DOI: 10.1007/978-1-84882-132-3_3.11, © Springer-Verlag London Limited 2010

Fig. 3.11.1 Typical appearance
of Exomphalos major

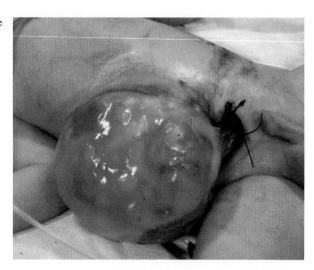

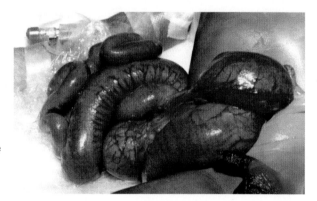

Fig 3.11.2 Typical appearance
of gastroschisis

3.11.1 Exomphalos (Fig 3.11.1)
3.11.1.1 Embryology

- At about 8 weeks gestation, the enlarging liver causes the displacement of other viscera outside the umbilical ring, to return by 10 weeks. Failure to do this results in *exomphalos*. Thus, it should be covered with sac and Wharton's jelly with insertion of the cord at its apex.
- The embryological defect of *gastroschisis* is disputed and appears to be a right-sided defect appearing by a normally inserted umbilicus. Even the timing is unclear although most are obvious from about 14 weeks gestation. Prolapse of uncovered viscera occurs thereafter.

3.11.1.2
Types

- Hernia of the umbilical cord – Small defect and sac may contain few loops of intestine.
- *Exomphalos minor* – Defect <5 cm.
- *Exomphalos major* – Defect >5 cm, and predominantly contains liver.

3.11.1.3
Clinical Features

Antenatal (80%) confirmation is possible from ~12 weeks gestation. At this stage the key steps are to establish presence of chromosomal anomalies (by chorionic villous sampling or amniocentesis) and/or other significant anomalies (by fetal echocardiography, etc.). There is a high rate of spontaneous intrauterine death, particularly if the anomalies are multiple. Third trimester US should evaluate the safest mode of delivery (C-section is indicated for major exomphalos – avoids sac rupture, and obstructed labor).

Postnatally, it is important to establish if the sac is intact or not. Typically intrauterine loss of the sac, leads to early labor and preterm delivery.

3.11.1.4
Investigations

Important to evaluate whole baby – not just an anterior abdominal wall sac. Look for other anomalies, and particularly if it could be B.W. syndrome (beware of hypoglycemia).

1. Echocardiogram
2. Renal ultrasound
3. Skeletal radiography

3.11.1.5
Management

There are a number of surgical options.

- *Elective primary fascial closure* – for exomphalos minor and most cases of exomphalos major
- *Staged closure (silo)* – where primary closure not possible, but reasonable-sized infant
  - Initial application of custom silo (± removal of sac)
  - Delayed fascial (± prosthetic patch) closure and skin closure (7–10 days)

For infants with an intact sac who are *small, preterm* (<32/40), or who have other *significant anomalies* then *conservative sac management* may be preferred. This involves epithelialization encouraged by various topical agents (e.g., silver nitrate, silver sulfathiazine). Fascial closure is performed at some later date (2–3 years), although the problem of viscero-abdominal disproportion still remains.

3.11.2
Gastroschisis (Fig 3.11.2)

- Most cases are all too obvious at birth – the only exception is that of a closed gastroschisis and "vanishing midgut," where the prolapsed bowel has died *in utero* and simply fallen off leaving the defect to close spontaneously.
- Mostly adjacent loops of bowel become adherent and matted together ("peel"). Some believe this response is an inflammatory one to waste products within amniotic fluid, others that it is ischemic in origin associated with the neck of the defect.

3.11.2.1
Clinical Features

Antenatal detection is possible from ~14 weeks gestation and most are normally picked up at the "fetal anomaly scan" at 18–20 weeks gestation. The main risk to the fetus at this stage is the possibility of "closed gastroschisis" (i.e., closure of ring around prolapsed midgut) as this can lead to complete loss of the midgut, or at the very least entry and exit intestinal atresias.

Most cases of gastroschisis can be delivered vaginally without undue harm to the gut. There is no benefit from too early delivery but most fetal medicine centers suggest planned delivery at ~38 weeks.

3.11.2.2
Management

First aid – Cover exposed bowel loops with "cling-film." Ensure no twist in midgut and consider if ring may be too tight. If so divide under local anesthesia.

3.11.2.3
Surgery

There are then a number of surgical options.

- *Primary fascial closure* (60%) – selected on basis of attempt under GA
- *Staged closure (silo)*
  - Delayed fascial (± prosthetic patch) closure and skin closure (7–10 days)

- *Preformed silo* – cotside application in *all* infants. No anesthesia
  - — Delayed fascial (± prosthetic patch) closure and skin closure (2–10 days)
  - — ↓ incidence of compartment syndrome
  - — Final "sutureless" closure possible without GA, using intact umbilical cord

3.11.2.4
Complications

Abdominal wall integrity is not usually a problem after the first 2 weeks; however, the acquisition of intestinal peristalsis is prolonged and parenteral nutrition is invariable.

- Average time to full enteral nutrition ~25 days
- ↑ risk of NEC (usually "benign" rather than "necrotizing")
- Intestinal atresia. Sometimes occur where bowel enters and leaves the closing ring. Best option is probably to leave anastomosis until final fascial closure when bowel quality has improved. Avoid stomas.
- Prolonged (>3 months) dysmotility – decreased transit time from small to large bowel. Consider distal ileostomy as solution to chronic pseudo-obstruction.

3.11.2.5
Outcome

- >95% survival in recent series
  - — Death usually due to midgut infarction and prolonged PN-induced liver disease

Further Reading

1. Lakasing L, Cicero S, Davenport M et al (2006) Current outcome of antenatally diagnosed exomphalos: an 11 year review. J Pediatr Surg 41:1403–1406
2. Rijhwani A, Davenport M, Dawrant M et al (2005) Definitive surgical management of antenatally diagnosed exomphalos. J Pediatr Surg 40:516–522
3. Houben C, Davenport M, Ade-Ajayi N et al (2009) Closing gastroschisis: diagnosis, management, and outcomes. J Pediatr Surg 44:343–347
4. Allotey J, Davenport M, Njere I et al (2007) Benefit of preformed silos in the management of gastroschisis. Pediatr Surg Int 23:1065–1069
5. Charlesworth P, Njere I, Allotey J et al (2007) Postnatal outcome in gastroschisis: effect of birth weight and gestational age. J Pediatr Surg 42:815–818
6. Cantrell JR, Haller JA, Ravitch MM (1958) A syndrome of congenital defects involving the abdominal wall, sternum, diaphragm, pericardium, and heart. Surg Gynecol Obstet 107:602–614

Part IV

Children's Surgery

Surgical Neck Pathology

4.1

Chandrasen K. Sinha, Meena Agrawal, and Mark Davenport

The anatomy of the neck is complex and the pathology derived from this is myriad. Despite this, consideration of the age of onset, and knowledge of natural history and typical behavior patterns can lead to the correct diagnosis in most cases of unknown swelling, lump, or sepsis.

Considered here will be

- Branchial pathology
- Thyroglossal cysts
- Cervical node pathology
- Sternomastoid "tumor"
- Lymphatic malformations
- Dermoid and epidermoid cysts (Fig. 4.1.1)

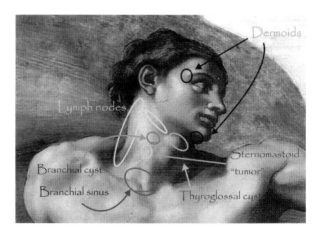

Fig. 4.1.1 Schematic of the differential diagnosis of a lump in the neck

C. K. Sinha (✉)
Paediatric Surgery Department, Kings College Hospital, London, UK

C. K. Sinha and M. Davenport (eds.), *Handbook of Pediatric Surgery*,
DOI: 10.1007/978-1-84882-132-3_4.1, © Springer-Verlag London Limited 2010

The anatomy of the neck is a good example of the principle of *recapitulation of ontogeny* (i.e., human evolution) as the branchial arches, obvious in the embryo, hark back to the gills of our fishy ancestors.

Embryology

Branchial[1] Arch Development

There are five pairs of branchial (or pharyngeal) arches evident from day 22, numbered I, II, III, IV, VI (V is missing in humans). Each has a cartilaginous center, a nerve, and an aortic arch-associated artery. They are separated externally by ectodermal clefts and internally by endodermal pouches. Derivatives of the first arch cartilage are the malleus and incus of the middle ear; the second arch forms the stapes, stylohyoid, and upper part of hyoid bone, and the third arch the remainder of the hyoid. Derivatives of the first pouch include the tympanic cavity and Eustachian tube; the second pouch leads to the tonsils, and the third pouch to the thymus gland and inferior parathyroid glands.

Thyroid Development

The thyroid precursor anlagen arises on the back of tongue (foramen caecum) and migrates caudally to lie in front of the proximal tracheal rings, leaving the potential for a track (should obliterate by fifth week) and cyst formation within (*thyroglossal cyst*).

4.1.1
Branchial Fistula/Sinus/Cyst (Rare)

4.1.1.1
Clinical Features

- Fistula > sinus > cyst

Although branchial remnants are congenital and therefore present since birth, there is some debate about the etiology of "branchial cysts," which is usually found in later childhood. Most cysts are located anterior to the sternomastoid muscle, posterior to the submandibular gland and lateral to the carotid sheath.

Most are usually second arch remnants and their external opening is usually sited near the insertion of the sternomastoid at clavicular level. Sinuses then ascend the neck along the carotid sheath to the level of the hyoid bone turning medially between the internal and external carotid artery, in front of the hypoglossal nerve to end in the region of tonsillar fossa.

Sometimes, there is mucoid discharge from this opening and occasionally it can become infected.

Cysts occur deep to the middle 1/3 of sternomastoid, and can be complicated by sepsis.

---

[1]*Branchial (*Greek*) – gills.

4.1.1.2
Investigation

- *Ultrasound* – looking for cystic change

4.1.1.3
Surgery

Elective excision of the complete tract or cyst. If infected, treat this first prior to definitive procedure. Transverse skin incision(s) with methylene blue to outline the sinus.

Recurrence ~3% after elective operation, ↑ if previous unsuccessful excision.

> *First branchial arch sinus* – rare, with external opening at the level of angle of jaw, and track ascending theoretically toward the middle ear.

4.1.2
Thyroglossal Cyst (Rare)

Unknown incidence

4.1.2.1
Clinical Features

- Most (80%) are related to and in contact with hyoid bone.
- Midline swelling (elevates with swallowing or protrusion of the tongue).

May be complicated by infection and if allowed to discharge a distal midline fistula often results.

4.1.2.2
Investigation

1. Cervical US – shows cystic nature and also confirms presence of normal thyroid gland.

Differential diagnosis includes nodal pathology, dermoid cyst, thyroid pathology, and if suprahyoid, a *ranula*[2].

---

[2]*Ranula* (Latin) "Little frog" – named for its appearance in floor of mouth.

4.1.2.3
Surgery: Sistrunk's Operation[3]

Skin crease incision with development of skin flaps.

1. Mobilize cyst from distal tract (if any).
2. Dissect and isolate the body of hyoid in continuity with the cyst.
3. Identify proximal track to base of tongue.
4. Repair in layers, approximate hyoid remnants.

If everything removed, then recurrence risk is low (~5%).

   A very small (<1%) risk of cancer has been described in these cysts.

4.1.3
Cervical Node Infections (Common)

Over 75% of lymphatic tissue is found within the head and neck, and this remains the commonest site of manifestation of lymphatic pathology. The ears, nose, mouth, pharynx, and upper airway remain the commonest portal for bacterial and viral entry and this is reflected in the huge incidence of lymphadenitis seen in childhood. Fortunately, most either goes without comment and subsides spontaneously or is dealt with in general practice by the liberal use of antibiotics. Table 4.1.1 illustrates the nature of the typical organisms by the age of the child.

4.1.3.1
Clinical Features

Whatever the cause, the usual scenario is to evolve (days) through an active inflammatory *cellulitic phase* with later central *cavitation and pus formation*. The disease process then resolves via discharge to the skin or by surgical intervention (I&D). In both NTM and TB,

Table 4.1.1 Common pathogens causing lymphadenitis

Age Group	Common pathogens
Neonate	*Staphylococcus aureus*, late-onset Gp B Strep
<5 years	Gp. A Strep, *S. aureus*, NTM
5–18 years	EBV, cytomegalovirus, toxoplasmosis, TB, infectious mononucleosis

NTM nontuberculous mycobacterium; *EBV* Epstein–Barr virus; *TB* tuberculosis

---

[3]Walter E. Sistrunk (1880–1933) – American surgeon at Mayo Clinic, MO.

the process is much more prolonged and "cold," and because of the inadequacy of the host cellular response, it is often not resolved by discharge or I&D.

4.1.4
Miscellaneous Nodal Pathology

4.1.4.1
Nontuberculous Mycobacterium (NTM)
(Aka Atypical Mycobacterium)

- *Mycobacterium avium – intracellulare (two species difficult to differentiate), M. kansasii, M. scrofulaceum*

Most enters via oropharynx, and is a feature in preschool (<5 years) children. Typical groups affected include cervical and submandibular. There tends to be obvious overlying skin changes, with ultimate discharge but very often fistula formation.

4.1.4.2
Investigation

1. *CXR* (usually negative)
2. Mantoux (i.e., PPD) test (usually negative), now specific NTM antigen skin test
3. Ziehl–Neilsen (ZN) stain and culture (takes up to 12 weeks)
4. (rapid) PCR (looking for mycobacterial RNA)

4.1.4.3
Management

- Surgical excision (if possible)
  - Beware of proximity to mandibular branch of Facial (VII) nerve and spinal Accessory (XI) nerve.
- Clarithromicin/azithromicin

4.1.4.4
Tuberculosis

This is now rare in developed countries but may occur in the Immunosuppressed (e.g., posttransplant).

Surgery is limited to diagnostic biopsy (or fine-needle aspiration cytology), or I&D of abscesses.

4.1.5
Cat Scratch Disease

- *Bartonella henselae – found in cats and kittens.*

4.1.5.1
Clinical Features

Usually causes regional lymphadenopathy (typical site is axillary or epitrochlear nodes) but can cause pre-auricular lymphadenopathy (and granulomatous conjunctivitis – Parinaud's syndrome[4]).

4.1.5.2
Investigations

- ELISA possible.
- Biopsy – granulomatous reaction. Visible on Warthin–Starry stain.
- PCR on sampled material possible.
- Most are self-limiting in immunocompetent children, but azithromycin for severe symptoms.

4.1.6
Kawasaki's Disease[5]

This is a vasculitic disease of unknown etiology, which principally affects

- Heart – coronary artery aneurysm.
- Skin and mucous membranes – "strawberry" tongue, red palms and soles with later desquamation.
- Lymph nodes – cervical adenopathy.

4.1.6.1
Investigation

No specific test – diagnosed on clinical criteria (5-day fever, erythema of lips, etc.)

---

[4]Henri Parinaud (1844–1905) – French opthalmologist.
[5]Dr. Tomisaku Kawasaki (b 1925) – Japanese pediatrician who described 50 cases in 1967.

4.1.6.2
Management

- High-dose immunoglobulin and salicylates ± steroids

4.1.7
Sternomastoid "Tumor" (Rare)

Uncertain etiology and unknown incidence

There has sometimes been a history of birth trauma or breech delivery suggesting that there has been hemorrhage within muscle, followed by fibrosis and muscle shortening.

4.1.7.1
Clinical Features

Typically presents with painless lump within sternomastoid muscle at 2–4 weeks of age with or without torticollis (head rotated and tilted away from the affected side). Initially, any abnormal head positioning can be corrected, but with time this becomes fixed. There is then secondary soft tissue changes and facial asymmetry.

4.1.7.2
Investigation

1. *US* may show focal or diffuse enlargement of the sternocleidomastoid muscle.
2. *Cervical radiography* – exclude vertebral anomalies (e.g., hemivertebra).
3. *MRI* – precise definition of cervical vertebral anomalies.

4.1.7.3
Management

- Cervical Physiotherapy – successful in >90% of cases.
    - Early diagnosis and intervention.
    - Passive neck movement and stretching exercises – avoid cot positioning, which exacerbate neck deformity.
- *Surgery* – division of sternomastoid muscle – achieves ↑ length.

4.1.8
Lymphatic Malformations (Rare)

- ~50% of these malformations are diagnosed at birth
- ~90% present before 2 years of age.
- Uncertain incidence – 1 in 6,000 live-births

4.1.8.1
Associations

- Chromosomal anomalies (e.g., Turner's (XO), Noonan's syndrome (single gene defect on Ch12q24.1), Down's syndrome (Trisomy 21)).

Lymphatic malformations are vascular malformations composed of primitive embryonic lymph sacs of varying sizes. Mostly found in relation to head and neck, but can be ubiquitous.

Cystic hygroma – term used to describe congenital neck lesions. Some are huge and can cause polyhydramnios, obstructed labor, and failure to establish an airway at birth.

They can be divided into three clinical types:

1. *Microcystic*
2. *Macrocystic*
3. *Mixed lesions*

They may also be described as *unilocular, multilocular; focal,* or *diffuse/infiltrative.*

4.1.8.2
Clinical Features

Lymphatic malformations typically increase in size as the child grows, and they may show rapid increase in size in association with upper respiratory tract infection or intralesional hemorrhage, causing compromise of airway if present in suprahyoid region.

4.1.8.3
Investigation

1. *US* – to determine cyst size and number.
2. *MRI* – defines anatomical relationship to cervical vessels and trachea.

Sometimes, lymphatic malformations may be a part of mixed vascular malformations (typically venous) (see Chap. 4.13-Vascular Anomalies).

4.1.8.4
Management

Contentious, confusing, and contradictory!

- *Chemotherapy – percutaneous injection/inflitration*
  - — OK-432 (Picabanil®) is a lyophilized mixture of *Streptococcus spp.*
  - — Absolute alcohol solution.
  - — Ethibloc® – combination of alcohol, mixed irritant proteins, and a radio-opaque marker.
  - — Cyclophosphamide – IV, reserved for life-threatening examples.
  - — Bleomycin – intralesional injection (total dose 5 mg/kg)
- *Surgery*
  - — Aim for complete excision – but this is easier said than done! May be difficult owing to nerve proximity, etc.

4.1.9
Dermoid Cysts and Epidermoid Cysts (Common)

Dermoid cysts represent superficial ectodermal elements, which have become trapped beneath the skin and occur at sites of ectodermal fusion. Typical sites include anywhere along the body's midline, or along the line joining upper ear to upper outer part of eyebrow (*external angular dermoid*).

- Dermoid cysts contain squamous epithelium and skin appendages such as hair follicles and sebaceous glands.
- Epidermoid cysts contain only squamous epithelium.

Further Reading

1. Acierno SP, Waldhausen JH (2007) Congenital cervical cysts, sinuses and fistulae. Otolaryngol Clin North Am 40:161–176
2. Bloom DC, Perkins JA, Manning SC (2004) Management of lymphatic malformations. Curr Opin Otolaryngol Head Neck Surg 12:500–504
3. Schoenwolf GC, Bleyl SB, Brauer PR, Francis-West PH (2009) Development of the pharyngeal apparatus and face. In: Larsen's human embryology, 4th edn. Churchill Livingstone, Philadelphia, pp 543–580

Developmental Lung Anomalies

4.2

Abid Q. Qazi, Chandrasen K. Sinha, and Mark Davenport

Once little regarded by pediatric surgeons. The advent of universal antenatal ultrasonography has opened a new field – the key is to sort out the cases that need treating and those that could be safely left alone.

4.2.1
Epidemiology

- Incidence for any of the anomalies described is not known.
- But, the increase in incidence of CCAM and sequestration seen in most institutions has been due to the advent of almost universal access to antenatal US.

Embryology

The laryngotracheal groove arises as ventral outpouching from the caudal end of primitive foregut. The trachea and lung bud originate from this groove, as it grows further caudally, into enveloping mesenchyme. It subsequently separates from dorsal foregut with the help of infolding lateral walls of foregut.

Further development of tracheo-bronchial tree can be divided into five phases comprising

- *Embryonic* (<5 weeks) – *division into bronchi and segments only.*
- *Pseudoglandular* (5–17 weeks) ~*16 generations to terminal bronchioles.*
- *Canalicular* (16–25 weeks) – *branching of cancaliculus and terminal acinus, in-growth of capillaries into mesenchyme.*

C. K. Sinha (✉)
Paediatric Surgery Department, King's College Hospital, London, UK

C. K. Sinha and M. Davenport (eds.), *Handbook of Pediatric Surgery*,
DOI: 10.1007/978-1-84882-132-3_4.2, © Springer-Verlag London Limited 2010

- *Saccular (25–40 weeks) – at birth only about 1/3 of final number alveoli are present.*
- *Alveolar (38 weeks – 1 year) – rapid ↑ number of alveoli.*

(Fetal lungs are a large source of amniotic fluid (~15 mL/kg/day)).
(Surfactant is produced by Type II pneumocytes from ~24 weeks).

Table 4.2.1 Classification of bronchopulmonary anomalies

Trachea and bronchi	Parenchyma
Agenesis	Pulmonary agenesis[a]
Bronchogenic cyst	Lung (aplasia to hypoplasia)
Enteric duplication cyst	Congenital cystic adenomatoid malformation (CCAM)
Tracheo-esophageal fistula	Bronchopulmonary sequestration
Vascular ring	Congential lobar/segmental emphysema
Tracheomalacia/bronchomalacia	

[a]Pulmonary agenesis is differentiated from lung aplasia by the absence of carina (in lung aplasia)

Table 4.2.1 illustrates two broad categories of pathology based on perceived origin.

4.2.2
Pulmonary Agenesis and Hypoplasia

True agenesis is rare, and can be bilateral (obviously fatal), but varying degrees of hypoplasia are not that uncommon.

- Spectrum varies from blind-ending main bronchus with no lung tissue to malformed bronchus and poorly developed lung tissue.
- Cardiac, GI, GU, or skeletal anomalies may be present in 50% of cases.
- Prognosis depends on the degree of hypoplasia, degree of development of contralateral lung, lung volume, and the prognosis of their associated anomalies.
- Treatment depends mostly on the underlying condition, but overall the mortality ranges from 70% to 95%.

4.2.3
Bronchopulmonary Sequestration (BPS)

Definition – Nonfunctioning mass of lung parenchyma, with no tracheo-bronchial communication and an independent arterial supply from systemic circulation.

Venous drainage is commonly to the azygous or hemiazygous veins. There is an exaggerated yet futile circulation through the BPS, out of proportion to actual volume of lung tissue supplied.

BPS is subdivided into two types

- *Extralobar sequestration* (75%) – separate investment of pleura.
- Lower > upper
- M > F
- Sometimes infra-diaphragmatic
- *Intralobar sequestration* (25%) – shared pleura with surrounding lung.

May be associated with CCAM, diaphragmatic hernia, and TEF.

4.2.3.1
Clinical Features

Most are detected by routine antenatal US (18–20 week) scan.
Uncommonly, they may cause prenatal symptoms such as hydrothorax due to the presence of futile circulation. Postnatally, most are probably asymptomatic, but may cause:

- Infection – despite lack of bronchial connection.
- Cardiac failure (high-output) – tachypnoea, ↑ heart rate, ↑ cardiac diameter.

4.2.3.2
Investigations

- *CXR* – typically solid, basal lesion.
- *CT* (IV contrast) scan.

4.2.3.3
Surgery

- Surgical resection (open or thoracoscopic).

4.2.4
Congenital Cystic Adenomatoid Malformation (CCAM)

(aka Congenital pulmonary airways malformation (CPAM))
Definition – multicystic mass of pulmonary tissue in which there is proliferation of the bronchial structures (terminal bronchioles) at the expense of alveoli.

Table 4.2.2   Stocker classification

Type	%	Features
0	<5	Acinar dysplasia – *solid bronchial-like structures – fatal*
1	20	Single or multiple cysts >2 cm in diameter Lined by *pseudostratified* columnar epithelium
2	75	Multiple small cysts <2 cm diameter Lined by *ciliated columnar or cuboidal* epithelium
3	<5	Solid lesions containing multiple very small (mm) cysts Lined by *cuboidal* epithelium
4	<2	Multiple thin-walled cysts lined with *alveolar* epithelium

Table 4.2.3   Adzick classification

Type	%	Features
Macrocystic	75	Single or multiple cysts >5 mm in diameter
Microcystic	25	Single or multiple cysts <5 mm in diameter

4.2.4.1
Stocker[1] Classification

Postnatal histological classification, originally with three types, now extended with two further types at either end (Table 4.2.2).

4.2.4.2
Adzick[2] Classification

Prenatal classification based on US measurements of cysts (Table 4.2.3).

4.2.4.3
Clinical Features

- R>L
- Upper > lower

Most are detected on routine antenatal US (18–24 weeks) scan, and remain static throughout the rest of the pregnancy. Possible complications at this stage include:

- Mediastinal shift (~20%), hydrops (~10%), fetal death (<5%).

---

[1]Col. J Thomas Stocker – American pathologist working at Armed Forces Institute of Pathology.
[2]Scott Adzick – American pediatric surgeon, currently at Children's Hospital of Philadelphia.

Fig. 4.2.1 (**a**) CT scan showing multicystic CCAM of right lung, (**b**) CT scan showing solid left basal lesion with feeding vessel, typical of an extralobar lung sequestration

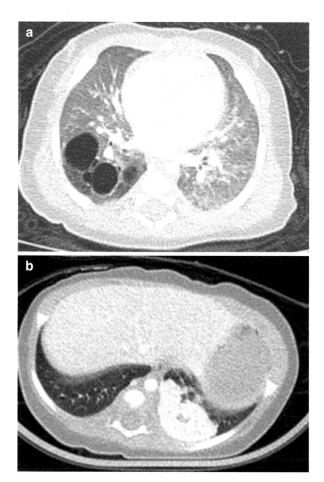

Postnatally, most will remain asymptomatic but ~25% will present with respiratory distress during the first week of life due simply to mass effect and displacement of functioning lung tissue. Thereafter, possible complications include lung infection, pneumothorax, mediastinal shift, and malignancy (see later) (Fig. 4.2.1).

4.2.4.4
Management

- Antenatal – if no evidence of hydrops, etc., then simply followed by serial US. Possible interventions (in the presence of signs of fetal distress) include
- Simple cyst aspiration and thoracoamniotic shunt (macrocyst).
- Percutaneous transamniotic laser ablation (microcyst) and fetal lung resection (currently only in USA).

- Postnatal management – symptomatic lesions should be surgically resected (open vs. thoracoscopic) usually lobectomy, but segmentectomy is possible for smaller discrete lesions.

Asymptomatic CCAM – although small lesions may well be managed using a conservative approach, most significant lesions should be probably resected in the first year. Currently, there is no prospective evidence-base for recommendations concerning those not surgically resected.

4.2.5
Mixed (Hybrid) Lesions

It is increasingly obvious that strict separation into BPS and CCAM is outdated, and the true situation is probably that of a spectrum-disorder with some overlap of pathology. Up to 20% of surgically resected composite series show features of both (e.g., aberrant systemic vessels with CCAM, synchronous CCAM and EPS, histological CCAM in obvious EPS, etc.).

Malignancy and CCAM

There is a predisposition toward the development of a variety of unusual malignancies, including
- Rhabdomyosarcoma (childhood)
- Bronchoalveolar carcinoma (adult)
- Pulmonary blastoma (childhood)

4.2.6
Congenital Lobar Emphysema (CLE)

Definition – bronchial pathology causing valve-like effect, resulting in overexpansion of lobe.
   May be congenital (e.g., bronchomalacia) or acquired due to extrinsic compression, or following respiratory tract infection.

4.2.6.1
Clinical Features

- LU lobe>RM lobe>RU lobe (classically)
- M:F 2:1

Presents during infancy with tachypnoea, especially during feeding, wheezing. Cyanosis may be seen. Signs include ipsilateral ↓ breath sounds, tracheal and mediastinal displacement.
   CXR – hyperlucent with faint bronchovascular markings. Sometimes, there is lung herniation into the mediastinum.

4.2.6.2
Surgery

Lobectomy – this is distinctly easier using an open thoracotomy and probably the thoraco-scopic option is contraindicated.

There is also a newly described variant affecting the distal segmental bronchus – here termed *congenital segmental emphysema*. All cases have been detected antenatally with a variety of features and some exhibited postnatal expansion, often after several years. There is often a central mucus-filled cavity termed a *bronchocele*. Treatment is surgical excision.

4.2.7
Bronchogenic Cysts

Definition – solitary, mucus-filled cyst with intimate (but noncommunicating) relationship with trachea or bronchus.

- M=F, Right=Left

Anatomically, they may lie in mediastinum (~85%) or within pulmonary parenchyma (~15%) with possible extrinsic compression of adjacent airways or even esophagus. Occasionally, they may be extrathoracic presenting as a subcutaneous cyst in the region of suprasternal notch.

4.2.7.1
Investigation

CXR, CT scan, or MRI is used to assess the size and anatomical relationship. Treatment is surgical excision.

4.2.8
Miscellaneous

Pulmonary isomerism is an anomaly of a number of lobes (i.e., right lung has two lobes and left has three)

    Azygous lobe – radiological finding – anomaly of RU lobe due to an aberrant azygous vein suspended by a pleural mesentery.

    Scimitar[3] *syndrome* – partial or total anomalous pulmonary venous drainage to inferior vena cava causing "scimitar-like" shadow on CXR. Important clinical features are conges-tive cardiac failure and pulmonary hypertension.

---

[3]*Scimitar* – Large curved sword, favored by Muslim warriors.

All antenatally detected lesions should be assessed radiologically (CT scan) in postnatal period irrespective of spontaneous "resolution."

Further Reading

1. Adzick NS, Harrison MR, Crombleholme TM, Flake AW et al (1998) Fetal lung lesions: management and outcome. Am J Obstet Gynecol 179:884–889
2. Davenport M, Warne SA, Cacciaguerra S et al (2004) Current outcome of antenatally diagnosed cystic lung disease. J Pediatr Surg 39:549–556
3. Azizkhan RG, Crombleholme TM (2008) Congenital cystic lung disease: contemporary antenatal and postnatal management. Pediatr Surg Int 24:643–57
4. Stanton M, Njere I, Ade-Ajayi N, Patel S, Davenport M (2009) Systematic review and meta-Analysis of the postnatal management of congenital cystic lung lesions. J Pediatr Surg 44:1027–1033

Gastro-Esophageal Reflux

4.3

Chandrasen K. Sinha and Benno Ure

About 85% of infants will vomit during the first week of life and another 10% have symptoms by 6 weeks of age. However, 60% of children will be asymptomatic by 2 years (due to upright posture and change to solid foods).

4.3.1
Normal Physiology

- Angle of His[1] (between esophagus and the fundus of stomach) is obtuse in newborns but decreases as infants develop. This ensures a more effective barrier against GOR.
- Pinch-cock action of right crus of diaphragm.
- Mucosal rosette – Redundant mucosal folds are present at gastro-esophageal junction only when a normal angle of His is present. These folds squeeze together to form a weak antireflux valve.
- *High-Pressure Zone* (manometric sphincter) – there is an area of increased muscular thickness near anatomical gastro-esophageal junction. Maturation of and hence ↑ in basal tone continues until ~45 days.
- *Intra-abdominal esophagus.*
- if >2 cm regarded as sufficient: <1 cm regarded as incompetent.
- Hiatus hernia may cause displacement of distal esophagus into the thorax (negative w.r.t. atmosphere).
- *Gastric outflow resistance* – causes ↑ intragastric pressure and exacerbates GER.

---

[1]Wilhelm His Sr (1831–1904) – Swiss anatomist, working in Basel and Leipzig, Germany.

C. K. Sinha (✉)
Paediatric Surgery Department, King's College Hospital, London, UK

C. K. Sinha and M. Davenport (eds.), *Handbook of Pediatric Surgery*,
DOI: 10.1007/978-1-84882-132-3_4.3, © Springer-Verlag London Limited 2010

Gastro-esophageal reflux (GER) can be divided into:

- Functional GER – common, rarely problematic
- Pathogenic GER (also termed gastro-esophageal reflux disease (GERD)) -is distinguished from functional GER by the frequency, ↑length of episodes and the presence of complications such as malnutrition, respiratory problems, erosive esophagitis, bleeding and strictures, Barrett[2] esophagus.
- Secondary GER – caused by the underlying conditions, e.g., hiatus hernia, gastric outlet obstruction, diaphragmatic hernia, etc.

4.3.2
Pathophysiology

- The major mechanism in infants and children is *transient LOS relaxation*, which accounts for about 95% of reflux episodes. Supine posture may promote reflux during periods of LOS relaxation phase.
- Fluid diet of infants facilitates the process of regurgitation when compared to the solid meals ingested by older children.
- ↓ Gastric emptying. Commonly seen in premature infants.

4.3.3
Associations and Predispositions

- Cerebral palsy, developmental delay.
- Down[3] syndrome and Cornelia de Lange[4] syndrome (genetic mutation, microcephaly, characteristic facies, ↑body hair).
- Drugs, e.g., benzodiazepines, theophylline.
- Diet and dietary habits (e.g., overeating, eating late at night, assuming a supine position shortly after eating), poor-quality foods (e.g., greasy, highly acidic).
- Food allergies.

---

[2]Normal Rupert Barrett (1903–1979) – Australian-born, British surgeon described columnar lined esophagus.
[3]John Langdon Down (1828–1926) – English physician, ascribed "racial" characteristics to various types of idiocy.
[4]Cornelia Catherina de Lange (1871–1950) – Dutch pediatrician, eventually professor in Amsterdam.

4.3.4
Clinical Features

There is an array of possible features, which can be dated to the first few months of life, and may be divided into.

- Regurgitation of food – one of the most common presentations in children, ranges from drooling to projectile vomiting. Most often, regurgitation is postprandial. Leads to weight loss and failure to thrive.
- Chest or abdominal pain – manifest as atypical crying and irritability in infancy.
- ENT – recurrent sore throat, stridor, hoarseness, and laryngitis.
- Sandifer[5] syndrome (i.e., posturing with opisthotonus or torticollis due to GER).

4.3.4.1
Relationship with Airway Problems

An infant's proximal airway and esophagus are lined with receptors that are activated by water, acid, or distension. Activation of these receptors by GER can produce laryngospasm, leading to obstructive apnea with resulting hypoxemia, cyanosis, and bradycardia – now termed an *Apparent Life-Threatening Event (ALTE).*

GOR may be a complicating factor in asthma, possibly due to microaspiration, and reflex bronchoconstriction. Suspect particularly if history of nocturnal wheezing is found.

4.3.4.2
Investigations

The diagnosis can be made in most cases on clinical grounds and conservative measures can be started empirically. However, if the presentation is atypical or if response to the therapy is inadequate, further evaluation is needed.

- *Upper GI contrast study* – GER is an episodic event and reflux may not be demonstrated initially. Hiatus hernia, strictures, esophagitis, and an impression of dysmotility can be appreciated.
- *24-h pH study* – quantification of reflux and its relationship to atypical symptoms and events (pathological – acid (<pII 4) exposure ≥4%).
- *Upper GI endoscopy (± biopsy)* – indicated in children, who are unresponsive to medical therapy.

---

[5]Paul H. Sandifer – English neurologist, worked at Great Ormond Street Hospital, London.

- Mucosal visualization of the mucosa – diagnosis of peptic esophagitis, peptic ulcer disease, *H. pylori* infection, and strictures.
- Histology – peptic esophagitis is suggested by basal cell hyperplasia, extended papillae, and mucosal eosinophils. (NB if >20 per high-powered field may be allergic (eosinophilic) esophagitis).

- Gastric scintiscan (not routine) – imaging can assess gastric emptying, observe reflux, and evaluate aspiration. Its disadvantages are the need for immobilization and that it cannot detect late postprandial reflux readily in the brief period it takes for evaluation.
- Esophageal manometry (not routine) – used to assess esophageal motility and LES function.

4.3.5
Management

4.3.5.1
Medical

- Conservative measures (although not definitely proven) include: upright positioning after feeding, elevating the head of the bed, providing small frequent thickened feeds, and thickening of formula. Feeding through nasojejunal or gastrojejunal tube are helpful in some cases. Functional GOR should need only reassurance.
- Drugs
  - Metoclopramide (dopaminergic antagonist – ↑LOS tone, ↑gastric emptying.
  - Antacids (↑gastric pH >4 and inhibits proteolytic activity of pepsin).
  - H_2 receptor antagonists (e.g., ranitidine) – similar inhibition of pepsin, together with ↓acid refluxate. (All medicines are more or less equipotent when used in equivalent doses).
  - Proton pump inhibitors (e.g., omeprazole) are suggested in children needing complete acid suppression (e.g., chronic respiratory disease or neurological impairment).

(N.B. Therapeutic response may take up to 2 weeks. If successful then ↑weight and ↓vomiting episodes).

4.3.6
Surgery: fundoplication (Fig. 4.3.1)

4.3.6.1
Indications

- *ALTE* associated with confirmed GER.
- Failure of medical therapy (persisting symptoms, failure to thrive).

- Oropharyngeal and esophageal complications, e.g., peptic stricture, Barrett esophagus.
- Anatomical GER, e.g., hiatus hernia.
- Severe GER in retarded children, where medical treatment has failed. (In these children, gastrostomy is often a useful addition.)

Many of these children have malnutrition, chronic aspiration, pneumonia, or pulmonary dysfunction; so assessment and optimizing these patients' nutritional and pulmonary status preoperatively is important.

The *principles of surgery* are

- Lengthening of the intra-abdominal esophagus
- Accentuation of the angle of His
- ↑ High-pressure zone at the esophago-gastric junction
- Approximation of the crura

Fundoplication achieves all of the above, although there are many variants, and comparative studies are rare. Partial wrap may be preferred in esophageal dysmotility disorders because these are less likely to cause obstructive symptoms.

All now include a crural repair and may be performed laparoscopically. Laparoscopic fundoplication has been well studied and accepted as equivalent (or even better by some studies) to open procedures in children.

4.3.6.2
Procedure (Nissen and Toupet) (Fig. 4.3.1)

1. Mobilization of fundus and distal esophagus – division of short gastric vessels.
2. Definition of hiatus – anterior vagus, separate posterior vagus.
3. Post-esophageal window – enough space to allow fundus though.
4. Crural repair (nonabsorbable suture) ± bougie (to prevent too much narrowing).
5. Wrap (variants as above).
6. ±Gastrostomy.

4.3.6.3
Complications

Variable but may be functional (e.g., retching, bloating), or related to recurrent reflux (unwrapping or displacement into chest).

Delayed gastric emptying (DGE) is common in children with neurological impairment. This may be looked for prior to surgery and a gastric emptying procedure (antroplasty, pyloroplasty) may be added. Dumping syndrome (e.g., diarrhea) can be a potential complication of such an addition though.

Fig. 4.3.1 Schematic illustration of different types of fundoplication: **(a)** Nissen, **(b)** Thal, **(c)** Toupet

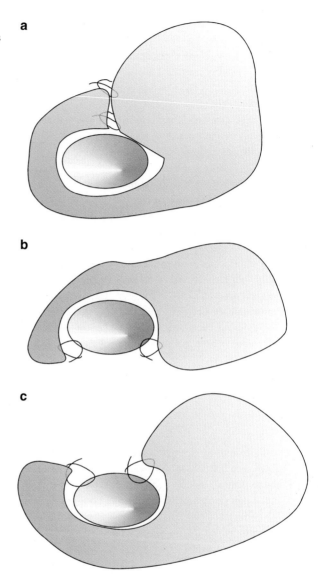

4.3.6.4
New Antireflux Endoscopic Procedures

- *Endoscopic gastroplication* (EndoCinch®) tightening of gastro-esophageal junction area by endoscopic suturing and knotting.
- *Stretta procedure* (application of radiofrequency energy to the LOS to augment lower esophageal sphincter pressure and increase the gastric yield pressure). Introduced in 2000, but pediatric experience limited.
- *Endoscopic submucosal injections* (of bovine collagen, Teflon, or nonbiodegradable polymer like ethylene vinyl alcohol at the level of cardia to increase LOS pressure).

- Nissen[6] fundoplication (commonest)
  - 360° circumferential wrap around the distal esophagus
- Thal [7]
  - 180° anterior wrap
- Toupet[8]
  - 270° posterior wrap

4.3.7
Outcome

- About 60-80% of GOR resolve by 18-24 months (~50% resolve by 12 months). Some infants require lifestyle modifications, and others require medications to control the symptoms of GOR.
- Surgery is required in a minority of cases and it controls reflux in about 90% (95% in neurologically normal/85% in neurologically abnormal).

[6]Rudolf Nissen (1896–1981) – German surgeon – posts in Turkey and USA, before finishing as Professor of Surgery in Basel, Switzerland.
[7]Alan P. Thal – American thoracic surgeon, worked in Minneapolis, MN.
[8]Andre Toupet (b1915) – French surgeon who worked at Hopital Bichat, Paris.

Further Reading

1. Fonkalsrud EW, Ashcraft KW, Coran AG et al (1998) Surgical treatment of gastroesophageal reflux in children: a combined hospital study of 7467 patients. Pediatrics 101:419–422
2. Michail S (2007) Gastroesophageal reflux. Pediatr Rev 28:101–110
3. Schmidt AI, Gluer S, Ure BM (2005) Fundoplication in paediatric surgery: a survey in 40 German institutions. Eur J Pediatr Surg 15:404–408
4. Tovar JA, Luis AL, Encinas JL et al (2007) Pediatric surgeons and gastroesophageal reflux. J Pediatr Surg 42:277–283

Gastrointestinal Bleeding

4.4

Juan A. Tovar

GI bleeding is relatively common in children and may be life-threatening. Surgeons must have a clear diagnostic strategy to implement the correct therapeutic procedures.

Gastrointestinal (GI) tract bleeding may arise from any segment of its wall and from the digestive organs that communicate with its lumen (e.g., liver).

4.4.1
Clinical Features

A practical classification suggests dividing the cause of GI bleeding into *high* (those within the reach of the upper GI endoscope), and *low* (those beyond this level). Although colonoscopy and capsule endoscopy are useful diagnostic tools, the diagnosis in low GI bleeding tends to be the more difficult.

High GI bleeding usually causes hematemesis (blood-stained vomiting) followed by melena[2] (stools containing digested, black blood). Most episodes are painless, although epigastric or retroesternal pain may suggest mucosal ulceration (e.g., esophagitis, duodenal ulcer). There may also be signs of underlying liver disease and portal hypertension (e.g., splenomegaly).

Low GI bleeding is not preceded by hematemesis but may cause hematochezia (red, undigested blood in stool) or melena, depending on how much of the intestine the blood

---

[2]*Melena*, or *meluena* – Latin for "black," not as commonly misspelled "*malena*" and therefore assumed to be "bad"!

J. A. Tovar
Department of Pediatric Surgery, Hospital Universitario La Paz, Madrid, Spain

C. K. Sinha and M. Davenport (eds.), *Handbook of Pediatric Surgery*,
DOI: 10.1007/978-1-84882-132-3_4.4, © Springer-Verlag London Limited 2010

has had to travel through. Massive GI blood loss will also lead to features of hypovolemia (e.g., tachycardia, hypotension, oliguria, etc.). Chronic GI bleeding may also present with a hypochromic, microcytic (i.e., iron deficiency) anemia.

4.4.1.1
High GI Bleeding (Table 4.4.1)

- *Epistaxis* is easily detected usually because of a previous history, but sometimes the patient is brought to the emergency room after hematemesis and a number of tests are performed that could have been avoided by a well-taken history.
- *Esophagitis* does not usually cause severe bleeding, but rather "coffee-grounds" vomiting or, even more often, chronic blood loss that goes undetected until microcytic, iron-deficient anemia appears. Symptoms of gastroesophageal reflux (GER) are invariably present.
- *Extra- and intrahepatic portal hypertension* (due to portal vein obstruction and liver cirrhosis, respectively) cause formation of varices (initially in esophagus, but also in stomach and ano-rectum). If these rupture, bleeding is usually massive and life-threatening. Splenomegaly and superficial abdominal venous collaterals may be apparent in PHT of whatever cause. There may be additional signs of chronic liver disease (e.g., jaundice, ascites, spider naevi, etc.)– See Chap. 6.6.
- *Gastritis* is usually due to ingestion of drugs, like aspirin, steroids, or other anti-inflammatory medications, but it may also accompany portal hypertension.
- *Hemobilia* is exceedingly rare and occurs when trauma or other causes create intrahepatic blood loss in communication with the biliary tract. Bleeding may be severe.
- *Gastroduodenal ulceration* (usually in relation to *Helicobacter pylori*) may occur in children although less often than in adults. The same symptoms and signs may be present but the relatively older age of most patients facilitates history taking and diagnosis.

4.4.1.2
Low GI bleeding (Table 4.4.1)

- *Meckel's diverticulum*[3] is a common cause of bleeding in children below 2 years, but it remains a possibility throughout life. The actual cause of bleeding is ectopic gastric secretory tissue at the base of the diverticulum causing ulceration in the neighboring ileal mucosa. Melena is usually apparent although when bleeding is massive, the stools may be red or mauve.
- *Intussusception* is perhaps the commonest surgical cause of GI bleeding in infants (0.2 per 1,000 live births) and is due to enlargement of the mucosal lymphoid (Peyer's[4]) patches of the terminal ileum. This is due to viral infection and creates a leading point

---

[3]Johan F. Meckel the younger (1781–1833) – famous German anatomist.
[4]Johan Conrad Peyer (1653–1712) – Swiss anatomist.

for intussusception. The lead point can be also a Meckel's diverticulum, a duplication cyst, or tumors such as lymphoma. Bleeding is characteristically low and is often accompanied by mucous secretion ("red-currant jelly" stool) and, of course, the classical symptoms and signs of intussusception.

- *Inflammatory bowel disease* (Crohn's[5] disease or UC). Bleeding can be massive but more often is less dramatic. Usually accompanied by pus or mucus mixed with stool together with prolonged history of abdominal pain and often weight loss (See Chap. 4.9 and 4.10).
- *Colonic polyps* cause hemorrhage but are rarely profuse. Although mostly solitary (e.g., juvenile polyps), there are a number of polyposis syndromes. These include
- *Peutz–Jegher's[6] syndrome* (multiple intestinal hamartomatous polyps, usually small bowel, with lip and palatal pigmentation).
- *Familial Adenomatous Polyposis* (autosomal dominant condition, with development of hundreds of colonic polyps by adolescence, invariably malignant if left). Colonoscopy is the key investigation.
- The term *angiodysplasia* involves vascular malformations that may be relatively extensive and can bleed at any age. The level of the lesion accounts for its variable expression and its often diffuse nature makes diagnosis frustrating.

4.4.2
Investigations

- Contrast Barium Meal and/or Enema – These are rarely of help in the scenario of acute bleeding. Chronic GER and sometimes esophagitis may be detected with an Upper GI series and some polyps, duplications, or intraluminal tumors revealed with barium enemas. A contrast enema was the classical diagnostic tool in intussusception, but has been largely replaced by other procedures.
- *Ultrasonography* – Used for detection of intussusception, duplication cysts, and sometimes large polyps. Has minor role in evaluation of GER, varices, and hemobilia.
- *CT scan and MRI* – Newer imaging modalities (especially spiral CT and MR angiography) may help with diagnosis of angiodysplasia, hemobilia, and duplication cysts.
- *Scintigraphy* – Diagnosis of Meckel's diverticulum may be facilitated by scintigraphy using Technetium pertechnectate 99 m uptake by the ectopic gastric mucosa. Unfortunately, although specific if positive, the sensitivity is not particularly high (it ranges from 60 to 70%). Ectopic tissues in some duplication cysts may sometimes be detected.
- *Laparoscopy* – When a structural cause is suspected (e.g., Meckel's, duplication) but scintigraphy has been unhelpful, then laparoscopy offers a relatively easy way of visualizing the small and large bowel.

---

[5]Burrill B. Crohn (1884–1983) – New York gastroenterologist described "terminal ileitis" in 1932.
[6]Johannes Peutz (1886–1957) – Dutch physician. Harold Jeghers (1904–1990) – American physician.

4.4.2.1
Endoscopy

- *Esophago-gastro-duodenoscopy* – Current small caliber endoscopes (e.g., 9 mm OD) allow direct observation of the GI tract down to the duodenum and even to the angle of Treitz[7]. Endoscopy is the key investigation and esophagitis, gastritis, mucosal tears, varices, and ulcers are all diagnosed readily.
- *Recto-sigmoidoscopy and Colonoscopy* – Endoscopy from below has the same advantages, but it rarely goes beyond the ileo-cecal valve. Hemorrhoids, polyps, and inflammatory bowel disease can be observed and biopsies can be taken when necessary.
- *Capsule endoscopy* – The development of small-size endoscopic capsules promised much advancement in the inspection of the long "blind" segments of the GI tract (i.e., the small bowel). However, although there have been published reports of its use in bleeding in children, it is not definitive, and even if images are diagnostic, the level of the lesion is often difficult to establish.

4.4.3
Management of GI Bleeding

4.4.3.1
Medication

Mainly indicated in the treatment of reflux esophagitis, erosive gastritis, or gastroduodenal ulcers.

- Proton pump inhibitors (e.g., omeprazole) or H2 receptor antagonists (e.g., ranitidine). Both significantly inhibit acid secretion and volume.
- *H. pylori* eradication therapy (usually short-course triple or double antibiotics).
- Octreotide (short-term) – ↓ portal hypertension
- Propranolol (long-term) – ↓ portal hypertension

4.4.3.2
Endoscopy

- Acutely bleeding varices are better treated by endoscopic sclerotherapy (e.g., intravariceal ethanolamine) or in overwhelming hemorrhage by placement of a Sengstaken–Blakemore[8] pattern tube. In those not actually bleeding, endoscopic band ligation is quicker to achieve variceal obliteration and has less complications.

---

[7]Wenzel Treitz (1819–1872) – Czech physician who described a suspensory muscle ("ligament") of duodenum in 1853 – often used to demarcate the duodeno–jejunal junction.

[8]Robert Sengstaken and Arthur Blakemore – New York surgeons who described custom-made tube with esophageal and gastric balloons in 1950. The first patient was a 15-year-old girl with portal vein thrombosis.

- Endoscopic electrocoagulation may be used in selected cases of gastroduodenal ulceration, particularly where there is a visible vessel.

4.4.3.3
Radiological Treatment

Intussusception should be treated nonoperatively whenever possible. Barium enema reduction has been progressively replaced by saline enema reduction under ultrasound monitoring or by pneumatic reduction with insufflating balloon and a safety pressure valve.

4.4.3.4
Surgery

- Structural pathology such as Meckel's diverticulum and duplications should be excised and a laparoscopic approach may be adopted.

Table 4.4.1 Causes of GI bleeding

	Cause	Notes
High	Epistaxis	
	Esophagitis	GER, alkali ingestion, foreign body
	Mallory–Weiss tear[1]	Prolonged retching causing mucosal tear at GOJ
	Varices (gastroesophageal)	Commonest cause in *de novo* bleeding – portal vein thrombosis
	Gastritis	e.g., drugs
	Gastroduodenal ulcer	e.g., *Helicobacter pylori*
	Hemobilia	Associated with obstructive jaundice, caused by trauma (e.g., liver biopsy)
Low	Meckel's diverticulum	
	Intussusception	Usually in infants
	Infective enteritis	e.g., *Campylobacter spp. Salmonella spp. Shigella spp.*
	Crohn's disease	Adolescence
	Ulcerative colitis	Adolescence
	NEC	Commonest causes in neonates
	Angiodysplasia	
	Anal fissure	Commonest cause in children
	Polyps	Single or multiple
	Hemorrhoids	
	Varices (ano-rectal)	

---

[1]GK Mallory (1900–1986), S Weiss (1898–1942) – described this in 15 alcoholic patients in 1929.

- Definitive management of extrahepatic portal hypertension may require porto-systemic or meso-portal shunting if endoscopic management fails. The equivalent situation in end-stage liver disease due to cirrhosis requires consideration of liver transplantation.
- Inflammatory bowel disease may require surgery if bleeding is persistent or when medical treatment fails. The aim in Crohn's disease is to use limited intestinal resection or bowel-preserving strategies (e.g., stricturoplasty). An emergency colectomy (typically for UC) may be required if bleeding is ongoing and life-threatening.
- Inflammatory recto-sigmoid or colonic polyps can be safely excised endoscopically using diathermy snares. Sometimes, colectomy is indicated where polyps are multiple (e.g., FAP) and the risk of malignant change is high (usually postpuberty).

Further Reading

1. Gilger MA (2004) Upper gastrointestinal bleeding. In: Walker WA, Goulet O, Kleinman RE et al (eds) Pediatric gastrointestinal disease, vol. 1. BC Decker, Hamilton, pp 258–265
2. Justice FA, Auldist AW, Bines JE (2006) Intussusception: trends in clinical presentation and management. J Gastroenterol Hepatol 21:842–846
3. Menezes M, Tareen F, Saeed A et al (2008) Symptomatic Meckel's diverticulum in children: a 16-year review. Pediatr Surg Int 24:575–577
4. Swaniker F, Soldes O, Hirschl RB (1999) The utility of technetium 99m pertechnetate scintigraphy in the evaluation of patients with Meckel's diverticulum. J Pediatr Surg 34:760–764
5. Turck D, Michaud L (2004) Lower gastrointestinal bleeding. In: Walker WA, Goulet O, Kleinman RE et al (eds) Pediatric gastrointestinal disease, vol. 1. BC Decker, Hamilton, pp 266–280

Acute Abdomen

4.5

Pablo Laje and Marcelo Martinez-Ferro

An acute abdomen is usually defined as a rapid onset of abdominal pain that requires a prompt evaluation. Although the spectrum of possible causes is wide, the only initial issue that needs to be addressed is whether the patient has a medical or a surgical condition. In most, this distinction can be made with history, physical examination, and basic investigations, but there are some cases where surgery itself is the diagnostic tool.

4.5.1
Possible Causes

There are many different clasifications, but a reasonable approach divides the possible causes according to the age-group most likely affected (Table 4.5.1).

Some conditions occur almost exclusively in certain age-groups; for instance, most children who develop a midgut volvulus secondary to intestinal malrotation are below 1 year of age, but cases can be seen in older children, teenagers, and even adults. As a general rule, congenital conditions tend to become symptomatic early in life.

Alternatively, abdominal pain can be divided according to the underlying pathophysiology (Table 4.5.2).

- Infectious/inflammatory (pain, fever, leukocytosis, elevated C-reactive protein)
- Occlusive (pain, intestinal obstruction, no systemic signs of sepsis)
- Hemorrhagic (pain, paleness, acute anemia)

In general, each surgical condition can be clearly classified within one of these categories, but as the primary process evolves, the distinction becomes less clear. For example, an acute appendicitis during its early stages will have the features of an infectious acute abdomen, but if it turns into a generalized peritonitis, an occlusive component will appear. Furthermore, an occlusive acute abdomen due to postsurgical adhesions can turn into an inflammatory acute abdomen if a bowel loop becomes necrotic or perforates.

P. Laje (✉)
Department of Pediatric Surgery, The Children's Hospital of Philadelphia, Philadelphia, PA, USA

C. K. Sinha and M. Davenport (eds.), *Handbook of Pediatric Surgery*,
DOI: 10.1007/978-1-84882-132-3_4.5, © Springer-Verlag London Limited 2010

Table 4.5.1 Causes of abdominal pain during childhood

1–12 months	1–5 years	6–12 years	13–18 years
Infantile colic	Nonspecific abdominal pain		
Intussusception	Appendicitis		
	Mesenteric adenitis		
Gastroenteritis			
Incarcerated hernias			
Hirschsprung's	Constipation		
Metabolic diseases	Meckel's diverticulitis		Cholecystitis
Internal hernias			Crohn's disease/ulcerative colitis
Midgut volvulus		Omental torsion	
Urinary tract infections			PID
Pharyngitis			Ovarian torsion
	Urinary calculi		Pancreatitis

Table 4.5.2 Schematic of abdominal pain

Infection / inflammatory	Examples – appendicitis, cholecystitis, Crohn's disease
Occlusive	Examples – intussusception, incarcerated hernia, midgut volvulus
Hemorrhagic	Examples – trauma (solid organ), ectopic pregnancy, ruptured tumor

4.5.2
Clinical Features

A brief summary of each of the most frequent entities will follow.

4.5.2.1
Acute Appendicitis (See Chap. 4.7)

- Acute appendicitis is the most common surgical cause of the acute abdomen in children.

While a typical clinical picture is usually present, atypical presentations are very frequent, especially in younger patients. The most common presentation is that of vague abdominal pain that starts in the peri-umbilical area, and 12–24 h later migrates to the right lower quadrant. Fever, vomiting, and anorexia are typically part of the picture. As the disease progresses and involves the parietal peritoneum, signs of peritonism appear such as rebound tenderness and guarding. In older children, even without specific treatment, the infection usually tends to localize in the right lower quadrant first as a complex abdominal mass (phlegmon), then as an appendiceal abscess. In younger children, localization is not common and peritonitis with spreading infection occurs early.

- Laboratory signs of inflammation, e.g., ↑ WBC and ↑C-reactive protein.
- Plain radiography – usually nonspecific, but a radio-opaque fecalith or localized dilated ileal loops are suggestive findings.
- Nonselective ultrasound – increasingly popular in the work-up of a suspected acute appendicitis.
  - Signs – noncompressive, enlarged tubular structure, and peri-appendiceal fluid.
  - Valuable role in the evaluation of adnexal disease such as ovarian cysts/torsion in teenage girls with lower abdominal pain. .
- CT scanning – increasingly used to evaluate possible appendicitis – however, it should be appreciated that at least 24 h must elapse from the beginning of the pain before the inflamed appendix becomes large enough to be clearly distinguished from a normal appendix.

In general, there is no test that can replace the physical exam of an experienced surgeon to diagnose an acute appendicitis.

4.5.2.2
Intussusception (See Chap. 4.6)

- Peak incidence occurs between 6 and 18 months of age with an ileo-cecal intussusception being the most common type.

The typical clinical presentation is of colicky abdominal pain, vomiting, and eventually bloody diarrhea. Most infants are lethargic in between the episodes of pain with signs of dehydration if diagnosis is delayed. Plain radiographs may show signs of a soft-tissue mass in the right upper quadrant or signs suggestive of small bowel obstruction with central, dilated intestinal loops. Ultrasound remains the key investigation in suspected cases and is highly sensitive and specific. CT scan is also sensitive, but is rarely necessary.

4.5.2.3
Incarcerated Inguinal Hernia

- This is a clinical diagnosis, and no further tests are required.

Most can be safely reduced in the emergency department (with or without sedation), after which the child should be admitted for observation and scheduled for an early repair. Ideally, at least 24 h should elapse before the repair to allow the tissue edema to settle.

Sometimes, the incarcerated viscus may be suspected to be nonviable or at least severely compromised. Consider this if the history is more than a day, there are peritoneal signs, or free air is visible on radiography. External reduction should not be attempted, and urgent open exploration should be expedited.

4.5.2.4
Ovarian Torsion

- Solid or cystic masses arising in the ovaries are common in teenage girls, and are at risk of ovarian torsion.

These are usually simple functional cysts, followed by hemorrhagic cysts and then tumors (benign > malign).

Torsion usually causes severe acute abdominal pain that can be intermittent. Ultrasound remains the ideal diagnostic tool and Doppler evaluation can assess the viability of the torted ovary prior to surgical exploration.

Intussusception

4.6

Prema Ambalakat Menon and Katragadda L. N. Rao

Intussusception is a condition largely peculiar to infants with, typically, telescoping of a proximal loop of distal ileum into the adjoining ascending colon.

4.6.1 Epidemiology

- 1–4 cases of intussusception[1] per 1,000 live-births (in UK)
- Seasonal variation – suggested to parallel gastroenteritis, i.e., spring/summer
- No racial variation
- Rotavirus vaccine (RotaShield®, but not RotaTeq®)
- M:F ratio is 3:2

4.6.2 Pathogenesis

Can be divided into two types

- Primary (or idiopathic) – (common)
  - Principally in infants (9–18 months). Unknown underlying but assumed to be hypertrophic Peyer's[2] patch in distal ileum. Recent viral infection (e.g., adenovirus or rotavirus) may have precipitated hypertrophy.

---

[1]*Intussusception* (Latin) - Intus meaning "within" and suscipere meaing "to receive."
[2]Johan Conrad Peyer (1653–1712) – Swiss anatomist.

P. A. Menon (✉)
Pediatric Surgery Department, Post Graduate Institute of Medical Education and Research, Chandigarh, India

C. K. Sinha and M. Davenport (eds.), *Handbook of Pediatric Surgery*,
DOI: 10.1007/978-1-84882-132-3_4.6, © Springer-Verlag London Limited 2010

- Secondary – (~5%) – due to a specific lead point

  – Meckel's diverticulum
  – Polyps (rarely Peutz[3]–Jeghers[4] syndrome, familial adenomatous polyps, etc.)
  – Duplication cysts
  – Lymphoma
  – Intramural hematoma (e.g., Henoch–Schonlein purpura, blunt abdominal trauma)

Whatever the cause, there is invagination of the proximal part of the intestine into the distal part. The inner and middle cylinders or the intussuscepted bowel constitutes the *intussusceptum*, while the outer cylinder is termed the *intussuscepiens*. The constrained bowel becomes ischemic due to impairment of venous and lymphatic drainage, leading ultimately to necrosis (hence, mucus production and sloughing of mucosa to produce classic "redcurrant jelly stool").

- Ileocaecal region (~80%)
- Ileoileal (~10%)
- Colocolic or ileoileocolic (<10%)

(Very rarely, there is retrograde progression – <1% in authors' series over 14 years.)

4.6.3
Clinical Features

Typically, a pale, lethargic infant (otherwise well-nourished) presents with intermittent attacks of colicky pain associated with pulling up of the legs. Vomiting is almost invariable.

- A sausage-shaped mass is palpable in the RUQ with the RLQ often distinctly empty of palpable bowel loops (Dance's[5] sign).
- In some environments, there may be diagnostic delay due to a coincident diarrheal illness (especially dysentery). Progression of the condition leads to the mass moving even further along the GI tract. Thus, it may be palpable per rectum or even visible as a prolapse. In this scenario, the gloved finger can pass between the prolapsing bowel and the anus while in a true rectal prolapse this is not possible.
- Mucoid or bloody stool ("red-currant jelly").
- Hypovolemia and septic shock may be seen due to the gangrenous bowel (± perforation).

---

[3]Johannes Peutz (1886–1957) – Dutch physician first described features in 1921.
[4]Harold Jeghers (1904–1990) – American physician.
[5]Jean Baptiste Dance (1797–1832) – French pathologist and physician.

4.6.3.1
Investigations

- *AXR* – dilated small bowel loops or a soft-tissue mass.
- *US* – "target" sign, or "pseudokidney" sign (Fig. 4.6.1).
- *Contrast enema* still diagnostic (and therapeutic) option.
- *CT scan* – usually in the older child where there are irregular features and their associated pathology is suspected (e.g., lymphoma) (Figs. 4.6.2 and 4.6.3).

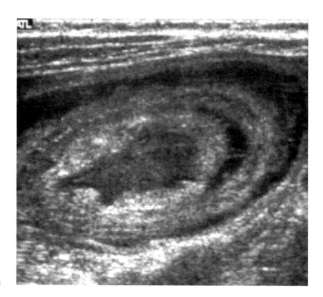

Fig. 4.6.1 Ultrasound showing a multilayered "target" appearance suggestive of intussusception

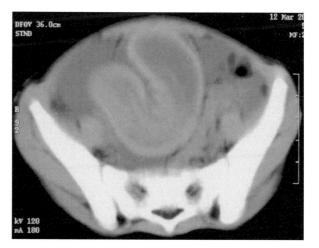

Fig. 4.6.2 Noncontrast abdominal CT showing hyperdense bowel in intussuscepted loop suggestive of intramural hematoma

Fig. 4.6.3 Film taken
during barium enema
reduction of intussusception
in transverse colon

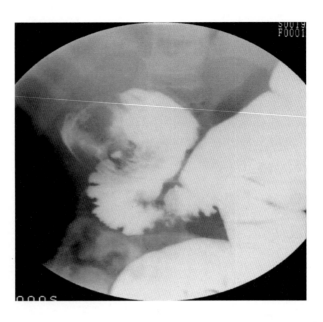

4.6.4
Management

Includes age-appropriate resuscitation and correction of fluid deficits together with NG tube, aspiration, and broad-spectrum antibiotics.

- *Radiology-directed reduction (air, saline, or barium)* – initial method of choice in the absence of perforation or peritonitis.
  - Highly variable reported success rate (50–90%).
  - Confirmation of success includes reflux of contrast into the terminal ileum – most units should achieve >60% success rate.
  - Recommended pressures (<120 cm H_2O for air enema, or 1 m above the level of buttocks for barium or other contrast).
  - If partial reduction – repeat procedure after 3 h.
  - Perforation is the most important complication (usually due to ischemia of bowel and an inexperienced radiologist) – if obvious pneumoperitoneum – use of needle puncture to decompress.

Therapeutic contrast enema is not useful in ileoileal intussusception and is relatively contraindicated in the older atypical group who tend to have secondary pathology and therefore require surgical management. Occasionally, children with medical conditions (e.g., Henoch–Schonlein purpura) may respond to steroid therapy.

4.6.5
Surgery

Indications

- Peritonitis
- Bowel perforation (during enema reduction)
- Failure of contrast enema
- Secondary pathology suspected

Incision – right transverse close to the umbilicus

1. Deliver mass into wound – cecum is usually mobile in most cases making this easy. Warm saline compresses are applied and the *intussusceptum* gently *pushed* out of the *intussuscepiens*.
2. A segmental resection (and anastomosis) is performed in the presence of perforation, suspected lead point, or if there is persistent ischemia and lack of peristalsis in any part of the bowel.

4.6.5.1
Outcome

1. Recurrence – postcontrast enema, 5–10% within the first 72 h
2. Ischemic stricture

Laparoscopic Reduction

Reasonable alternative in some centers and can be advantageous if there is doubt about adequacy of reduction postcontrast enema. Nonetheless, safe manipulation of ischemic bowel is not easy, and *pulling out* the intussusceptum rather than pushing has been advocated (but is contentious).

Acknowledgment The authors thank Dr. Akshay Kumar Saxena, Consultant Pediatric Radiologist, PGI, Chandigarh, India, for the photographs.

Further Reading

1. Daneman A, Navarro O (2004) Intussusception. Part 2: an update on the evolution of management. Pediatr Radiol 34:97–108
2. Kia KF, Mony VK, Drongowski RA (2005) Laparoscopic vs open surgical approach for intussusception requiring operative intervention. J Pediatr Surg 40:281–284
3. http://www.who.int/vaccines-documents/DocsPDF02/www640.pdf

Appendicitis

4.7

Ciro Esposito

Appendicitis is the most common surgical cause for the acute abdomen in childhood.

4.7.1
Epidemiology

- *Twentieth century disease* – barely described in the nineteenth century with escalating incidence in the twentieth century. Ascribed to reciprocal fall in infantile gastrointestinal diarrheal diseases and, paradoxically, improvements in hygiene/living standards.
- Lifetime risk ~7% (in Western populations).

4.7.1.1
Pathology

Progressive inflammatory disease

1. Obstruction of lumen – e.g., fecolith, lymphoid hyperplasia virus for instance, rarely foreign body.
2. Catarrhal inflammation and luminal distension. Transmural bacterial migration by resident flora (aerobic and anaerobic; *E. coli and Bacteroides spp, etc.*).
3. Ulceration of mucosa and fibrinopurulent exudates.
4. *Gangrene* eventually occurs as a result of progressive bacterial invasion and vascular impairment.
5. *Perforation* (20–40%), causing peritonitis and/or abscess formation.

C. Esposito
Pediatrics Department, "Federico II" University of Naples, Naples, Italy

C. K. Sinha and M. Davenport (eds.), *Handbook of Pediatric Surgery*,
DOI: 10.1007/978-1-84882-132-3_4.7, © Springer-Verlag London Limited 2010

(a) ↑ incidence in younger children (>80% for <5-year olds; ~100% in 1-year olds)
(b) Reasons
   1. Caused by impaired communication and a poorer history than in older children.
   2. Parents and caregivers assume "gastroenteritis" based on the common features of anorexia, vomiting, diarrhea, and fever.
   3. Increasing perforation rates may be due to socioeconomic factors such as ethnicity, access to healthcare, insurance status, and patient referral patterns.

4.7.2
Clinical Features

The key features are abdominal pain, nonbile-stained reflex vomiting, and anorexia.

1. Pain is initially periumbilical or poorly localized and correlates with luminal distension and early inflammation. Progressive transmural inflammation and serosal exudates cause localized irritation of the overlying parietal peritoneum and a distinct *shift* of the pain to the RLQ (or wherever the appendix is).
2. Nausea and vomiting – after the onset of pain and may be short-lived.
3. Anorexia – almost invariable. If child is hungry, the diagnosis could be in doubt.

Examination shows a child who appears acutely ill, often with a slight flush of the cheeks.

1. Typical maximum point of tenderness – McBurney's[1] point *(2/3 along line drawn from umbilicus to anterior iliac spine).* Peritonism limits walking and some children adopt a legs-flexed posture when lying down.
2. Hierarchy of abdominal muscle reflex response – from rebound tenderness, through guarding to rigidity – depending on the degree of parietal peritoneal involvement.

(N.B. *Obturator Sign (internal rotation of flexed hip exacerbates pain)* and *Psoas sign (leg extension exacerbates pain)* are usually seen in retrocecal appendicitis.)

3. Fever is usually moderate (38–39°C), and indeed if higher it suggests the presence of perforation or another diagnosis (e.g., viral mesenteric adenitis).
4. Rectal examination (older children) may show right-sided tenderness and is key to clinical diagnosis of pelvic appendicitis (where RLQ tenderness may be absent).

Only about half of the patients demonstrate the typical pattern of symptoms described here.

---

[1]Charles McBurney (1845–1913) – Surgeon at Roosevelt Hospital, New York City, USA. During 1880s and 1890s, he was a leading advocate for surgery in appendicitis, describing clinical features and incision.

4.7.2.1
Investigations

Laboratory tests are of limited value in the diagnosis of appendicitis.

1. A mild leukocytosis (11,000–15,000) with left-shift is typical but not universal. A high WBC (20,000) in a patient with minimal findings suggests that another condition is responsible for the symptoms.
2. Elevated C-reactive protein is typical but does not increase discrimination.

Clinical scoring systems (e.g., Alvarado) incorporating elements of the history, examination, and lab studies have been used but realistically sensitivity and specificity are still only modest (70–80%).

Diagnostic accuracy can be improved in equivocal cases by *repeating* the examination and lab studies over a period of 12–24 h following admission – this so often simplifies the decision to discharge or proceed to appendectomy.

4.7.2.2
Imaging

Unnecessary if the diagnosis is obvious, and should be reserved for equivocal cases.

1. Abdominal X-rays – RLQ soft-tissue mass displacing bowel loops. Fecolith (<10%).
2. *US* – looking for fluid collection, abscess cavity, soft-tissue mass, etc. Excellent specificity (~90%), but variable sensitivity (50–90%) for the disease. Highly operator (and patient) dependent.
3. *CT scans* – probably offer no further improvement in accuracy in children but can be useful for those with prolonged or atypical features.

As perforated appendicitis leads to increased morbidity, length of hospitalization, and cost, negative laparotomy rates of 10–20% were considered appropriate to keep perforation rates low. However, most of the current authors have criticized such a tolerant attitude, citing the risks and expense of unnecessary surgery.

4.7.3
Surgery

Includes correction of fluid, electrolyte, and acid/base imbalance (due to vomiting, etc.), together with antibiotics (effective against anaerobes and Gram-negative coliforms) to combat features of systemic bacterial sepsis.

Antibiotic regimen – selected for effect against likely pathogens

(a) Nonperforated appendicitis – single agent, e.g., second-generation cefalosporins, ampicillin/sulbactam, ticarcillin/clavulanate, or piperacillin/tazobactam.
(b) Perforated appendicitis – "triple" antibiotic regimen (e.g., ampicillin, gentamycin, and clindamycin or metronidozole) or a combination (e.g., ceftriaxone/metronidozole or ticarcillin/clavulante and gentamycin).

(Personal practice – nonperforated appendicitis (three perioperative doses) with those having perforated appendicitis an IV regimen is continued until normally fed and apyrexial. Then discharge with oral antibiotic to complete a 10-day course.)

4.7.3.1
Timing

- *Short-history, nonperforated appendicitis* – prompt appendectomy. But no real increase in perforation rates or morbidity if delayed to following morning, etc.
- *Short history, perforated appendicitis* – full IV fluid resuscitation and antibiotic loading with appendectomy after clinical improvement.
- *Longer history, palpable mass* – continuation of nonoperative management with deferred appendectomy (8–12 weeks) if clinical resolution. If no clinical improvement (24–72 h), then laparotomy is indicated. [Some recent studies have not recommended interval appendicectomy].

4.7.3.2
Open appendectomy

Muscle-splitting RLQ incision centered on McBurney's point (or point of maximum tenderness). Ensure that skin incision follows normal skin crease (Langer's lines) for improved cosmesis.

1. Ligation/coagulation of meso-appendix.
2. Excision of appendix, typically with stump inversion into cecum using a purse-string suture.
3. ±Peritoneal lavage depending on the degree of soiling.

4.7.3.3
Laparoscopic appendectomy (three ports)

1. Umbilical (Hasson[2]) access + 5-mm LLQ and 10 mm RLQ
2. Coagulation of meso-appendix (unipolar hook)

---

[2]Harrith Hasson – American gynecologist – described open access technique in 1971.

3. Ligation/transection of appendix (double endo-loop)
4. Excision of appendix (withdrawal through umbilical port)
5. Peritoneal lavage depending on degree of soiling

4.7.3.4
One trocar appendectomy (one port)

1. Umbilical (Hasson) access – (11 mm operative optic with 5 mm operative channel)
2. Ligation of meso-appendix (outside the abdominal cavity)
3. Ligation/transection of appendix (outside the abdominal cavity)
4. Repositioning of the appendiceal stump into the abdominal cavity
5. Peritoneal lavage if necessary

The choice of approach is variable throughout the world; however, most pediatric studies generally conclude that LA is comparable with OA in most crucial aspects (incidence of complications, etc.) (Fig. 4.7.1).

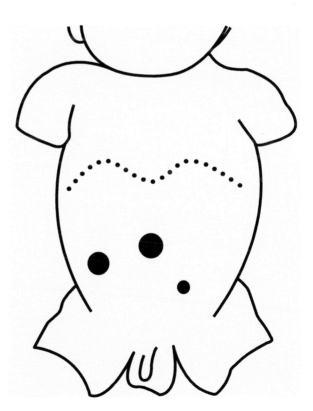

Fig. 4.7.1 Trocar position in laparoscopic appendectomy

4.7.4
Outcome

The complication rate in most current series should be <10%, but may consist of:

- Abscess formation (interloop, pelvic, rarely subdiaphragmatic, or subhepatic).
- Intestinal obstruction – early or late but >90% occur within the first 3 months. It is caused by inflammation and adhesions, and may be severe after perforated appendicitis.
- Sterility – due to inflammatory obliteration of the Fallopian tubes in girls with perforated appendicitis. Literature is conflicting and incidence is controversial.

Further Reading

1. Addiss DG, Shaffer N, Fowler BS (1990) Tauxe RV The epidemiology of appendicitis and appendectomy in the United States. Am J Epidemiol 132:910–925
2. Esposito C (1998) One trocar appendectomy in pediatric surgery. Surg Endosc 12:177–178
3. Esposito C, Borzi P, Valla JS et al (2007) Laparoscopic versus open appendectomy in children: a retrospective comparative study of 2, 332 cases. World J Surg 31:750–755
4. Fishman SJ, Pelosi L, Klavon SL, O'Rourke EJ (2000) Perforated appendicitis: prospective outcome analysis for 150 children. J Pediatr Surg 35:923–926
5. Morrow SE, Newman KD (2007) Current management of appendicitis. Semin Ped Surg 16:34–40

Mark Davenport

Although conditions such as acute appendicitis and intussusception are relatively common causes of acute abdominal pain, neither is as common as the *"nonspecific abdominal pain" (NSAP),*[2] which is seen in children of all ages and all places for which no diagnostic test or specific remedy exists. Clinical acumen and experience are the usual diagnostic tools, with reassurance and perhaps temporary relief from food as bedside remedies.

Children will suffer from classical surgical pathology such as *uro-sepsis* (Chap 6.5), *uro-calculi*, and *intestinal volvulus*. Additionally, girls will suffer from *pelvic inflammatory disease*, *torted ovaries*, *mittleschmerz*[1], etc.

Children will also suffer from classical metabolic pathology (e.g., *diabetic ketoacidosis* and *hypercalcemia)* and hematological disorder (e.g., *sickle cell anemia*). In all these, abdominal pain will feature and, particularly with de novo cases, confusion can occur as to what is going on.

Apart from the first subject, this chapter is therefore devoted largely to minutiae.

4.8.1
Helicobacter pylori

- Gram –ve, spiral bacterium, acquired in childhood (~5% overall).
- Increasingly prevalent with age.
- May be ↓ in prevalence (at least in West).

---

[1]Mittleschmerz (German) for "middle pain," i.e., pain felt in middle of period due to ovulation.
[2]NSAP – "No sweat abdominal pain!"

M. Davenport
Paediatric Surgery Department, Kings College Hospital, London, UK

C. K. Sinha and M. Davenport (eds.), *Handbook of Pediatric Surgery*,
DOI: 10.1007/978-1-84882-132-3_4.8, © Springer-Verlag London Limited 2010

4.8.1.1
Clinical Features

- Mostly asymptomatic
- Gastritis, duodenal, and gastric ulceration
- Malignant change (possible in adults)

4.8.1.1.1
Investigation

1. Serology (anti–*H. pylori* antibodies) – nonspecific
2. Stool antigen
3. Urea breath test (e.g., PYtest®)
4. Mucosal biopsy and "CLOtest®" – rapid urease test for Campylobacter-like organism

4.8.1.1.2
Eradication

- Triple therapy (amoxicillin, clarithromycin/metronidazole, omeprazole) for 1 week
- Bismuth preparations – more effective, less palatable

4.8.2
Yersinia[3] Infections

Yersinia enterocolitica, Yersinia pseudotuberculosis,

- Gram –ve cocco-bacillus, which can be a specific cause of mesenteric adenitis, acute ileitis, appendicitis, and even enterocolitis.
- Prevalent in Scandinavia, may be related to ingestion of undercooked pork, and tends to affect young (<5 years) children.

Sensitive to third-generation cephalosporins, gentamicin but DOC probably Septrin® (sulfa/trimethoprim). Resistant to co-amoxyclav.

4.8.3
Lead Poisoning (Painter's Colic)

Chronic exposure, usually ingestion, may lead to poisoning. Found in paint (toys), petrol, plumbing (both pipes and solder) – particularly that of previous centuries, and some herbal preparations. Sometimes due to ingestion of contaminated soil.

---

[3]AEJ Yersin, Swiss bacteriologist who discovered the cause of bubonic plague *(Y. pestis)*.

4.8.3.1
Clinical Features

- Abdominal colic
- Neurocognitive symptoms – lethargy, hyperactivity, seizures
- ↑ Blood pressure

4.8.3.1.1
Investigation

Blood lead level should be <10 µg/L.

4.8.4
Porphyrias[4]

Family of metabolic defects within the synthetic pathway of heme. This leads to tissue accumulation of toxic precursors in the skin, liver, nervous system, etc.

Example – acute intermittent porphyria.

4.8.4.1
Clinical Features

Most present in adolescence, or have +ve family history.

- *Recurrent abdominal pain* – typical feature in AIP, can be triggered by certain drugs (e.g., phenobarbitone), hormones, infection, and fasting. Can be extreme, with minimal abdominal signs, usually lasts for days.
- Discolored urine – red, brown, purple.
- Autonomic neuropathy – ↑ heart rate, ↑BP – peripheral neuropathy.
- Anemia.
- Skin sensitivity – sunlight.
- Psychiatric and neurological symptoms (e.g., seizures).

4.8.4.1.1
Investigations

- ↑↑ porphyrins in urine, feces, and blood.

Treatment is medical and supportive and involves loading with carbohydrate (IV glucose) and hematin supplementation to suppress heme synthesis.

---

[4]*Porphyria* (Greek – *porphura*) – purple pigment. Denoting one of the characteristic features – discoloration of urine.

4.8.5
Familial Mediterranean Fever

One of the autoinflammatory conditions of childhood, this is a hereditary condition (single gene mutation *(MEFV)* on Ch16) afflicting characteristic groups clustered around Mediterranean (Armenian, Greeks, Turkey, Sephardi Jews, etc.). There is a deficit in the protein *pyrin*, a key part of the inflammatory cascade.

4.8.5.1
Clinical Features

- Abdominal pain – childhood onset, often prolonged over period of days. Probably caused by intrinsic peritonitis.
- Other inflammatory membranes – e.g., pleuritis/pericarditis/tunica vaginalis (acute scrotum).
- Joint pain.
- Fever (~25%).

4.8.5.1.1
Investigation

- Nothing specific acutely but ↑↑ CRP and ESR.
- Mutational analysis possible.

Treatment is supportive but colchicine may have a role in ↓ attacks.

Further Reading

1. Daugule I, Rowland M (2008) Helicobacter pylori infection in children. Helicobacter 13(suppl 1): 41–46
2. Blakelock RT, Beasley SW (2003) Infection and the gut. Semin Pediatr Surg 12:265–274
3. Henry K, Harris CR (2006) Deadly ingestions. Pediatr Clin North Am 53:293–315
4. Ahmed I (2002) Childhood porphyrias. Mayo Clin Proc 77:825–836
5. Gattorno M, Federici S, Pelagatti MA et al (2008) Diagnosis and management of autoinflammatory diseases in childhood. Clin Immunol 28(suppl 1):S73–S83

Crohn's Disease

4.9

Chandrasen K. Sinha and Arnold G. Coran

Burrill Bernard Crohn, a gastroenterologist, and two surgeons, Leon Ginzburg and Gordon Oppenheimer, presented 14 cases of a granulomatous inflammation of the terminal ileum in 1930. Initially naming it "terminal ileitis," but changing it to "regional ileitis" for the paper to avoid the morbid implications of the word "terminal."

4.9.1
Epidemiology of Inflammatory Bowel Disease

(*Crohn's*[1] *disease (CD) and Ulcerative colitis (UC)*)
- Incidence
    - ~5 per 100,000 (CD adults and children)
    - ~2 per 100,000 (UC children) (4–6 per 100,000 in adults)
- Prevalence ~200 (adults and children)/100,000 – for both CD and UC
- ~20% of cases occur before the age of 20 years
- Peak age of onset
    - Young adult and older adolescents (~5% of new cases occur in children <5 years)
- M = F
- *Racial variation* – ↑ Caucasian, ↑ Ashkanazi jews, ↓ Japanese, and Chinese
- *Geographical variation* – North > South (Europe and North America)
- ~15% of cases have +ve family history

---

[1]Burrill Bernard Crohn (1884–1983) – American gastroenterologist working at Mount Sinai Hospital, New York.

C. K. Sinha (✉)
Paediatric Surgery Department, King's College Hospital, London, UK

C. K. Sinha and M. Davenport (eds.), *Handbook of Pediatric Surgery*,
DOI: 10.1007/978-1-84882-132-3_4.9, © Springer-Verlag London Limited 2010

4.9.2
Etiology

Multifactorial – but best summarized as "infectious and environmental factors activating the immune system in a genetically predisposed individual."

4.9.3
Pathology

- Can involve all GI tract but commonest site is terminal ileum (~60%).
- Typical endoscopic findings include patchy areas of inflammation separated by normal bowel ("skip lesions"). Intially, aphthous ulcers progress to form linear ulcers, which cross transverse folds to give typical "cobblestone" appearance.
- Histological features include the characteristic (but not pathognomic) lesion of noncaseating granulomata. There is transmural inflammation; mucosa – cryptitis, crypt abscesses, basal plasmacytosis, and crypt ulcers; stromal proliferation and nodular inflammatory changes leading to fibrous strictures.

(N.B. About 10% of the patients have *indeterminate colitis* with features of both CD and UC. On long-term follow-up, these patients develop features of Crohn's in their small bowel.)

4.9.4
Clinical Features

- Abdominal pain, diarrhea, and weight loss/failure to thrive.

Sometimes, patients may present with complications such as

- Small bowel obstruction
- Intra-abdominal abscess – leading to enteric fistula/bowel perforation
- Toxic megacolon (rare in CD but commoner in UC)
- Perianal pathology – e.g., anal fissure (dominant symptom in 5–10%)

CD is also characterized by a variety of extra-intestinal features, involving

- Buccal mucosa – e.g., aphthous ulcers
- Skin – e.g., *erythema nodosum, pyoderma gangrenosum*
- Hepato-biliary – e.g., chronic hepatitis, *sclerosing cholangitis*, gall stones
- Joints – e.g., *ankylosing spondylitis*
- Eye – e.g., iritis, uveitis

Failure to thrive is an important extra-intestinal manifestation in children, which is due to the effect of decreased caloric intake and cytokines produced by the disease process.

Growth failure is an important determining factor for surgical intervention.

4.9.4.1
Differential Diagnosis

Key differential is with UC but other possibilities need to be considered such as infections (e.g., bacterial/viral gastroenteritis, amoebiasis), granulomatous disease (e.g., tuberculosis). Appendicitis may create confusion in diagnosis and in many occasions definitive diagnosis is made at the operating table.

4.9.4.1.1
Investigations

- Laboratory
  - FBC for evidence of anemia caused by iron, vitamin B12, or folic acid deficiency
  - Albumin and prealbumin levels, trace elements (e.g., zinc, selenium, copper) and electrolytes (e.g., calcium and magnesium) levels for evidence of malnutrition
  - Prothrombin times and vitamin A and vitamin D levels due to fat malabsorption
  - C-reactive protein levels – degree of inflammation
  - Liver function tests – evidence of sclerosing cholangitis, etc.
  - Stool cultures – exclude infective diarrhea
  - ASCA (anti–*Saccharomyces cerevisiae* antibodies)
    +ve in 60% cases with CD (cf ~10% in UC)
- *Radiology*
  - *CT scan* (preferable in acute stage). It may show bowel-wall thickening, mesenteric edema, abscesses, and fistulas.
  - *Small-bowel contrast-enhanced studies* may show the disease process (e.g., mucosal fissures, bowel fistulas, strictures, obstructions).
  - *MRI* – gaining in popularity for both the diagnosis and assessment of severity of CD.
- *Endoscopy*
  - Colonoscopy with intubation of the terminal ileum is now the standard diagnostic procedure. It evaluates the extent of disease, strictures, fistulas, and also obtains biopsy material for tissue diagnosis.
  - Upper-gastrointestinal endoscopy should exclude gastroduodenal disease.

4.9.5
Management

The aim of treatment is to control active symptoms and achieve a state of disease remission.

- Medical management of Crohn's disease includes *corticosteroids, 5-aminosalicylates, 6-mercaptopurine, azothioprine, methotrexate,* and *cyclosporine.* In addition, both *metronidazole* and *ciprofloxacin* have a supportive role in disease flares. Most recently, *infliximab* (chimeric monoclonal antibody against TNF-α) has shown significant success in refractory CD.
- Nutritional therapy plays an important role in reversing growth retardation and nutritional deficiencies.

Surgery in Crohn's cannot cure the disease – in contrast to UC.

Indications for Surgery

- Failure of medical therapy.
- Growth retardation.
- Complications such as strictures, bowel obstruction, perforation, perianal abscess and fistula, intra-abdominal abscess, bowel fistula, and rarely megacolon.

4.9.5.1
Surgical Aim and Options

The surgical procedures performed for CD are dictated by the site of involvement and complications.

- *Localized terminal ileal disease* (better prognosis than when associated with colonic disease).
  - *Ileocecectomy with primary anastomosis* is indicated for local perforation with abscess, persistent fistula, or obstructive symptoms secondary to refractory inflammation. Although localized perforation and abscess formation may initially be managed with intravenous antibiotics and bowel rest, ileocecal resection is often required for complete resolution of terminal ileal disease. Resection margins should

---

[2]Walter Heineke (1834–1901) – German surgeon, describing this technique in context of a pyloroplasty.
[3]Jan Mikulicz-Radecki (1850–1905) – Polish surgeon.

extend to only just beyond the area of gross disease – resection to microscopically clear margins offers no protection against recurrence.

- *Multisegment disease and stricture formation.* In the past, multiple strictures were managed with multiple intestinal resections, which often led to short-bowel syndrome. Current standard of care limits resection to patients with perforation, fistula formation, areas of severe bowel-wall thickening, and long-segment areas of disease.

  - *Strictureplasty* is a safe and effective surgical alternative and has become the operation of choice. Strictures of up to 10 cm in length may be treated with a Heineke[2]–Mikulicz[3] strictureplasty, while involved segments up to 30 cm may be treated with a Finney[4] side-to-side anastomosis. Strictureplasty is recommended for all strictures in which the inner diameter is ≤2 cm but may also be beneficial when the lumen is less compromised.

- *Colorectal disease*

  - *Total colectomy with ileorectal anastomosis* is probably the best option where there is rectal sparing (normal sphincter function and distensibility) and the terminal ileum is not involved. Partial colectomy is no longer recommended as it has been shown to have a recurrence rate of up to 60% at 5 years.[1] Fibrosis in the area of the rectal canal is a known complication of Crohn's colitis, and may require the child to undergo a permanent diverting ostomy.

  - *Total colectomy with ileostomy and Hartmann's[5] pouch* as the first-stage procedure, (later ileorectal anastomosis) if associated with significant perianal disease but the rectum appears normal.

  - *Total proctocolectomy with permanent ileostomy* – now reserved for children with severe, refractory rectal, or perianal CD, failed ileorectal anastomosis, or carcinoma.

(NB Total proctocolectomy with ileoanal pouch anastomosis is currently not recommended in patients with CD as over half of these patients will require their pouch to be excised or defunctionalized.[2])

- *Severe perianal disease* – while many will respond to medical therapy, surgery is often required.
- Small, superficial abscesses respond well to incision and packing.
- Large abscesses involving the deeper ischiorectal space often require fluoroscopically guided placement of bulky drains. These drains are left in place for several weeks to create controlled sinus tracts, which can then be treated with silver nitrate or fibrin glue. Recent reports have documented some success in using local injection of infliximab into perianal fistulae, but this strategy remains experimental.

---

[4]John Miller Turpin Finney (1863–1942) – American surgeon at Johns Hopkins, Hospital, Baltimore.

[5]Henri Hartmann (1860–1952) – Chief of Surgery at Hotel Dieu, Paris, France.

- *Fistula-in-ano*.
- Fistulotomy and fistulectomy, if below the sphincters.
- Seton suture or debridement of the tract followed by instillation of silver nitrate or fibrin glue if suprasphincteric.

(Recent reports have demonstrated that the use of Surgisis plugs (bioabsorbable xenograft made of lyophilized porcine intestinal mucosa) is successful in closing deep anorectal fistulae in 80% of Crohn's patients.)

- *Anal fissures* are best managed with medical therapy as fissurectomy is complicated by poor wound healing, loss of sphincteric control, and a high rate of recurrence. Severe fissures may be managed medically with dietary restriction and TPN or surgically by proximal diversion with an end colostomy.
- *Lateral internal sphincterotomy* is reserved for the rare patient with a classic posterior midline fissure and documented anal sphincter hypertonia on manometry.

Less severe perianal CD may be manifested by anal strictures and skin tags. The skin tags may become swollen and inflamed in the setting of diarrhea, but are best managed with sitz baths and control of the inciting diarrhea. Excision of skin tags is not recommended due to poor wound healing. Strictures are generally asymptomatic but on occasion lead to urgency and tenesmus. Short symptomatic strictures may be gently dilated either in the operating room or at home using Hegar dilators. Long strictures or those that do not respond to dilatation are usually associated with more aggressive disease that often leads to diversion or proctocolectomy.

4.9.6
Outcome

Short-term complications include:

- Wound infection – e.g., ~10% post open ileocecectomy, ↓ if laparoscopic-assisted procedure.
- Anastomotic leak – e.g., ~10% poststrictureplasty, ~3% post-IR anastomosis, with sepsis, recurrent stenosis, fistula formation, etc.
- Small bowel obstruction (~8% in laparoscopic ileocectomy). ↑ Risk if a re-operation.
- Postoperative hemorrhage – from the anastomosis.
- Urinary tract infection.

Long-term complications:

- Recurrence
- possible long-term risk in male patients – retrograde ejaculation and impotence.

Table 4.9.1 Long-term recurrence rate in Crohn's disease

	Recurrence rate		Notes
Ileocecectomy	5y	60% (children)	
	5y	25% (adults)	
Stricturoplasty	5y	35–50%	↑ Risk if young age at first operation
Proctocolectomy	10y	20%	
Perianal procedures	2y	50%	Transsphincteric and ischiorectal fistulae Poorest outcome, only ~30% will see disease resolution, even if diversion/resection used

Perianal disease

Short-term complications of perianal disease are mostly due to persistence or recurrence (table 4.9.1). Initial healing for perianal fistulae occurs in ~80% of patients, but many have recurrence after initial healing. Fecal incontinence following management of transsphincteric fistulae has been documented at <1%, although incontinence of liquid stool or flatus may be slightly higher.

Further Reading

1. Crohn BB, Ginzburg L, Oppenheimer GD (1932) Regional ileitis; a pathologic and clinical entity. J A M A 99:1323–1329
2. Fichera A, McCormack R, Rubin MA et al (2005) Long-term outcome of surgically treated Crohn's colitis: a prospective study. Dis Colon Rectum 48:963–9
3. Brown CJ, Maclean AR, Cohen Z et al (2005) Crohn's disease and indeterminate colitis and the ileal pouch-anal anastomosis: outcomes and patterns of failure. Dis Colon Rectum 48:1542–1549
4. Cintron JR, Park JJ, Orsay CP et al (2000) Repair of fistulas-in-ano using fibrin adhesive: long-term follow-up. Dis Colon Rectum 43:944–999
5. Asteria CR, Ficari F, Bagnoli S et al (2006) Treatment of perianal fistulas in Crohn's disease by local injection of antibody to TNF-alpha accounts for a favourable clinical response in selected cases: a pilot study. Scand J Gastroenterol 41:1064–1072
6. O'Connor L, Champagne BJ, Ferguson MA et al (2006) Efficacy of anal fistula plug in closure of Crohn's anorectal fistulas. Dis Colon Rectum 49:1569–1573
7. Longo WE, Oakley JR, Lavery IC et al (1992) Outcome of ileorectal anastomosis for Crohn's colitis. Dis Colon Rectum 35:1066–1071
8. Williamson PR, Hellinger MD, Larach SW, Ferrara A (1995) Twenty-year review of the surgical management of perianal Crohn's disease. Dis Colon Rectum 38:389–392
9. Michelassi F, Melis M, Rubin M, Hurst RD (2000) Surgical treatment of anorectal complications in Crohn's disease. Surgery 128:597–603

Ulcerative Colitis

4.10

Chandrasen K. Sinha and Arnold G. Coran

- Cases of chronic bloody diarrhea with ulceration were first recognized by (the appropriately named) Soranus of Ephesus in the second century AD.
- In 1875, Samuel Wilks and Walter Moxon, physicians at Guy's Hospital in London, were able to distinguish "idiopathic colitis" cases from the usual cases of *"bloody flux."*

Ulcerative colitis (UC) is a chronic inflammatory disorder of the intestine, which involves rectum and extends proximally in a continuous manner and presents commonly with colicky abdominal pain and bloody diarrhea. The entire colon may be involved in advanced cases (Table 4.10.1).

4.10.1
Pathology

The etiology of UC is not known and a multifactorial pathogenesis has also been postulated.

1. Loss of normal mucosal pattern – broad-based ulcers cause islands of normal mucosa to appear as *pseudopolyps.*
2. Inflammation is limited to mucosa and submucosa. Acute and chronic infiltrate in lamina propria and villous atrophy are present. Granulomas are not found in UC.
3. In severe cases, *toxic megacolon* may develop owing to the involvement of muscularis propria, which leads to damage in the nerve plexus, causing colonic dysmotility, dilation, and eventually gangrene.

C. K. Sinha (✉)
Paediatric Surgery Department, King's College Hospital, London, UK

C. K. Sinha and M. Davenport (eds.), *Handbook of Pediatric Surgery*,
DOI: 10.1007/978-1-84882-132-3_4.10, © Springer-Verlag London Limited 2010

Table 4.10.1 Key differences between Crohn's disease and ulcerative colitis

Features	Ulcerative colitis	Crohn's disease
Site	Colon only involved	Pan-intestinal (ileocecal region most common site)
Pathology	Continuous inflammation extending proximally from rectum	Skip-lesions with intervening normal mucosa
	Inflammation in mucosa and submucosa only	Transmural inflammation
	No granulomas	Noncaseating granulomas
Clinical features	Bleeding is common	Bleeding is uncommon
Complications	Fistulae are rare	Fistulae are common
Investigation	pANCA (anti-neutrophil cytoplasmic antibodies) +ve	ASCA (anti-*Saccharomyces cerevisiae* antibodies) +ve
Surgery	Often curative	Palliative

4.10.2
Clinical Features

- Colicky abdominal pain with bloody diarrhea.
- Systemic complaints (e.g., fatigue, arthritis, failure to gain weight, and delayed puberty) may be seen.
- Fulminant UC – severe diarrhea, pyrexia, abdominal distention, and raised inflammatory markers (more common in children).

Primary sclerosing cholangitis (PSC) is an important extra-intestinal manifestation of UC. About 5% of cases with UC have cholestatic liver disease, and 40% of these patients have PSC. Alternatively, ~75% of cases with PSC have associated inflammatory bowel disease.

Other extra-intestinal manifestations are similar to CD (e.g., *uveitis, pyoderma gangrenosum, erythema nodosum, ankylosing spondylitis*).

4.10.2.1
Investigations

Laboratory work-up is similar to CD. But,

- pANCA (perinuclear antineutrophil cytoplasmic antibodies) assay.
  — +ve in 60–80% of cases with UC. Positivity is also associated with an earlier need for surgery.
- Endoscopy and biopsy (except in the acute presentation with active sepsis).
  — Colonoscopy and multiple biopsies are the diagnostic investigations of choice.

- Radiology (nil specific).
  - *CT scan* may show dilated and thickened colon, and mesenteric inflammatory changes are suggestive of UC (cf. small-bowel thickening is suggestive of CD).
  - *MRI* (popular alternative to CT).
  - Technetium 99m (^{99m}Tc)-labeled white blood cell scan may be used to show the site of inflammation (whether small or large bowel and whether contiguous or noncontigous lesions).

4.10.3
Management

Medical treatment for UC includes 5-aminosalicylate-based anti-inflammatory agents (e.g., *sulfasalazine*) and immunosuppressive agents (e.g., *corticosteroids, azathioprine, 6-mercaptopurine, cyclosporine*). However, many children remain refractory to these medications and require frequent hospitalizations as well as long-term use of steroids. The result is that children with chronic UC may have delayed growth and puberty, cushingoid features, hypertension, cataracts, and osteopenia.

While medical therapy may lead to remission for variable periods of time, it cannot truly be cured without removal of the colon and rectum. Given the long-term problems associated with immunosuppression and steroid therapy in children, surgery should be considered in any child with UC before permanent disability develops.

Indications for Surgery

- Persistent symptoms despite maximal medical therapy.
- Growth retardation.
- Inability to participate in school, sports, or social activities secondary to disease.
- To prevent compromise of final stature by removing the colon prior to closure of the growth plates.
- Emergency surgery is indicated for a small subset of patients with acute, fulminant disease characterized by extensive rectal bleeding, toxic megacolon, or systemic sepsis.
- Risk of cancer.

4.10.3.1
Surgical Aim and Options

The aim of surgery is to remove the entire colon and rectum. The simplest way to do this is a *standard proctocolectomy with end-ileostomy*. However, a permanent stoma may be unacceptable to many children and their families.

Currently, the two most common operations performed are:

- *Total colectomy with rectal mucosectomy and ileoanal pouch procedure (IAPP)*
- *Colectomy with subtotal mucosectomy and stapled ileorectal anastomosis (less popular nowadays)*

Option

- *Ileoanal endorectal pull-through without an ileal reservoir*

In most cases, a temporary diverting ileostomy is added to protect the distal anastomosis.

Advantages of performing an endorectal dissection include minimal disruption of the extrarectal space with a subsequent decreased risk of injury to the sphincter muscle and surrounding deep pelvic nerves. This approach also maintains continence by preservation of the anorectal angle, levator muscle complex, anal sphincters, rectal ampulla, and anorectal sensation.

In acute life-threatening disease, initial emergency surgery consists of *colectomy and end-ileostomy*. This may later be followed by an ileoanal pull-through ± pouch to restore intestinal continuity. This second operation is usually performed with a diverting ileostomy, which would be closed in a third and final procedure.

Recently, there have been two new trends in operative management of UC. One is the use of a double-stapled technique in restorative proctocolectomy. Rather than performing a hand-sewn ileoanal anastomosis, the distal 1.5 cm of rectal mucosa is preserved and utilized for a double-stapled end-to-end anastomosis using the circular stapler. It is a safe technique and comparable with the hand-sewn approach. The second trend is toward the use of laparoscopic or lap-assisted subtotal colectomy. Although operative times may be longer, perioperative clinical outcomes are similar to open subtotal colectomy and cosmesis is improved.

4.10.4
Outcome

4.10.4.1
Short-Term

The complication rate following the IAPP may reach as high as 65%, but the mortality is less than 1%.

- Anastomotic strictures – minimized by serial Hegar dilation (twice/week) for several months. Predisposes to pouch distention and stasis.
- Pouch fistula (5–10%) – to the perianal skin or vagina. These will often require operative intervention, including a protective ostomy as well as a revision of the pull-through.
- Pelvic abscess or sepsis (up to 10%) – usually secondary to anastomotic leak.
- Wound infection (~10%) and incisional hernia (~5%).
- Small-bowel obstruction (~25%).
- Severe incontinence (~5%).
- Pouch hemorrhage (2%).

4.10.4.2
Long-Term

The expectation is that children treated with ileoanal pouches have an average number of about four bowel movements per day. The rate of twice-weekly nocturnal stooling or soiling is about 5% at 6 months.

Up to 45% of patients eventually require reoperation for complications following ileoanal pull-through, and up to 10% experience pouch failure requiring ileostomy with or without pouch excision.

* *Pouchitis*
  — Incidence – up to 50% in patients followed for more than 10 years.
  — Most common in the first few years; episodes are more frequent and severe in children.
  — Characterized by a constellation of symptoms including low-grade fever, lower abdominal pain, diarrhea, bloody stools, and malaise or fatigue. It is hypothesized that stasis of fecal matter within the ileal reservoir leads to bacterial overgrowth and subsequent mucosal inflammation.
  — Children with +ve pANCA serology and preoperative "backwash ileitis" have ↑ risk.

Pouchitis is treated with antibiotics (*ciprofloxacin* and *metronidazole*), *steroid enemas*, and dilatation of any ileoanal strictures. Probiotics (e.g., *lactobacillus spp.*), after acute therapy may reduce recurrent episodes. If recurrent, endoscopy and biopsy need to be performed to exclude Crohn's disease.

(NB pouchitis rarely seen in patients who undergo IAPP for familial polyposis – underlying UC is therefore thought to play an important role in its development).

* *Risk of cancer*
  — Increases at a rate of 1% per year (after 10 years of disease).
  — A long-term, retrospective study from the Cleveland Clinic, USA, found that colorectal cancer developed in ~2% of adolescents with UC.
  — In procedures where any rectal mucosa is left behind, routine surveillance should be established within 8–10 years after initial diagnosis of the disease.
  — Both adenocarcinoma and squamous cell carcinoma occurring in the anorectal epithelium below the ileorectal anastomosis have been reported.
  — Carcinoma of the pouch has been reported, although dysplastic transformation of the ileal pouch mucosa is rare.
  — Patients at highest risk are those with either dysplasia or carcinoma in the resected colon or those with long-standing disease.

(NB: Colectomy and ileoanal anastomosis can also lead to problems with fertility in women.)

Further Reading

1. Robb BW, Gang GI, Hershko DD et al (2003) Restorative proctocolectomy with ileal pouch-anal anastomosis in very young patients with refractory ulcerative colitis. J Pediatr Surg 38:863–867
2. Gionchetti P, Rizzello F, Helwig U et al (2003) Prophylaxis of pouchitis onset with probiotic therapy: a double-blind, placebo-controlled trial. Gastroenterol 124:1202–1209
3. Fonkalsrud EW, Thakur A, Beanes S (2001) Ileoanal pouch procedures in children. J Pediatr Surg 36:1689–1692

Short Bowel Syndrome

4.11

Mark Davenport

> Failure to maintain normal nutrition, body weight and internal physiology without external parenteral nutritional support.

The major consideration in this entity is how much (small) bowel is left and is it sufficient to meet the nutritional needs of the body. Residual length is important but there is no standard for its measurement and particularly in the extreme preterm it can mean little.

4.11.1
Normal Intestinal Length

Few detailed studies

- Term 250–300 cm (stretched – antimesenteric)
- Adult ~600 cm

Problems should be anticipated in term infants IF

(i)   ≤100 cms – invariable need for short-term PN but reconstruction unlikely to be needed.
(ii) <75 cms – invariable need for long-term PN ± reconstruction surgery. Possible bowel/liver transplantion.
(iii) <25 cms – invariable need for long-term PN ± reconstruction ± bowel/liver transplantation.

M. Davenport
Paediatric Surgery Department, Kings College Hospital, London, UK

C. K. Sinha and M. Davenport (eds.), *Handbook of Pediatric Surgery*,
DOI: 10.1007/978-1-84882-132-3_4.11, © Springer-Verlag London Limited 2010

4.11.2
Causes (Examples)

- Intestinal atresia, NEC, midgut volvulus, gastroschisis.
- Intestinal dysmotility syndromes – chronic pseudoobstruction.
- Microvillus inclusion disease (Davidson's[1] disease) – profuse watery diarrhea from neonatal period.
- Crohn's disease (older children) and trauma (older children).

4.11.2.1
Factors in Intestinal Failure

- Residual bowel length.
- Intact ileo-cecal valve (by implication preservation of at least the right colon).
- Functioning intestinal continuity.
- Degree of cholestasis.
- Age at the time of resection – premature infants have proportionally more growth of the remaining intestine.
- Type of bowel remaining – ileum adapts better than jejunum.
- Effective motility and integrity of the remaining small bowel.

Gut adaptation is the body's innate response to a deficit in the enterocyte mass and may last up to 18–24 months. It is controlled by complex network of GI hormones (e.g., growth hormone) and cytokines (GLP-2, EGF, HGF, IL-11). Improvements in gut function could be anticipated owing to an increase in surface area (lengthening villi, deepening crypts) and intestinal elongation.

4.11.3
Management

This can be divided into three elements

- *Provision of safe parenteral nutrition*
- *Medical techniques to improve gut adaptation*
- *Surgical techniques to promote gut function*

---

[1]Davidson GP, Cutz E, Hamilton JR, Gall DG (1978) Familial enteropathy: a syndrome of protracted diarrhea from birth, failure to thrive, and hypoplastic villus atrophy. *Gastroenterology* 75:783–790

4.11.3.1
Medical

1. Enterocyte stimulation
   - Glutamine acts as enterocyte fuel
   - Short-chain triglycerides
   - Pectin
2. Peristalysis – ↑transit time
   - Loperamide (1–2 mg TDS, in children)
3. Bind bile-salts (cause of secretory diarrhea)
4. Cholestyramine
5. Suppress bacterial overgrowth
   - Enteral antibiotics (e.g., cyclical neomycin/metronidazole)
   - Octreotide
6. Hyperacidity
   - E.g., ranitidine, proton-pump inhibitors

Parenteral Nutrition-Associated Cholestasis (PNAC)

This, together with sepsis, is the usual cause of mortality, although the actual mechanism is obscure. Incidence is much higher in infants and children on long-term PN than adults, exacerbated by recurrent line sepsis, overprovision, and possibly type of lipid solutions. Treatment options have included ursodeoxycholic acid and cholecystokinin, but most recent (and encouraging) progress has been with substituting usual soy-bean-derived lipid emulsions with those derived from fish oil (e.g., Omegaven®).

4.11.4
Surgery

The aim of surgery is to maximize the potential of the native bowel and this is best achieved by creation of an *intestinal tube capable of effective prograde peristalsis.*

- *Restore intestinal continuity*
  - Early closure of stomas
  - Refeed intestinal content into distal limb
  - Maintains mucosal integrity
  - ↑ Nutrient absorption (by colon and bacterial fermentation of CHO)
- *Improve native bowel propulsive efficiency*
  - Tapering enteroplasty
  - Imbrication
  - Bianchi lengthening (Fig. 4.11.1a)
  - STEP (Fig. 4.11.1b)

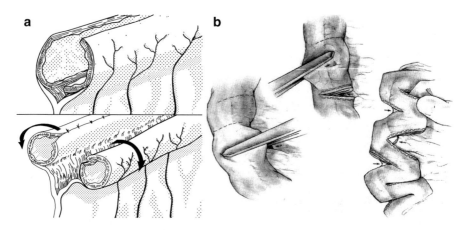

Fig. 4.11.1 (a) Bianchi bowel lengthening. (b) Serial transverse enteroplasty (STEP) procedure. (Reprinted with permission from Kim et al (2003) Serial transverse enteroplasty (STEP): a novel bowel lengthening procedure. J Pediatr Surg 38(3):425–429.)

4.11.4.1
Bianchi[2] Longitudinal Intestinal Lengthening

The typical indication is a nonpropulsive *dilated* proximal segment (e.g. jejunal atresia).

1. Working from the most distal part of jejunum – identify inverted "triangle of dissection," where base is the mesenteric border of intestine and apex is the point where end-vessels arise from mesenteric arcades. Usually, they alternate to right and left side. Separate the vessels and divide the mesenteric bowel. Divide the antimesenteric bowel and repeat in about 5–10 cm lengths.
2. Continue proximally until a point is reached where there is no longer enough bowel dilatation.
3. Tubularize – continuous longitudinal suturing almost buried in mesentery.
4. Restore continuity – ensure *prograde tube orientation* – a mesenteric window will be required.

4.11.4.2
Serial Transverse Enteroplasty

The aims of both Bianchi and STEP are to reduce luminal diameter and increase luminal length, thus increasing effective propulsion and (hopefully) improving nutritional absorption. Again, dilated bowel is mandatory.

---

[2]Adrian Bianchi – Malteste surgeon, working in Manchester, UK. Described technique in pig model, before applying to infants.

1. The stapler is applied sequentially from the right and then left.
2. Small mesenteric windows are created to allow the stapler to cross the midline.
3. Oversew potential leak-points at the apex of staples.

(NB: Neither procedures increase mucosal surface area.)

Further Reading

1. Andorsky DJ, Lund DP, Lillehei CW et al (2001) Nutritional and other postoperative management of neonates with short bowel syndrome correlates with clinical outcomes. J Pediatr 139:27–33
2. Bianchi A (2007) Autologous gastrointestinal reconstruction for short bowel syndrome. Br J Hosp Med (Lond) 68:24–27
3. Modi BP, Ching YA, Langer M, Donovan K, Fauza DO, Kim HB, Jaksic T, Nurko S (2009) Preservation of intestinal motility after the serial transverse enteroplasty procedure in a large animal model of short bowel syndrome. Pediatr Surg Int 44:229–235
4. Wales PW, de Silva N, Langer JC, Fecteau A (2007) Intermediate outcomes after serial transverse enteroplasty in children with short bowel syndrome. J Pediatr Surg 42:1804–1810
5. Gura KM, Lee S, Valim C et al (2008) Safety and efficacy of a fish-oil-based fat emulsion in the treatment of parenteral nutrition-associated liver disease. Pediatrics 121:e678–e686

Intestinal Transplantation

4.12

Alastair J. W. Millar and Girish Gupte

4.12.1
Intestinal Failure

4.12.1.1
Incidence

- 1–2 per million population (children)

4.12.1.2
Etiology

Causes of intestinal failure can be subdivided into three categories: short bowel syndrome, disorders of bowel motility, and primary mucosal disease (Table 4.12.1).

4.12.1.3
Primary Motility Disorders

Chronic intestinal pseudo-obstruction (CIP) is a heterogeneous group of rare disorders, presenting with symptoms and signs of intestinal obstruction, but without a mechanical basis. They result from a variety of abnormalities in the enteric nervous system or musculature and can affect variable segments of the GI tract, sometimes with other hollow viscera involved, such as the bladder. Most patients present in infancy. The diagnosis is usually by exclusion. Exploratory laparotomy should be avoided unless there is clear evidence of mechanical obstruction.

A. J. W. Millar (✉)
University of Cape Town Health Sciences, Red Cross War Memorial Children's Hospital,
Cape Town, South Africa

C. K. Sinha and M. Davenport (eds.), *Handbook of Pediatric Surgery*,
DOI: 10.1007/978-1-84882-132-3_4.12, © Springer-Verlag London Limited 2010

Table 4.12.1   Causes of intestinal failure

Short bowel syndrome	*Neonatal period* Gastroschisis Necrotizing enterocolitis (NEC) Small bowel atresia Malrotation with volvulus Total intestinal aganglionosis	*Older children* Crohn's disease Mesenteric infarction Radiation enteritis Tumors Trauma
Motility disorders	Hirschprung's disease Hollow visceral myopathy Neuronal intestinal dysplasia Megacystis-Microcolon-Hypoperistalsis syndrome Abnormalities of interstitial cells of Cajal Chronic intestinal Pseudo - obstruction	
Mucosal disorders	*Primary epithelial abnormalities* Microvillous inclusion disease Tufting enteropathy (primary epithelial dysplasia) Congenital disorders of glycosylation	*Immune mediated* Underlying immunodeficiency states, e.g., SCID, pan-hypo-gammaglobulinemia Autoimmune enteropathy

Children with CIP will need gastrostomy, gastro-jejunal tube, or a jejunostomy for advancing low-fiber, low-lactose, low-residue, and low-fat feeds. Indicators of poor prognosis are the onset of symptoms before 1 year of age; involvement of the urinary tract; midgut malrotation or a myopathic histology. The prognosis of children with CIP has improved substantially over recent years with the advent of home PN and meticulous care of central venous catheters.

4.12.1.4
Primary Mucosal Disorders

Recent advances in molecular biology and immunology have led to a better understanding of the enteropathies associated with intractable diarrhea. *Microvillous inclusion disease*, a probable disturbance in the apical targeting mechanism for microvilli, *tufting enteropathy*, and *primary epithelial dysplasia* usually present in the first few months of life as intractable diarrhea.

4.12.1.5
Isolated Liver Transplantation (LT) in Children with SBS

Some infants and young children with SBS and adequate length of bowel who fail to achieve maximal adaptation because of early-onset end-stage liver disease may benefit from LT.

Current practice suggests that LT should be offered to children who show

1. ≥50% of daily requirements enterally
2. Weight gain
3. ≥30 cm residual small bowel and IC valve or ≥70 cm residual bowel alone

Following LT, weaning from PN to full enteral feeds may take from several months to years.

4.12.2
Intestinal Transplantation

Intestinal transplantation (IT) has evolved from an experimental procedure in the late-1980s to a life-saving option for children who develop major complications of intestinal failure.

4.12.2.1
Indications and Contraindications

- Indications are irreversible intestinal failure and one of the following:

1. Impaired venous access (reduced to two suitable veins for placement of feeding catheters)
2. Progressive liver disease with coagulopathy, ascites, and encephalopathy
3. Life-threatening episodes of catheter sepsis

Contra-indications Can Be Further Subdivided into

Absolute

1. Profound neurologic disabilities
2. Life-threatening and other irreversible disease not related to the digestive system
3. Nonresectable malignancies

Relative contraindications are:
Severe congenital or acquired immunologic deficiencies,
multisystem autoimmune diseases
insufficient vascular patency to guarantee vascular access for up to 6 months after transplantation
and chronic lung disease of prematurity.

4.12.2.2
Types of Operation (Fig. 4.12.1)

Complete multivisceral allograft specimen consists of the

- Liver and biliary system with duodenum and pancreas
- Intestine up to the mid-transverse colon (supplied by the celiac axis and the SMA)

The *severity of the liver disease* determines the organs to be transplanted, so that patients with mild liver disease (no evidence of portal hypertension, mild hepatic fibrosis on liver biopsy) can be offered an isolated intestinal, or a modified multivisceral graft, including stomach if dysmotility of the foregut is a prominent clinical problem. In patients with moderate to severe liver disease, a liver and small bowel (±right colon) transplant is recommended.

The precise method of implantation of the organs can be varied, but the preferred technique is a *composite graft* where the liver and intestine with bile ducts, duodenum, and head of pancreas can be implanted en bloc with minimal disruption to the vascular and other structures connecting the organs. Organs can be retrieved from the donor, separated, and implanted individually, which is known as *noncomposite combined liver and small bowel transplantation*. Venous drainage of an isolated intestinal graft may be either into the portal vein or inferior vena cava of the recipient (no documented adverse effects). Indeed, portal venous drainage is contra-indicated if there is liver fibrosis and portal hypertension. *Multivisceral transplantation* is the term applied to any intestinal transplant, in which more than the liver and small bowel are transplanted (usually including the whole pancreas) and is offered to patients with extensive disease, e.g., motility disorders or desmoid tumor.

Problem: large adult donors for small children – En bloc graft reduction using liver and small bowel with excision of right lobe liver and mid-section of small bowel. Tissue expanders may be required to allow for skin cover after transplant where the abdominal domain is compromised.

Living-related ITx – beneficial in monozygotic twins, but does not seem to confer any immunologic benefit in other situations.

4.12.2.3
Surgical Technique

Blood group identical and size-matched donor (blood group compatible and size mismatch of up to 3:1 acceptable) is required. Tissue expansion pretransplant, graft size reduction, staged abdominal closure, and prosthetic replacement of the abdominal wall have been effective.

- *Isolated intestine graft* (absence of liver disease and portal hypertension in the recipient): only the small bowel on its vascular pedicle is procured as part of a multiorgan procurement.
  - Recipient upper jejunum anastomosed end-to-end with the donor jejunum.

– Distal graft is joined to distal recipient bowel with more proximal venting and stoma is brought out as access for biopsy and for stoma effluent monitoring – or end stoma if recipient residual bowel is unusable. The stoma may be closed months to years later when rejection is controlled.

- *Combined liver and intestinal transplant*
  – Portal venous drainage of the residual foregut is diverted first with a porta-caval shunt prior to the removal of residual diseased bowel and hepatectomy. Some centers have advocated a total abdominal exenteration including most of the foregut, pancreas, spleen, and all of the residual gut to increase the abdominal domain and facilitate replacement by a composite liver and intestinal graft.

Immunosuppressant protocols include tacrolimus, steroids, mycophenylate mofetil (MMF), an anti-CD 25 monoclonal antibody (IL2 receptor antagonist), or antilymphocyte globulin. Maintenance of immune suppression may include rapamycin, which is not toxic to the kidneys. Rejection episodes, suspected by fever, malaise, gut dysfunction, and biopsy findings of cellular infiltrate and apoptotic bodies on histology are treated in the same way as for other solid organ transplants with steroid bolus doses and increased immune suppression. The level of immune suppression required to prevent rejection is greater than that with other solid organ transplants and the tendency for rejection to occur persists for longer time after transplantation. It is important to achieve a balance between adequate immune suppression and maintenance of graft health and avoidance of excessive recipient immune compromise resulting in debilitating opportunistic bacterial, fungal, and viral infections.

Waiting times usually >3 months with expected >50% mortality for those ≤10 kg weight.

4.12.3
Outcome

Complications following ITx include

- Moderate to severe acute rejection.
- Opportunistic infections (cytomegalovirus and Epstein–Barr virus infections).
- Graft ischemia, intestinal perforations, intestinal obstruction, biliary tract dilatation, and abdominal compartment syndrome.

The incidence and severity of rejection has improved considerably after the advent of IL2 blockers and other immunosuppression strategies. An appropriate CMV prophylaxis regimen (ganciclovir) and Epstein–Barr virus (EBV) PCR monitoring techniques for the prevention of quasi-neoplastic posttransplant lymphoproliferative disease (PTLD) has reduced the incidence of these dreaded complications. Advances in surgical techniques, particularly the avoidance of abdominal compartment hypertension along with the use of newer

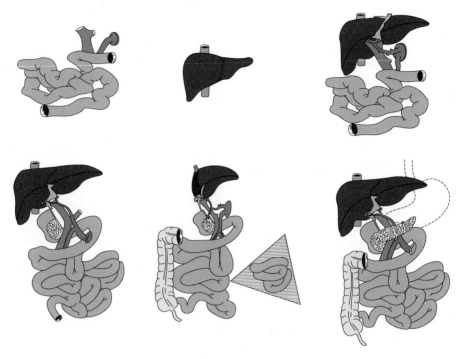

Fig. 4.12.1 Types of grafts for intestinal failure: Isolated intestine, Isolated liver for short bowel syndrome, composite liver and intestine, multivisceral grafts including pancreas and stomach and reduced size composite grafts

immunosuppressive regimens, have resulted in improved outcomes with increased optimism that it offers a real opportunity for cure (Fig. 4.12.1).

Quality of life is equivalent to healthy children of the same age, although their parents remain more anxious than the parents of healthy children. The catch-up growth seen in children following LT has not been demonstrated in children with IT. This is probably related to the severity of the illness at the time of presentation and the use of high-intensity immunosuppression including the use of long-term steroids.

Most recipients achieve enteral autonomy by the first month post transplantation. Those transplanted for dysmotility syndromes, who have never learnt to enjoy eating, may require prolonged support to establish a normal feeding pattern.

Retransplantation has a much poorer outcome, especially if the first graft failed because of rejection. However, there are now a significant number of children who have lived for prolonged periods with normal graft function.

- Current one-year survival is >80%.

- Three- and five-year survivals are 60% and 40%, respectively – due to the more delicate balance required in keeping the graft healthy and free of rejection, but at the same time avoiding over immune suppression with all its consequences.

Further Reading

1. Gupte GL, Beath SV, Kelly DA et al (2006) Current issues in the management of intestinal failure. Arch Dis Child 91:259–264
2. Millar AJ, Gupte GL (2007) Small bowel transplantation in children. Br J Hosp Med (Lond) 68:19–23
3. Sauvat F, Fusaro F (2008) Lacaille F et al Is intestinal transplantation the future of children with definitive intestinal insufficiency? Eur J Pediatr Surg 18:368–371
4. Reyes JD (2006) Intestinal Transplantation. Seminars in Pediatric Surgery 15(3):228 - 234
5. Intestinal Failure: Diagnosis, Management and Transplantation. Eds. Langnas AN, Goulet O, Quigley EMM, Tappenden KE (2008) Blackwell Publishing

Vascular Malformations

4.13

R. V. Patel and J. I. Curry

It has been estimated that up to 60% of all vascular anomalies are misdiagnosed.

Congenital vascular anomalies is an all-inclusive term for vascular malformations, vascular tumors, and other congenital vascular defects.

There are two basic types (Table 4.13.1).

- *Hemangiomas* have plump endothelia, increased mast cells, and multilaminated basement membranes and are superficial, deep or combined and may be proliferating or involuting.
- *Vascular malformations* have flat endothelia, normal mast cell numbers, and a thin basement membrane and may be capillary, venous, arterial, lymphatic, or a combination of these.

4.13.1
Pathology

Infantile hemangiomas are not inherited.
1. Mutation in a primitive stem cell responsible for developing blood vessels.
2. Hemangioma is a model of pure, unopposed angiogenesis with common expression of immunohistochemical markers including *glut-1, Fcy RII, Lewis Y antigen*, etc.
3. Possible derivation from or sharing a common precursor with placenta.
4. Angiogenic peptides.
   (a) Proliferating phase – expression of vascular endothelial growth factor (VEGF), basic fibroblast growth factor (bFGF) and type IV collagenase are
   (b) Involution phase – tissue inhibitor of metalloproteinases (TIMP-I) and mast cell secreted modulators.

Vascular malformations are usually sporadic but can also be inherited in a family as an autosomal dominant trait. They are a manifestation of many different genetic syndromes

R.V. Patel
Paediatric Surgery Department, Great Ormond Street Children's Hospital, London, UK

C. K. Sinha and M. Davenport (eds.), *Handbook of Pediatric Surgery*,
DOI: 10.1007/978-1-84882-132-3_4.13, © Springer-Verlag London Limited 2010

Table 4.13.1 Biological classification

Hemangiomas Tumors with Proliferation	Vascular Malformations Developmental errors
Common infantile hemangiomas Rapidly involuting congenital hemangiomas (RICH) Noninvoluting congenital hemangiomas (NICH) Kaposiform hemangioendothelioma (KHE) Tufted angiomas Intramuscular hemangiomas (rare)	*High-Flow Lesions* Arteriovenous malformations (AVM) Arteriovenous fistulas (AVF) *Low-Flow Lesions* Capillary malformations (CM) – port wine stain Venous malformations (VM) - cavernous lesion Lymphatic malformations (LM) Lymphatic-venous malformations (LVM)
Combined rare syndromes	
Kasabach-Merritt syndrome – see Sect. 4.13.2.1 *Diffuse neonatal hemangiomatosis* Multiple, small, cutaneous lesions, dome shaped, uniform in size, may be associated with visceral lesions, liver, GI, CNS. May be asymptomatic, high-output cardiac failure, hemorrhage, obstructive jaundice, coagulopathy, involution of cutaneous and visceral lesions by age 2 years, US or MRI studies are indicated. Treat symptomatic patients *PHACE(S) syndrome*: *P*osterior fossa CNS malformations (Dandy-Walker), *H*emangioma, *A*rterial anomalies, *C*ardiac anomalies, *E*ye anomalies and (*S*ternal defects), lumbosacral lesions, spinal anomalies, GU anomalies	*Klippel-trenaunay syndrome (KTS)* – see Sect. 4.13.2.2 *Parkes-Weber Syndrome (PWS)* – see Sect. 4.13.2.3 *Sturge-Weber syndrome (SWS)* – see Sect. 4.13.2.4 *Proteus syndrome*: PWS with partial gigantism, macrocephaly, epidermal nevi *Maffucci's syndrome*: venous malformations, enchondromas – distal extremities *Blue-Rubber Bleb Nevus syndrome*: venous malformations of skin and GI tract – compressible, painful lesions – GI hemorrhage is common cause of death
Rare Lesions: *Sinus pericranii* *Glomovenous malformation* *Bannayan riley ruvalcaba syndrome* *CMTC*-cutis marmorata telangiectatica congenita-marbled (cutis marmorata) patches of skin caused by widened (dilated) surface blood vessels (livedo reticularis telangiectases) *Multifocal lymphangioendotheliomatosis* with thrombocytopenia *Hyperkeratotic cutaneous capillary-venous malformation*	*Gorham's syndrome* – venous and lymphatic malformations involving skin and skeleton-osteolytic bone disease *Bannayan-Zonana syndrome*: subcutaneous/ visceral venous malformation, lipomas, and macrocephaly *Cobb syndrome*: Spinal cord vascular birthmarks or lesions – venous malformations of spinal cord, truncal PWS *Wyburn-Mason syndrome*: retinal and CNS AVM, facial PWS *Riley-Smith syndrome*: cutaneous venous malformation, macrocephaly

that have a variety of inheritance patterns and chances for reoccurrence, depending on the specific syndrome present.

4.13.2
Specific Examples

4.13.2.1
Kasabach-Merritt Syndrome

Characterized by the combination of a rapidly growing vascular tumor, thrombocytopenia, microangiopathic hemolytic anemia and a consumptive coagulopathy. The coagulopathy results from platelets and other clotting factors from the blood being "used up" within the tumor. Seen in extremties and in some viscera (e.g., liver) There is a high mortality rate in untreated cases.

Treatment: surgical excision, interferon, systemic corticosteroids.

4.13.2.2
Klippel-Trenaunay Syndrome (KTS)

Characterized by soft tissue hypertrophy and bony overgrowth of extremity (usually single and lower limb). Overgrowth not present at birth and significant limb length discrepancy possible later with prominent hypertrophy of foot and toes.

No CNS or visceral anomalies,

Treatment: premature epiphyseal closure of longer leg. Surgical debulking not usually feasible.

4.13.2.3
Parkes-Weber Syndrome (PWS)

Similar to KTS except that an arteriovenous malformation (AVM) which occurs in association with a cutaneous capillary malformation and skeletal or soft tissue hypertrophy.

4.13.2.4
Sturge-Weber Syndrome (SWS)

Facial port wine stain in region of trigeminal cranial nerve.

V1 lesions – may cause of seizures, mental retardation. Look for "railroad track" calcifications and eye lesions (ipsilateral choroidal angiomatosis, glaucoma can be seen with V2 lesions involving eyelid).

4.13.3
Clinical Features

Vascular anomalies manifest with very wide clinical spectrum of lesions ranging form small skin discoloration to very large life-threatening conditions (Table 4.13.2).

4.13.3.1
Investigations

Most vascular anomalies can be diagnosed clinically without biopsy but imaging studies are required for the assessment of the lesion:

Table 4.13.2 Summary of clinical features

Criteria	Hemangioma	Vascular malformations
Age, Sex	Only occurs in infants, F:M 5:1	All ages, both sexes
Incidence	Most common benign tumor of infancy of proliferative endothelium	Result of vascular morphogenesis of capillary, venous, arterial, lymphatic channels or combination thereof
Appearance	Variety – raised, flat, smooth, bosselated, superficial, deep-blue subcutaneous	Most thin and deep, diffuse, focal or fruit-like appearance
Age of onset	Not visible at birth, appear at 1–2 weeks, More common in preterm and low birth weight, more in whites	Usually visible and always present at birth, appear suddenly after an illness, trauma/times of hormonal changes
Growth	Rapid for 0–9 months, stop growing between 6 and 18 months	Most grow slowly after birth or sudden onset and slow/intermittent growth
Involution	Almost all, slow may take up to 10 years, often with a cosmetic deformity	Essentially none, usually grow with individual with growth spurts
Lesions	80% solitary, 20% multiple	Can be in brain, liver, intestines, spine, stomach, or organs
	80% in head and neck	
	Outside/inside body-e.g., brain, liver, intestine	
Complications	Ulceration, infection, bleeding	Bleeding, bony distortion, hypertrophy
Characteristics	Stay same when sick, feels spongy, warm, compressible, rapid refill, pulsatile, bruit	Lymphatic swell/shrink with respiratory illness. Venous fill when dependent, arteriovenous have pulse when pressed. Transilluminate
Intervention timing	Not necessary in majority, Early intervention in complicated cases	Early intervention recommended to minimize extent of surgery
Prognosis	Generally good	Variable depends on type

Table 4.13.3   Multimodal therapy for common vascular lesions

Criteria	Hemangioma	Vascular malformations
Steroid therapy	Systemic/intralesional ↑ regression in 33% Stabilization in 33% No response in 33%	Responses, at best, are limited to occasional case reports
Angiogenesis inhibitor therapy (α-interferon)	Induces involution in almost all, but reserved for lesions that pose threat to life, vital functions or tissue due to its serious potential toxicity in infants.	Essentially no response
Laser therapy	Some respond to laser	Some respond to laser
Sclerotherapy	Not indicated	Intralesional for venous/lymphatic lesions
Embolization	In complicated large lesions, internal	For arterial malformations
Surgical therapy	For residual lesion, complications	Excision, contouring or debulking

1. *Laboratory*: CBC, Hb, Platelets, CRP, Coagulation profile, genetic studies
2. *Imaging*
   (a) *US and Doppler-flow* – best initially.
   (b) *MRI* – confirms the suspected diagnosis and evaluates the extent of the lesion. Also plays a major role in decision making (surgery vs. embolization/sclerotherapy etc).
   (c) *MRA and MRV*: supply additional information on the rate of flow of the vascular anomaly lesion.
   (d) *CT and plain radiography* – phleboliths, calcification, limited role. Some multidetector CT scanners may be used for vascular imaging (CT angiography) in selected patients, particularly in patients with high-flow vascular lesions (AVM, hemangioma, arteriovenous fistula).
   (e) *Angiography*: The most invasive technique is used in association with therapeutic superselective embolization. Venous angiography (phlebography) still has a place in the assessment and management of certain venous malformations.
3. *Biopsy* – rarely indicated but if malignancy cannot be excluded e.g., infantile fibrosarcoma, teratoma, siloblastoma, plexiform neurofibromatosis, etc.

4.13.4
Complications

- Alarming hemangioma involving vital/important structures: eye, larynx, ear, distal extremities.

- DIC and coagulopathy with platelet trapping can occur (Kasabach-Merritt syndrome).
- Cosmetically sensitive regions: nose, lip, ear, large truncal.
- Minor complications include bleeding, infection, ulceration, calcification (microthrombia), thrombosis with rapidly growing lesions.

4.13.5
Management (Table 4.13.3)

Hemangiomas – depends upon their size, location, and severity.

- *Conservative treatment* – usually recommended for small, noninvasive hemangiomas, since they will involute on their own. However, hemangioma that causes bleeding problems, feeding or breathing difficulties, growth disturbances or sensory impairment may require multimodality treatment.
- *Medical Treatment.*
- *Steroid therapy* – topical, intralesional triamcinolone or systemic oral steroids i.e., prednisolone 3, 2.5, 1.2, 0.6, 0.3 mg/kg from week 1 to 5 and may be repeated up to 6–12 months and rebound is well known (Table 4.13.4).
- *Antiangiogenic drugs and immunomodulation* in selected cases.
- *Laser therapy*: CT/Fluoroscopy guided: Different lasers can be used for treatment.
  - Nd:YAG laser photocoagulation – particularly effective because of its deep penetration into tissue.
- *Interventional radiology* – embolization of the blood vessels in internal lesions.
- *Surgical removal* – Large and/or life-threatening lesions after evaluation by a multidisciplinary team of specialists.

Vascular malformations – depends upon the type of the malformation. Each type is treated differently. Most often, a combination of these various treatments is used for effective management of the lesion.

Treatment options include:

- *Laser surgery*: usually effective for capillary malformations or port wine stains.
- *Sclerotherapy* – direct injection of a sclerosing solution (e.g., ethanol, sodium tetradecyl sulfate (Sotradesol®)), doxycycline and OK 432.
- *Embolization*: abnormal vessels that are doing more harm than good are closed off with various substances (e.g., alcohol, glue and coil).

Surgical removal of the lesion: for cosmetic reasons /functional or development of complications.

Table 4.13.4 Typical Steroid schedule

Week 1	Week 2	Week 3	Week 4	Week 5
3 mg/kg	2.5 mg/kg	1.2 mg/kg	0.6 mg/kg	0.3 mg/kg

Further Reading

1. http://www.birthmark.org/hemangiomas.php
2. Bielenberg DR, Bucana CD, Sanchez R et al (1999) Progressive growth of infantile cutaneous hemangiomas is directly correlated with hyperplasia and angiogenesis of adjacent epidermis and inversely correlated with expression of the endogenous angiogenesis inhibitor, IFN-beta. Int J Oncol 14:401–408
3. Blei F, Walter J, Orlow SJ, Marchuk DA (1998) Familial segregation of hemangiomas and vascular malformations as an autosomal dominant trait. Arch Dermatol 134:718–722
4. Mulliken J, Glowacki J (1982) Hemangiomas and vascular malformations in infants and children: a classification based on endothelial characteristics. Plast Reconstr Surg 69:412–420
5. National Organization of Vascular Anomalies (NOVA): Hemangioma and vascular malformation: advocacy and support. [www.novanews.org, 11 July 2008]

Inguinal Hernias and Hydroceles

4.14

V. Scott, Mark Davenport, and Ross M. Fisher

A hernia may be defined as a protrusion of a portion or whole of an organ or tissue, through an abnormal opening.

4.14.1
Groin Hernia

Three types

- Inguinal
  - Indirect (only common one in childhood)
  - Direct
- Femoral

4.14.1.1
Epidemiology

- 1–5% of term males
- Male (80%) indirect type (99%)
- Right (60%), Left (30%), bilateral (10%)
- ↑ Incidence in preterm infants (e.g., 12% at 32 weeks)
- ↑ Incidence in conditions of increased intra-abdominal pressure
  - Abnormal content (e.g., ascites, peritoneal dialysis)
  - Abnormal abdominal wall configuration (e.g., exomphalos, gastroschisis, bladder extrophy)

M. Davenport (✉)
Paediatric Surgery Department, Kings College Hospital, London, UK

C. K. Sinha and M. Davenport (eds.), *Handbook of Pediatric Surgery*,
DOI: 10.1007/978-1-84882-132-3_4.14, © Springer-Verlag London Limited 2010

4.14.1.2
Embryology

The embryonic testis descends from the region of the deep inguinal ring through the anterior abdominal wall muscles to its final destination in the scrotum. It is preceded by a tongue of parietal peritoneum, which becomes the tunica and processus vaginalis. The processus normally obliterates at ~35 weeks of gestation, but failure is common and results either in a hydrocele or an inguinal hernia depending on the degree of patency. In girls, the canal is occupied by the round ligament, but sac formation from a putative processus may occur in the same way (Fig. 4.14.1).

Contents of the sac may commonly include omentum, small and large bowel intestine, and lateral corner of bladder, and in girls the ovary. Rare contents include the appendix (Amyand[1] hernia), Meckel's diverticulum (Littre[2] hernia), or only part of the small bowel (Richter[3] hernia).

Anatomy of Inguinal Canal

- *Entry – deep inguinal ring* (defect in transversalis fascia; medial border contains epigastric vessels).
- *Exit – superficial inguinal ring* (triangular defect in external oblique: base is body of pubis. Cord structures can be felt on underlying bone.)
- *Contents* – spermatic cord has three layers (external and internal spermatic fascia, sandwiching a layer of muscle – cremaster), three nerves (ileo-inguinal, genital branch of genito-femoral, and sympathetics), and three other structures (vas, vessels, and lymphatics).
- The processus envelopes the central structures (vas/vessels) anteriorly and is enveloped by the fascial layers. During open surgery, the fascial layers are teased off the anterior aspect and processus/sac unrolled to expose the posterior aspect – the route to the vas/vessels.

Fig. 4.14.1 Schematic illustrating cross-sectional anatomy of inguinal hernias. The processus or hernial sac envelopes the vas and vessels from front to back and is in turn surrounded by fascial layers taken from each layer of the abdominal wall

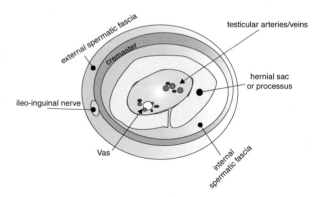

---

[1]Claudius Amyand (1681–1740) – English surgeon, Huguenot name! Reputed to be first surgeon to deliberately remove the appendix (because it was in an inflamed hernial sac, this being somewhat easier).

[2]Alexis Littre (1658–1726) – French surgeon who described this in 1700.

[3]August Gottlieb Richter (1742–1812). German surgeon.

4.14.1.3
Clinical Features

Intermittent swelling, noted during crying and descending toward the scrotum/labia. This may reduce either spontaneously or on gentle, lateral pressure. The bulge may be difficult to elicit in the outpatient setting, but examination should reveal unilateral thickening and slipperiness – the "silken cord sign." This, in conjunction with a good history, is adequate to proceed with surgery. The irreducible hernia presents as a firm, tender mass occupying the inguinal canal and possibly extending to the scrotum. Defining the testis as separate confirms the diagnosis.

4.14.1.4
Management

An acute obstructed hernia should be reduced typically by taxis with semi-elective repair when settled. If this fails, then emergency surgery is warranted.

4.14.1.5
Surgery: Inguinal Hernia

Skin-crease groin incision

1. Incise external oblique (to open canal).
2. Identify sac and separate from vas and vessels. This is often difficult with a flimsy sac in infants, but it is important to keep proximal parts together if possible.
3. Ligation of the sac at the deep inguinal ring (herniotomy).

Caveats

1. The bladder or the ovaries are the usual internal structures, which can form part of a *sliding hernia*. These need careful separation and probably a purse-string under vision to control neck of sac.
2. Sometimes, in small infants, there is a definite *posterior wall weakness* predisposing to recurrence. Perform Bassini [4]repair (suture conjoint tendon down to inguinal ligament) or use a modified darn (absorbable) to strengthen the area.

> *NB – female child with bilateral inguinal hernia – ? possible androgen insensitivity syndrome.*

There has been much recent debate around the value of exploration of the contralateral side (to prevent a metachronous hernia becoming symptomatic). Thus, factors increasing the

---

[4]Edoardo Bassini (1844–1924) – Italian surgeon.

Laparoscopic Hernial Repair – This is accomplished using 3 or 5 mm umbilical port and 3 mm working ports/instruments. The internal ring is usually closed as a purse-string or by a "Z" suture of nonabsorbable material. No real advantage apart from in bilateral repairs and perhaps recurrence.

chances of this have included gender (female>male), laterality (right>left), and age (pre-term>term). Some will insert a telescope via the hernial sac to assess the contralateral deep ring, although even this has problems. Despite this, our policy remains that of leaving surgery to the affected side only.

4.14.1.6
Outcome

- Complication rate should be <1%
  — Risk of damage to vas or vessels, recurrence, atrophy, or iatrogenic ascent of the testis.
- ↑↑ Risk following an episode of incarceration.

4.14.2
Hydrocele

- A collection of fluid in the space surrounding the testicle between the layers of the tunica vaginalis.

4.14.2.1
Classification

- Congenital – due to patency of processus vaginalis (usually children)
- Acquired (usually adults)
  — Idiopathic
  — Secondary (e.g., post-trauma, tumor, lymphatic infiltration (*W. bancrofti*, scrotal filariasis))

The processus vaginalis *should* obliterate by the time of birth (some studies suggest 80% are actually patent). Failure results in ingress of fluid from peritoneal cavity to fill tunica vaginalis.

An *abdominal-scrotal hydrocele* is a variant where there is a large sac extending from scrotum to retroperitoneum – this tends not to have an obvious connection with the peritoneal cavity.

A *hydrocele of the cord* is a fluid-filled cavity within the processus and palpable between superficial inguinal ring and upper scrotum. This may feel like a third testicle.

4.14.2.2
Clinical Features

Hydroceles are usually seen as asymptomatic swellings with diurnal variation (absent in morning). They may also be present only intermittently. The key sign on examination is the ability to get above (i.e. differentiates from hernia) and transilluminate (showing fluid nature). Sometimes, if communicating, the swelling can be reduced slowly by sustained pressure.

4.14.2.3
Management

Management is predominantly noninterventional, as most will resolve spontaneously by 1–2 years of age. Some giant examples do need surgery even in infancy, as they tend to bury the penis.

4.14.2.4
Surgery: Hydrocele

Skin-crease groin incision

1. Canal usually left intact, with separation of cremaster fibers at the level of superficial inguinal ring to identify deeper processus vaginalis.
2. Separation from vas and vessels.
3. Ligation – usually combined with the opening of distal sac to drain all the fluid.

We do not support office aspiration of hydrocele either as diagnostic process or even as an attempt at treatment (unless postoperative).

Recurrence (<5%) is uncommon, but its risk is increased if it is long-standing and its sac is thick-walled. If confident that previous surgery did indeed ligate the PPV, then redo surgery should aim to obliterate tunica vaginalis by excision or eversion (Jaboulay[5]) or plication (Lord[6]).

---

[5]Mathieu Jaboulay (1860–1913) – French surgeon, also performed first attempts at xenotransplants by anastomosing kidneys from sheep and pig into patients dying of renal failure.
[6]Peter H. Lord. English surgeon.

Further Reading

1. Cox JA (1985) Inguinal hernia of children. Surg Clin North Am 65:1331–1342
2. Davenport M (1997) ABC of general paediatric surgery. Inguinal hernia, hydrocele, and the undescended testis. Brit Med J 312:564–567
3. Kumar VH, Clive J, Rosenkrantz TS et al (2002) Inguinal hernia in preterm infants. Pediatr Surg Int 18:147–152
4. Ron O, Eaton S, Pierro A (2007) Systematic review of the risk of developing a metachronous contralateral inguinal hernia in children. Br J Surg 94:804–811 (review)

The Acute Scrotum

4.15

Mark Davenport

Testicular torsion - a True Surgical Emergency!

The "acute scrotum" describes a clinical scenario of recent onset scrotal pain with obvious local tenderness or discomfort. There are a number of possibilities and in no particular order, these include

- Torsion
  - Testis
  - Testicular appendages (e.g., hydatid of Morgagni)
- Infection
  - Orchitis (e.g., mumpsvirus)
  - Epididymo-orchitis (bacterial)
- Trauma (includes vaginal delivery and the effects of forceps!)
- Varicocele
- Inguinal hernia (either de novo or incarcerated) and acute hydrocele (including that of cord)(Chapter 4.14)
- Idiopathic scrotal edema
- Tumor – rare, orchidoblastoma (young), and teratoma (adolescent)
- Referred pain from loin pathology (testis and kidney – shared heritage)

4.15.1
Torsion of the Testes

4.15.1.1
Epidemiology

- 1 in 4,000 (males <25 years) (UK)
- Winter > summer (UK, Nigeria, Kuwait, USA)

M. Davenport
Paediatric Surgery Department, Kings College Hospital, London, UK

C. K. Sinha and M. Davenport (eds.), *Handbook of Pediatric Surgery*,
DOI: 10.1007/978-1-84882-132-3_4.15, © Springer-Verlag London Limited 2010

- Latitude (North > South)
- Bimodal age distribution – small neonatal peak, then inexorable rise during adolescence. Rare >30 years.

May be divided into

- *Intravaginal* – torsion within tunica due to "bell-clapper" arrangement. Presents in adolescence.
- *Extravaginal* – torsion at the level of spermatic cord. It occurs in neonates and is presumed to be owing to failure of fixation of newly arrived testicle.

4.15.1.1.1
Clinical Features

Neonatal torsion presents with a firm scrotal mass, often inflamed but typically not tender. It is probably prenatal in origin and almost always the testis is beyond salvage. In adolescence, the scenario is a painful one with sudden onset and often reflex vomiting. Pain may be referred to the loin and fool the examiner as to its origin.

Examination should show a tender high-lying transverse testis without cremasteric reflex. There may be local reaction (edema and erythema) depending on the time from onset.

4.15.1.1.2
Investigations

- *Open surgery – delay is not an option; if it could be torsion explore!*
- *Urine microscopy and Gram stain* – for casts and organisms.
- *US and Doppler* (possible) – may show ↓ perfusion (up to 95% sensitive).
- *Radioisotope* (possible) – may show ↓ perfusion (up to 95% sensitive).

The latter options are rarely available when you want them.
Differential includes

1. Torsion of appendages (see below)
2. UTI – usually toddlers, ?underlying anomalies
3. Idiopathic scrotal edema – young children, *painless,* marked erythema
4. Epididymo-Orchitis (mumps, coliforms, klebsiella, Chlamydia, gonococci, etc.)
5. Tumor, e.g., teratoma, orchidoblastoma
6. Trauma – history is key. Breech delivery in neonates

4.15.1.2
Surgery: Torsion

Scrotal incision (unless tumor a real possibility)

1. Deliver testis out of scrotum
2. Untwist – leave 15 min, within warmed, wet packs
3. If necrotic – excise; if OK return; if debatable return
4. Fixation – 3-point nonabsorbable. REPEAT on the other side

In neonatal torsion, time to exploration in not so much of an issue, as orchidectomy is almost invariable and neonatal anesthesia must be safe. Contralateral fixation is still recommended.

4.15.2
Outcome

Time since onset is a key to testicular survival.
1. <6 h → 90% testicular salvage
2. 6–18 h → 40% testicular salvage
3. >18 h → <0%

Torsion of Testicular Appendages (of Morgagni[1])

There are two small Mullerian remnants on the upper pole of the testis and one on adjacent epididymus, which can also tort. Typically, the pain and swelling is much less acute, leading to later presentation (days) and the thing itself may be visible as the "blue dot sign." If diagnosis is secure, then treat with either excisional surgery or simply analgesia until tenderness settles.

Further Reading

1. Davenport M (1996) ABC of general paediatric surgery. Acute problems of the scrotum. Brit Med J 312:435–437
2. Davenport M, Bianchi A, Gough DC (1989) Idiopathic scrotal haemorrhage in neonates. BMJ 298:1492–1493

[1]Giovanni Battista Morgagni (1682–1771) – Italian anatomist working in Padua.

The Undescended Testes

4.16

Chandrasen K. Sinha and John. M. Hutson

Failure of the testis is to descend along its normal pathway into the scrotum is the commonest endocrine disorder in the male.

4.16.1
Epidemiology

Incidence

- Preterm boys – ~30%.
- Term 3–5%.
  — Falling to <1% at 6 months
- An undescended testis (UDT) is associated with 4–5-fold increased risk of cancer and a risk of infertility (*vide infra*).

4.16.1.1
Associated Anomalies

- Patent processus vaginalis, inguinal hernia, and abnormal epididymis
- Hypospadias
- Abdominal wall defects, e.g., gastroschisis, exomphalos
- Cerebral palsy, mental retardation
- Prune belly syndrome
- Wilms' tumor

C. K. Sinha (✉)
Paediatric Surgery Department, King's College Hospital, London, UK

C. K. Sinha and M. Davenport (eds.), *Handbook of Pediatric Surgery*,
DOI: 10.1007/978-1-84882-132-3_4.16, © Springer-Verlag London Limited 2010

4.16.2
Embryology

Testes develop from the gonadal ridge (antero-medial to the mesonephros) and within the coelomic cavity behind the peritoneum and below the developing kidneys.

1. 3–5 weeks – undifferentiated gonad develops along gonadal ridge.
2. 6 weeks – primodial germ cells migrate from the yolk sac into the gonadal ridges and differentiate into *gonocytes*. Determination of a testis is controlled by the *SRY* gene[1] (together with *WT-1, SF-1, SOX9*).
3. 7–8 weeks – Sertoli[2] cells develops and start secreting MIS (Mullerian[3] Inhibiting Substance) or antimullerian hormones, which causes regression of mullerian derivatives.
4. 9 weeks – Leydig[4] cells form and start secreting testosterone, which induces both the differentiation of the Wolffian[5] ducts into male internal accessory reproductive organs and masculinization of the external genitalia.

   Testicular descent then occurs in two phases.

5. 10–15 weeks – *Transabdominal phase* – controlled by the Leydig cell hormone (insulin-like hormone [INS3]).

By the third month, testes occupy a position immediately above the internal inguinal ring.

6. 24–35 weeks – *Inguino-scrotal phase* – regulated by androgens and the genitofemoral nerve.

Most (75%) infants born with UDT will have spontaneous descent by 4–6 months postnatally (corrected for term), thought to be due to a postnatal surge of testosterone.

4.16.3
Etiology

The precise cause is unknown but possible causes include:

- Defects in testosterone, INS3, and MIS.
- *HOXA10*[6] and *HOXA11* (developmental genes) may have some role.

---

[1] *SRY* – Sex determining Region Y: *WT-1*– Wilms' tumor; *SF-1*– Splicing Factor.

[2] Enrico Sertoli (1842–1910) Italian histologist, working in Milan.

[3] Johannes Peter Muller (1801–1858) German anatomist with posts in Bonn and Berlin.

[4] Franz von Leydig (1821–1908) German anatomist – interstitial cells first recognized in 1850.

[5] Caspar Friedrich Wolff (1733–1794) German embryologist and inventor of three germ layer principle.

[6] *HOX* gene family – Homeobox gene clusters (1–4).

- Hypogonadotrophic hypogonadism: Absence of gonadotrophin surge, which is normally seen at 60–90 days after birth, is an important sign of abnormal testicular function. This surge is called mini-puberty. If this surge is absent, Leydig cells do not proliferate and germ cells do not mature, leading to infertility.
- Differential body growth in relation to spermatic cord/gubernaculum.
- ↓ Intra-abdominal pressure – UDT is seen in a number of conditions with this feature (e.g., prune belly syndrome, exstrophy, exomphalos, gastroschisis).

4.16.4
Clinical Features

- Unilateral ~75% right > left
- Nonpalpable testes ~20%
- About 10% of total UDT have blind-ending vessels above the internal ring

Palpable testes may be found:

- Above tubercle 10–15%
- At the pubic tubercle 35–40%
- Upper scrotum 15–20%
- Ectopic 5–8%

4.16.4.1
Investigations

- For unilateral UDT without hypospadias, no further investigations are required.
- For unilateral UDT with hypospadias or bilateral nonpalpable UDT, investigation to rule out a disorder of sex development (DSD) is necessary.

Examination

Examine supine, and with crossed legs and if required in the upright position. Asymmetry of the scrotum suggests unilateral UDT, whereas a bilateral hypoplastic scrotum suggests bilateral UDT. If the testis is not obviously palpable, the fingers should be kept near the iliac crest and gently milked toward the scrotum. The fingers of one hand feel the testis while the other hand keeps the testis in that position. Even if it comes down to the bottom of the scrotum, it is important to assess whether it remains over there for some time after release to differentiate it from a retractile testis. An enlarged contralateral testis suggests either ipsilateral atrophy or absence. Perineal, penile, and femoral regions should be examined for ectopic testes.

- — LH (lutinizing hormone)
- — FSH (follicle-stimulating hormone)
- — hCG (human chorionic gonadotrophin) stimulation test

A negative testosterone response after hCG stimulation, in the presence of ↑LH and ↑FSH, is suggestive of bilateral absent testes (*anorchia*).

(NB: MIS can also be assayed for the presence of sertoli cells.)

- *US, CT*, and *MRI* have high false-negative results, so should be done only in difficult situations.
- Abnormalities of the upper renal tract may be ruled out by US if associated with hypospadias or bilateral UDT.
- A genitogram is helpful if an intersex problem is suspected.

4.16.5
Management

4.16.5.1
Role of Hormone Therapy

Hormonal (hCG, GnRH) treatment has been practiced in Europe for about 40 years. On the basis of some recent studies, the "Nordic consensus," however, has recommended against the use of hormones, considering the poor immediate benefits and the possible long-term adverse effects on spermatogenesis (hormones induce increased apoptosis of the germ cells). This recommendation remains controversial.

4.16.5.2
Orchidopexy

As descent is uncommon after 6 months, according to the *Nordic consensus on treatment of UDT*, orchidopexy is recommended soon after 6 months of age (corrected for term) or upon diagnosis, if it occurs late.

Operative intervention is not required for normally retractile testes.

4.16.5.2.1
Palpable UDT

1. Skin-crease groin incision
2. Mobilization of testis
3. Opening of inguinal canal
4. Hernial sac or processus vaginalis dissected free and transfixed at its neck

5. Mobilization of testis on vas and vessels up to and beyond the level of deep ring
6. Tension-free placement in dartos pouch

4.16.5.2.2
Nonpalpable Testis

Studies have suggested that even abdominal testes are histologically normal up to 6 months, but then show a sharp decrease in spermatogonia with age.

- *EUA* and *diagnostic laparoscopy* – if actually palpable convert to simple orchidopexy.
- *Two-stage Fowler[7]–Stephens[8] operation.*

This is indicated for high or intra-abdominal testis and can be performed open or laparoscopically (latter now more popular). Early decision is needed to avoid unnecessary devascularization of the blood supply coming along the vas deferens and cremaster muscles.

1. First stage – the testicular blood vessels are ligated or clipped, so that the testis develops its blood supply from vessels along the vas and cremaster muscle.
2. Second stage (>6 months after) – division of ablated testicular vessel pedicle and mobilization entirely on vas overlying peritoneum.

All children should be followed up at 3 months and after 1 year to check the testes for viability, size, and location.

4.16.5.2.3
Complications

- Testicular atrophy
  - 1–5% cases after open orchidopexy
  - 20–30% after FS orchidopexy
- Vas injury-1–5%
- Recurrence, reascent
  - Up to 10% is usually due to inadequate mobilization and inadequate hernial sac dissection. Revision orchidopexy is indicated.
- About half of acquired (previously not operated) UDT may come down on their own; hence, a conservative approach until puberty is indicated by some authors, although there is a risk to fertility, with lower sperm counts being reported in this group. Many authors would recommend orchidopexy in this situation.

---

[7]Robert Fowler (b1928) – Australian pediatric surgeon.
[8]Frank Douglas Stephens (b1913) – Australian pediatric surgeon.

4.16.6
Outcome

Fertility (difficult to predict).
- Bilateral UDT – ↓↓ fertility (~25% have adequate sperm counts).
- Unilateral UDT: ↓ fertility (~ 90% with ~ 75% have normal sperm counts after surgery at a mean age of 10 years).
- Subfertility – waiting time to pregnancy is longer in bilateral UDT.
- Fertility according to the preoperative site of the testis is difficult to predict.
    - Bilateral – ↑ position of the testes ↓ lower the fertility.
    - Unilateral – preoperative site is not a major determinant.

Further Reading

1. Hutson JM (2007) Treatment of undescended testes – time for a change in European tradition. Acta Paediatrica 96:608–610
2. Kolon TF, Patel RP, Huff DS (2004) Cryptorchidism: diagnosis, treatment, and long term prognosis. Urol Clin N Am 31:469–480
3. Murphy F, SriParan T, Puri P (2007) Orchidopexy and its impact on fertility. Pediatr Surg Int 23:625–632

Mark Davenport

4.17.1
Penile Problems

4.17.1.1
Natural History of Foreskin Separation

At birth, the foreskin is naturally adherent to the glans. From about 2–4 years of age, there is a dissolution of the bond presumably with the formation of pockets of sebaceous material (smegmal "pearls"), allowing it to retract. From about 5 years, most boys should have the ability of full unimpeded foreskin retraction.

Phimosis[1] may be defined as a condition where the foreskin is unable to be retracted to expose the glans. It can be divided into

- Physiological phimosis – simply the normal state in the first years of life
- Pathological phimosis
  - Primary – true congenital phimosis with pin-hole meatus present and symptomatic in the first year of life is very uncommon. Typically, urine accumulates in a distended preputial sac, needing to be expressed.
  - Secondary – recurrent infection and/or urine irritation leads to scarring and cicatrization.

Paraphimosis is that condition where the foreskin is able to be retracted but becomes stuck in that position resulting in distal congestion and edema of glans.

---

[1]*Phimosis* (φίμωσις Greek) – muzzling, as in the muzzle of dog's jaw.

M. Davenport
Paediatric Surgery Department, Kings College Hospital, London, UK

C. K. Sinha and M. Davenport (eds.), *Handbook of Pediatric Surgery*,
DOI: 10.1007/978-1-84882-132-3_4.17, © Springer-Verlag London Limited 2010

4.17.1.2
Clinical Features

Phimosis usually causes consistent difficultly with voiding due to obstruction; often the foreskin "balloons" with force of the stream. True retention is rare. Secondary bacterial infection may lead to *balanitis*[2] (inflammation of the glans) or *posthitis* (inflammation of the foreskin). *Balanitis xerotica obliterans* is a descriptive term for long-standing chronic inflammation and has a dead-white appearance of glans and foreskin with typically a pin-hole meatus.

4.17.1.3
Management

1. Conservative – reassure, gentle self-retraction
   (a) Topical steroids (e.g., betamethasone 0.1%)

2. Surgery
   (a) Preputial "stretch"
   (b) Preputioplasty – foreskin conservation with mini incisions around phimotic ring. Needs active retraction after otherwise high recurrence rate.
   (c) Circumcision

Paraphimosis – this is a real surgical emergency and treatment shouldn't be delayed. A number of techniques have been described to reduce a paraphimosis in the emergency room including compresses with ice or sugar (to reduce the swelling and allow protraction) or multiple needle punctures (again to allow fluid to be squeezed out). If everything else fails, then a dorsal slit of the tight band under a short GA will work.

4.17.1.4
Circumcision

History-Circumcision

Emerged in the prehistoric era from desert-dwelling semitic[3] people. It is an act of faith in both Jewish and Muslim religions for males to be circumcised: the former with a very precise chronology (eighth day of life) and liturgy (*Bris milah*); for the latter, the actual timing is less important and it tends to be done as more of a rite of passage from boy to man. Although in general, it is not a necessary part of most Christian faiths, various West African churches still encourage it.

---

[2]*Balanitis* (Greek) – the word balanos refers to resemblance of the glans to an acorn!

[3]*Semitic* – the word refers to one of the sons of Noah – Shem, and implies all the people of that part of the world.

Surgical Freehand

1. Complete foreskin retraction and division of adhesions.
2. Dorsal slit – then circumferential incision around outer skin. Hemostasis with bipolar (not monopolar) cautery. Specific attention to frenular artery.
3. Similar incision on inner preputial skin leaving 3–4 mm cuff at corona.
4. Reconstruction (absorbable suture) – ensuring that the skin is neither too lax nor too tight.

There are also a number of aids to allow a "non-surgeon" approach including the Plastibell® and the Gomko clamp®.

Complications

- Bleeding
- Infection
- Meatal stenosis

4.17.2
Varicocele

There is still an unresolved debate as to the causal relationship between varicoceles and infertility.

4.17.2.1
Epidemiology

- Common – 15% of adolescents (10–20 years)
- 95% left-sided
- Association with left renal tumors (e.g., Wilms' tumor) (rare)

Anatomy

The venous drainage from the testis is distinctly unusual with an initial venous pampiniform plexus (countercurrent flow) within the layers of the spermatic cord, gradually reducing to one or two testicular veins at the level of internal ring. These then ascend on posterior wall to join the renal vein on the left and the inferior vena cava on the right. The angle of entry is supposed to have a valve-like effect, and therefore, varicoceles "only" occur on the left.

4.17.2.2
Etiology

- Failure of the venous valve mechanism and reflux associated with standing posture
  — Left-side preference
- Occlusive left-sided renal vein encroachment.

This seems to be associated with ↑ testicular temperature and ↓ spermatogenesis – still a matter of dispute.

4.17.2.3
Clinical Features

Usually asymptomatic, but some have "dragging" sensation. Described in all books as a "bag of worms"!
 Examined in standing position with Valsalva[4] maneuver to allow clinical grading.

1. Palpable only on Valsalva
2. Palpable but not visible at rest
3. Palpable and visible at rest

4.17.2.4
Investigations

- *US (with color-flow Doppler)* – for confirmation, estimation of testicular volume (1–2 ml prepubertal), and exclusion of renal masses.
- *Prader orchidometer.*
- *Seminal analysis* (where appropriate).

4.17.2.5
Management

The indications are still somewhat controversial particularly with low-grade varicoceles in younger children. But clear ones include (1) symptoms, (2) infertility (3) evidence of testicular growth failure (w.r.t. contralateral testis).

---

[4] Antonio Maria Valsalva (1666 – 1723) – Italian anatomist working in Bologna. Main interest was that of middle ear and this tested patency of the Eustachian tube.

4.17.2.6
Surgery

The principle is diversion of venous drainage; and is achieved by ligation of testicular veins allowing subsidiary venous channels to open up (via cremasteric or vasal veins into the external iliacs).

Alternatives

- Laparoscopy (trans or retroperitoneal)
  - ○ Clips/bipolar to testicular vein(s)
    - — Testicular artery ± lymphatics

- Open
  - — Deep inguinal ring – Paloma approach
  - — Within canal – Ivanissevich
  - — Intrascrotal ligation

Venous embolization under radiological control is possible, and in some regions, direct injection of the varicocele has also been performed.

4.17.2.6.1
Complications

- Hydrocele (↓ by deliberate lymphatic sparing) (5–10%)
- Testicular atrophy – ↑ with lower level of surgery
- Recurrence – attributed to multiple testicular veins

Further Reading

1. Paduch DA, Skoog SJ (2001) Current management of adolescent varicocele. Rev Urol 3:120–133
2. Diamond DA (2007) Adolescent varicocoele. Curr Opin Urol 17:263–267
3. Cayan S, Woodhouse CR (2007) The treatment of adolescents presenting with varicocele. BJU Int 100:744–747
4. Davenport M (1996) Problems with the penis and prepuce – *ABC of Paediatric Surgery series*. Brit Med J 312:299–301

Miscellaneous Surgical Issues

4.18

Jean W. L. Wong, Chandrasen K. Sinha, and Mark Davenport

4.18.1
Tongue Tie (Ankyloglossia)

This is defined as short lingual frenulum, which restricts tongue movement and may interfere with tooth development.

• Incidence is ~3% in infants.

4.18.1.1
Clinical Features

The disease is mostly asymptomatic but may cause difficulty with breast feeding and speech impediment.

Protrusion of the tongue causes its tip to become notched and not extend past the incisors or touch roof of the mouth. In severe cases, the tongue is completely immobile and fixed.

4.18.1.2
Management

In the newborn with breast feeding problems, intervention (without anesthetic) is reasonable. After this period, it is judicious to wait for a reason (e.g., speech therapy defined problem) rather than pre-empt matters. A proportion will revert to normal by stretching or spontaneous rupture.

Division of frenulum is straightforward, but should avoid the submandibular ducts on either side.

C. K. Sinha (✉)
Paediatric Surgery Department, King's College Hospital, London, UK

C. K. Sinha and M. Davenport (eds.), *Handbook of Pediatric Surgery*,
DOI: 10.1007/978-1-84882-132-3_4.18, © Springer-Verlag London Limited 2010

4.18.2
Umbilical Issues

The umbilicus is the last link with fetal life and contains many peculiar embryonic vestiges.

Embryology and Anatomy

Vascular connection to the placenta is maintained by single large umbilical vein (to the porta hepatis) at 12 o'clock and two inferior umbilical arteries from the internal iliac artery at 5 and 7 o'clock, respectively. At birth, these structures close and obliterate but leave a potential space through the umbilical ring, which also has to close by a cicatrizing process. Failure to achieve this leads to the development of *umbilical herniation*. Two further structures may lead to vestigial-related problems

- *Vitello-intestinal duct* – communication from the apex of the midgut to the yolk sac of embryonic life. It should vanish, but remnants may include a *Meckel's diverticulum,* a fibrous connection to underside of umbilicus, or a completely patent duct.
- *Urachus* – connection between apex of bladder and allantois[1].

4.18.2.1
Umbilical Hernia

- Afro-Caribbean (particular of West African origin) » Caucasian
- 13% (vs. 2%) at 1 year of age (USA study)
- Low birth weight
- M = F

4.18.2.1.1
Associations

- Congenital hypothyroidism (defective cicatrization)
- ↑ Intra-abdominal fluid (e.g., ascites, VP shunts)

4.18.2.2
Clinical Features

Umbilical herniation is unique among hernias in that it may spontaneously reduce and repair overtime. They have a low risk of irreducibility and intestinal obstruction (<5%). Most would advise repair if they persist beyond the toddler stage.

4.18.2.3
Surgery

Subumbilical skin crease incision

1. Dissect around whole circumference of the neck of sac and reduce contents.
2. Dissect off overlying skin and then excise sac back to fascial ring.
3. Repair defect (usually transverse).
4. Umbilicoplasty – mostly skin is tacked to repair and cavity obliterated by pressure. Sometimes, so much skin is left that excision of a triangle and "swirling" the subsequent suture line is a better form of cosmesis.

4.18.3
Rectal Prolapse

Abnormal protrusion of rectal wall (or just mucosa) through the anus.

4.18.3.1
Epidemiology

- Common during infancy
- ↑ Incidence in tropical latitudes

4.18.3.1.1
Associations

- Acute diarrheal illness
- Cystic fibrosis
- Neuromuscular weakness (e.g., spina bifida, sacral agenesis)
- Malnutrition
- Ehlers–Danlos syndrome

4.18.3.2
Clinical Features

Usually nontender, mucosal mass protruding from the anus, initially only on straining. It may become irreducible and present all the time.

---

[1] *Allantois* (Greek – sausage) – is a diverticulum of cloaca within connecting stalk to placenta – main function in reptiles and birds (both lay eggs) is as a repository of nitrogenous waste.

Differentiate from

1. Intussusception – much more severe symptoms, ± intestinal obstruction. Finger or probe can freely be passed around all circumferences between anus and intussusceptum.
2. Prolapsed rectal polyp.

4.18.3.2.1
Investigations

- Exclude underlying condition, which may be overt (spina bifida) or covert (cystic fibrosis).
- If diarrhea – stool microscopy, culture and sensitivities, and screening for ova and parasites.
- Lower GI endoscopy – to exclude rectal polyps. There is usually little evidence of anything abnormal in prolapse.

4.18.3.3
Management

- Manual reduction with adequate sedation. Firm compression to reduce edema, then reduction of innermost mucosal lead-point first.

Thereafter, most would advocate a simple conservative policy of treating the underlying condition (e.g., diarrhea) and avoidance of straining. Most children (< 4 years) recover spontaneously.

Intervention is more likely to be needed in older children and those with neuromuscular etiology.

4.18.3.4
Surgery

- *Sclerotherapy*, e.g., oily phenol, hypertonic saline. This often needs multiple injections. Avoid anterior needle placement.
- *Thiersch[2] operation* – circumferential (typically absorbable) suture.
- *Rectopexy*, e.g., although many of them are described, usually these are for elderly women. In children, consider rectal fixation to sacral hollow from above (± prosthetic interposition).

---

[2]Karl Thiersch (1822 – 1895) – German surgeon who also pioneered use of split-skin grafts.

Further Reading

1. Antao B, Bradley V, Roberts JP, Shawis R (2005) Management of rectal prolapse in children. Dis Colon Rectum 48:1620–1625
2. Lalakea ML, Messner AH (2003) Ankyloglossia: does it matter? Pediatric Clin North Am 50:381–397
3. Pomeranz A (2004) Anomalies, abnormalities, and care of the umbilicus. Pediatr Clin North Am 51:819–827

Basic Pediatric Laparoscopy and Thoracoscopy

4.19

Steven S. Rothenberg and Suzanne M. Yoder

Over the last decade, an increasing number of reports have documented the safety and efficacy of such procedures as appendectomy, fundoplication, and splenectomy in the children, showing the same benefits as in the adult population. With the development of pediatric specific instrumentation and advanced skills, there has been a large push in the implementation of pediatric specific procedures such as pyloromyotomy for pyloric stenosis, colon pull-throughs for Hirschsprung's[1] disease and imperforate anus, repair of intestinal atresias, and advanced thoracoscopic procedures in both neonates and children.

4.19.1
General Principles

4.19.1.1
Positioning of the Patient and Port Placement

Ergonomics plays a strong role in dictating successful choices for positioning.

- Central (cross table) – infants (e.g., pyloromyotomy and pull-through). It gives the surgeon equal access to the head and foot of the patient while keeping them closer to the anesthesiologist during the case.
- Foot of table – (e.g., Nissen fundoplication). Surgeon stands at the patient's feet.
- Thoracoscopic procedures take advantage of lateral positioning to allow safe access to all structures within the thoracic space and use gravity to aid in retraction of the lung.

---

[1]Harald Hirschsrpung (1830–1916) – Danish pediatrician, who described key clinical features.

S. S. Rothenberg (✉)
Pediatric Surgery Department, Rocky Mountain Hospital for Children, Denver, CO, USA

C. K. Sinha and M. Davenport (eds.), *Handbook of Pediatric Surgery*,
DOI: 10.1007/978-1-84882-132-3_4.19, © Springer-Verlag London Limited 2010

4.19.1.2
Pneumoperitoneum

- *Closed Veress[2] needle technique* – special spring-loaded needle.
- *Open Hasson[3] technique* – dissection through fascia, visual identification of cavity.

Initial concerns suggested the need for decreased insufflation pressures in infants and children, but subsequent physiologic data does not support this. There is an increase in end tidal CO_2 with insufflation, but this can be remedied by increasing the minute ventilation. Hypotension and other physiologic effects have not been shown to be significant in most cases.

4.19.1.3
Pneumothorax

- CO_2 insufflation and valved trocars
- Single lung ventilation is by mainstem intubation of the contralateral bronchus
- Double lumen endotracheal tube (adolescents)

The slight tension pneumothorax created by the CO_2 helps to provide complete collapse in most cases, creating an adequate working environment.

4.19.1.4
Instrumentation

Pediatric specific (<10 kg)

- Shorter length shafts (18–20 cm)
- Smaller diameter (2.5–3 mm)

These instruments improve the ergonomics and allow the surgeon to perform fine dissection and suturing in a relatively confined space.

- Smaller scopes (3 and 4 mm) of shorter lengths (20 cm).

These may compromise light retrieval; therefore, a good light source and digital camera are imperative.

---

[2]Janos Veress (1903–1979) – Hungarian chest physician who used this needle for inducing pneumoperitoneum in the treatment of TB.
[3]Harrith M. Hasson. American gynecologist, working in Chicago, who first described this in 1971.

Standard Working Pressures

- Children (12–15 mmHg).
- Infants (10–12 mmHg) (NB in neonates, some insufflators are not sensitive enough to detect the rapid changes in pressure in their smaller peritoneal cavities, and this lack of sensitivity may result in over-insufflation).
- Initial flow 0.5–1 L/min.

4.19.2
Pyloromyotomy for Pyloric Stenosis (see Chap. 3.4)

Laparoscopic pyloromyotomy was probably the first truly pediatric laparoscopic procedure. Many felt that a laparoscopic approach added little advantage over a standard RUQ or supra-umbilical incision, but the ease and quickness of the procedure along with the superior cosmetic result has made it one of the most commonly adopted MIS procedures.

1. Crossways placement on the table.
2. Umbilical incision, trocar, and a 3 or 4 mm 30° telescope lens.
3. RUQ and epigastrium stab wounds (R side of falciform ligament, at approximately the liver edge).

   (a) Grasp the duodenum using 3 mm atraumatic grasper (Babcock or bowel clamp) through the RUQ incision.
   (b) Place retractable arthroscopy blade through the epigastric incision.

4. Advance blade 2–3 mm past the shield and make longitudinal myotomy. The blade is then retracted back into the sheath and the blunt sheath is used to deepen and widen the myotomy. The myotomy is then completed by either grabbing the upper muscle rim with the Babcock and detracting the lower muscle rim using the blunt sheath or by using a laparoscopic pyloromyotomy spreader.

The surgeon can visualize the muscle fibers splitting and can tell when the myotomy is complete by the bulging mucosa and the ability of the upper and lower muscle rims to slide tangentially to each other. If a mucosal perforation is noted, it should be suture closed and the pylorus rotated 90° and another myotomy made.

Postoperatively, feeds are started one to two hours after surgery and volumes are rapidly increased. Most patients are discharged within 24 h.

4.19.3
Laparoscopic Fundoplication and Gastrostomy Button (see Chap. 4.3)

Lap. fundoplications have routinely been performed in infants and children for 15 years and a number of large series show excellent results and recurrence rates at 10 year follow-up better than that achieved with traditional open surgery. There is also a striking decrease in morbidity, especially in terms of pulmonary complications and the incidence of postoperative bowel obstructions.

The most commonly performed procedure is the Nissen[4] fundoplication.

4.19.3.1
Five-Port Nissen Technique

Instrumentation and trocars are 5 or 3 mm in size depending on the size of the patient. Either a standard length 5 mm 30° telescope or a short wide-angle 4 mm 30° telescope is chosen based on patient size.

1. Umbilicus – camera port
2. The R and L mid-quadrants – working ports
3. R mid or upper-quadrant – liver retractor
4. LUQ – stomach retractor and gastrostomy tube site (Fig. 4.19.1).

4.19.3.1.1
Procedure

1. The left lobe of the liver is retracted superiorly, using a locking Babcock clamp, to expose the gastro-esophageal junction. This is placed through the RUQ incision (just to the surgeon's right of the falciform ligament at the liver edge). The shaft of the clamp hooks the falciform helping to elevate the liver and the clamp is used to grasp the diaphragm above the esophageal hiatus, thus allowing the shaft of the instrument to act as a self-retaining retractor. In some cases with an extremely large liver, it is necessary to place a *snake* or *fan retractor*.
2. Divide the esophagogastric and phrenoesophageal ligaments and identify the R and L diaphragmatic crura.
3. Divide/coagulate short gastric vessels (using hook cautery in patients <10 kg or one of the 5-mm sealing-dividing instruments in >10 kg).

---

[4]Rudolf Nissen (1896–1981) – German surgeon who worked in also Turkey, USA, and ultimately in Basel, Switzerland.

Fig. 4.19.1 Trocar position
for Laparoscopic Nissen
procedure

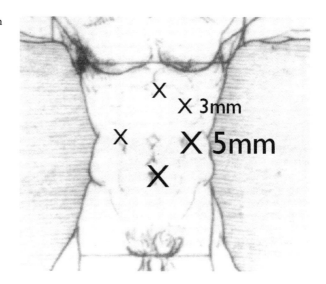

4. Develop a retro-esophageal window – taking care not to injure the posterior vagus nerve.
5. Crural repair in all cases – using a braided nonabsorbable suture.
6. Fundal wrap – formed around an intra-esophageal stent (size dependent on the size of the patient).

   (a) 1.5–3 cm in length and consist of 2–3 sutures going from stomach, to the anterior wall of the esophagus, to the retro-esophageal portion of the stomach.
   (b) The anterior portion of the wrap should lie at the 11 o'clock position to prevent tension or torsion of the esophagus, decreasing the incidence of dysphagia. The first stitch can also include the anterior diaphragmatic rim and some surgeons choose to place multiple collar stitches between the wrap and crus.

7. ±Gastrostomy button (if the patient is a poor eater or has primary aspiration).

   (a) In infants and smaller children, this is most easily accomplished by bringing the stomach up through the LUQ trocar site. The button is secured with a purse string suture and the stomach is tacked to the anterior abdominal fascia with two stay sutures, all placed through the trocar site (Fig. 4.19.2).
   (b) A Seldinger technique with a guide wire and dilators could be used (alternative). This technique utilizes full thickness sutures through the abdominal wall and anterior gastric wall to temporarily secure the button.

If the patient undergoes a fundoplication alone, liquids are started 2 h postoperatively and most patients are discharged on the first postoperative day. They are kept on a soft diet for approximately 1 week. In patients with gastrostomy buttons placed, feeds are started the next morning.

Fig. 4.19.2 Siting a
gastrostomy through
working port

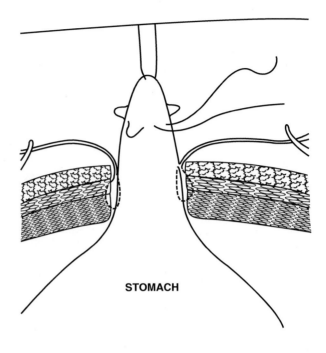

STOMACH

4.19.4
Malrotation (Ladd's [5] Procedure) (see Chap. 3.5)

Malrotation can present as a partial proximal bowel obstruction, or in cases of volvulous, as surgical emergency. Generally, the diagnosis of malrotation is made by upper GI contrast study, which shows an incomplete or abnormal C-loop. Once the diagnosis is made, the patient is explored. The duodenum is examined and an attempt is made to identify a normal ligament of Trietz [6]. If the ligament of Trietz is present but the cecum is not fixed, this is an incomplete rotation but not a malrotation, and no intervention is necessary.

If the diagnosis of malrotation is confirmed, the adhesions (Ladd's bands) overlying the malpositioned duodenum are divided. These are often draped over the duodenum extending to the right colon, causing external compression and partial obstruction. Once these bands are divided, the duodenum is mobilized and straightened so that it lies in the right gutter. The bowel is then run from proximal to distal, untwisting the bowel and dividing any congenital adhesions. During this process, the small bowel mesentery is widened. Once the colon is reached, it is positioned along the patient's left gutter and an appendectomy is performed. In infants, it is often easy to bring the appendix up through the umbilical incision and ligate and divide it extracorporeally.

---

[5]William Edwards Ladd (1880–1967) – American surgeon, widely regarded as the father of pediatric surgery in North America.
[6]Vaclav Wenzel Treitz (1819–1872) – Czech pathologist.

More advanced laparoscopic procedures are beyond detailed description in this text. Procedures such as duodenal atresia repair, laparoscopic-assisted pull-thorough for Hirschsprung's, and laparoscopic repair of imperforate anus are all routinely performed at many institutions. Further description of these procedures may be found in the sources listed at the end of this chapter.

4.19.5
Thoracoscopic Procedures

4.19.5.1
Empyema

Previously, empyema has been treated with antibiotics, prolonged chest tube drainage, and, if this failed, open thoracotomy for debridement. The minimal morbidity associated with thoracoscopy makes it ideal for the early treatment of empyema in children resulting in much shorter hospitalizations and a quicker resolution of respiratory symptoms.

4.19.5.1.1
Technique

1. Single lung ventilation – mainstem intubation of the contralateral bronchus (typically) – helps keep the lung collapsed during the procedure as the peel and effusion are removed. If not tolerated, then a standard tracheal intubation is acceptable.
2. Lateral decubitus position with the affected side up.
3. Effective support (axillary roll and appropriate protective padding secured with tape or straps). In an older child, support can be provided by a beanbag. The upper arm is extended upward and outward and secured in position. If the patient does not tolerate this position, because of persistent desaturation, they may be placed more supine.

As the surgeon will need to access the entire chest cavity, he may stand on either side of the patient. The surgical assistant is usually positioned on the opposite side of the table to hold the camera. Two monitors are used with one placed on each side of the patient at the level of the patient's chest near the shoulders to allow unobstructed views by the surgeon and assistant.

4. A Veress needle is placed just anterior to the mid-axillary line at approximately the fourth or fifth interspace after infiltrating the site with local anesthetic and making a small transverse incision. If there is an identified site on ultrasound or CT with a big fluid pocket close to one of the proposed port sites, this should be chosen as the point of entry. Insufflation with low-flow CO_2 to a pressure of 4–5 mmHg may help collapse the lung and improve visualization as the fibrinous adhesions are taken down. A 5-mm

trocar is then placed and the 30° scope is introduced. The endoscope may be used initially to take down adhesions and break up loculations, and allow for the placement of the second trocar under thoracoscopic vision.

5. Second 5-mm port is placed posteriorly and inferiorly at approximately the sixth inter-space along the posterior axillary line.

6. A suction-irrigator is introduced to aspirate the free pleural fluid and further break down loculations with blunt dissection. A sample of the fluid can be collected at this time. Grasping forceps or a bowel clamp can then be used to peel off and remove the fibrin-ous debris through the trocar. The scope and operating instrument can be interchanged from one port site to another to ensure that all of the pleural surfaces are reached.

Once the lung has been completely freed, the entire pleural fluid is drained, and most of the fibrinous peels are removed, the thoracic cavity is irrigated with warm normal saline that is subsequently aspirated out. The lung is allowed to expand fully with the help of positive pressure breaths from the anesthetist. Once full expansion is confirmed, the lower trocar is removed and a chest tube, appropriate to the child's size, is placed and positioned postero-inferiorly under thoracoscopic vision. The scope and remaining trocar are removed.

7. Port sites closed in two layers.

8. The chest tube is attached to a Pleurovac® (initially at −10 to −20 cm H_2O pressure).

Once drainage becomes minimal, there is no evidence of an air leak, and the child is improving; the chest tube can be removed, usually after a trial of underwater seal.

The patient is usually discharged on antibiotics, after he has been afebrile for 48 h.

4.19.6
Esophageal Atresia Repair (see chap 3.3)

In 2000, the first successful repair of an esophageal atresia (EA) with tracheo-esophageal fistula (TEF) in a newborn using a completely thoracoscopic approach was preformed, and the operation has now become the standard in many major pediatric centers across the world. The greatest advantage of this technique is the avoidance of the major morbidity associated with a formal thoracotomy in a neonate.

4.19.6.1
Technique

1. General endotracheal anesthesia with low-peak pressures (until the fistula is ligated to prevent over distension of the abdomen).

Initially, attempts were made to obtain a left mainstem intubation; however, this can be difficult and time-consuming in a compromised newborn. We now perform the procedure with just a standard tracheal intubation, as excellent right lung collapse in newborns can be achieved with CO_2 insufflation alone. Wasting even minutes trying to place a bronchial blocker or other manipulations can compromise the eventual success of a thoracoscopic approach.

2. Modified prone position with the right side elevated approximately 30–45°. If there is a right-sided arch, then the approach is left-sided.

This positioning gives the surgeon access to the area between the anterior and posterior axillary line for trocar placement while allowing gravity to retract the lung away from the posterior mediastinum. This arrangement gives excellent exposure of the fistula and esophageal segments without the need for an extra trocar for a lung retractor.

3. The surgeon and the assistant stand at the patient's front and the monitor is placed at the patient's back. Because fine manipulation is necessary, the surgeon and the assistant should position themselves so that they are in the most ergonomic and comfortable position.
4. Three-port technique (Fig. 4.19.3).

(a) The initial camera port (3–5 mm) is placed in the fifth intercostal space at approximately the posterior axillary line. A 30° lens is used to allow the surgeon to "look down" on his instruments and avoid "dueling."
(b) Two instrument ports are placed in the mid-axillary line 1–2 interspaces above and below the camera port. Upper port is 5 mm to allow for the clip applier and suture. Lower port is 3 mm in size. Ideally, these ports are placed so that the instrument tips will approximate a right angle (90°) at the level of the fistula. This positioning will facilitate suturing the anastomosis.

Once the chest has been insufflated and the lung collapsed, the surgeon must identify the fistula. In most cases, the fistula is attached to the membranous portion of the trachea just above the carina. This level is usually demarcated by the azygous vein.

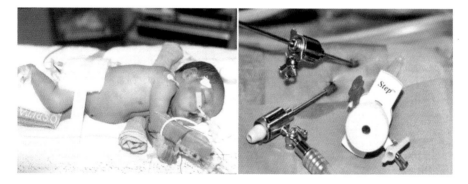

Fig. 4.19.3 Infant and trocar position for repair of esophageal atresia

5. Azygous vein mobilization (using a curved dissector or scissors), cauterization, and division (small hook cautery although bipolar cautery or other sealing devices can be used). Ties or clips are generally not necessary and could interfere with the dissection of the fistula.

With the vein divided, the lower esophageal segment is identified and followed proximally to the fistula. Because of the magnification afforded by the thoracoscopic approach, it is easy to visualize exactly where the fistula enters the back wall of the trachea.

6. Clip the TEF using a 5-mm endoscopic clip. Care should be taken to avoid the vagus nerve. The fistula is divided with scissors. As the distal segment may retract making it difficult to visualize, it may be preferable to wait until the upper pouch is dissected out before completely dividing the fistula.

Attention is now turned to the thoracic inlet. The anesthesiologist places pressure on the naso-gastric tube to help identify the upper pouch.

7. Identify the upper pouch by incising the pleura and mobilizing with blunt and sharp dissection. The plane between the esophagus and trachea can be seen well and the two should be separated by sharp dissection. Mobilization of the upper pouch is carried on up into the thoracic inlet. Once adequate mobilization is achieved, the distal tip of the pouch is resected with a generous enough opening to prevent later stricture formation.

8. Anastomosis is performed using 4-0 or 5-0 monofilament absorbable suture on a small taper needle in an interrupted fashion.

(a) The back wall is placed first with the knots intraluminal.
(b) Pass a naso-gastric tube into the lower pouch and on into the stomach.
(c) The anterior wall is then completed with the NG tube acting as a stent to prevent incorporation of the posterior wall and ensure patency of the anastomosis. Adequate bites should be placed to prevent the sutures from tearing out and, just as in the open procedure, it is important to get mucosa with all bites.

On completion of the anastamosis, a chest tube is placed under direct vision through the lower trocar site with the tip lying near the anastomosis. The other ports are removed and the sites are closed with absorbable suture.

Generally, the patient is left NPO for 4–5 days at which time an esophagram is obtained to check for any leak. If none are found, oral feeds are started and the chest tube is removed.

Thoracoscopic procedures including mediastinal mass resections, lobectomies, wedge resections, and lung biopsies are all being performed successfully in the pediatric population. These procedures are described in greater detail in the sources listed in suggested readings.

Further Reading

1. Avansino JR, Goldman B, Sawin RS, Flum DR (2005) Primary operative versus non-operative therapy for pediatric empyema: a meta-analysis. Pediatrics 115:1652–1659
2. Bax NM, Van der Zee DC (1998) Laparoscopic treatment of intestinal malrotation in children. Surg Endosc 12:1314–1316
3. Bax K, Georgeson KE, Rothenberg SS, Valla JS, Yeung CK (eds) (2008) Endoscopic surgery in infants and children. Springer, Berlin
4. Georgeson KE, Jona JZ, Rothenberg SS et al (1999) Primary laparoscopic assisted endorectal colon pull-through for Hirschsprung's disease – a new gold standard. Ann Surg 229:678–683
5. Georgeson KE, Inge TA, Albanese C (2000) Laparoscopically assisted anorectal pull-through for high imperforate anus – a new technique. J Pediatr Surg 35:927–930
6. Holcomb GW, Rothenberg SS et al (2005) Thoracoscopic repair of esophageal atresia and tracheoesophageal fistula: a multi-institutional analysis. Am J Surg 242:1–9
7. Holcomb GW, Georgeson KE, Rothenberg SS (eds) (2008) Atlas of pediatric laparoscopy and thoracoscopy. Elsevier, Amsterdam
8. Laborde F, Folligut T, Batisse A et al (1995) Video-assisted thoracoscopic surgical interruption: the technique of choice for patent ductus arteriosus. Routine experience in 230 pediatric cases. J. Cardiovasc Surg 110:1681–1684
9. Levitt MA, Rothenberg SS, Tantoco JG et al (2003) Complication avoidance in miniature access pyloromyotomy. Pediatr Endosurg Innov Tech 7:291–296
10. Partrick DA, Rothenberg SS (2001) Thoracoscopic resection of mediastinal masses in infants and children; an evolution of technique and results. J Pediatr Surg 36:1165–1167
11. Rothenberg SS (1998) Thoracoscopy in infants and children. Semin Pediatr Surg 7:213–219
12. Rothenberg SS (2002) Laparoscopic duodeno-duodenostomy for duodenal obstruction in infants and children. J Pediatr Surg 37:1088–1089
13. Rothenberg SS (2005) First decades experienced with laparoscopic fundoplication in infants and children. J Pediatr Surg 40:142–147
14. Rothenberg SS, Bealer J, Chang J (1999) Primary laparoscopic gastrostomy button for feeding tubes. Surg Endosc 13:995–997

Part V

Principles of Pediatric Urology

Urinary Tract Infection

5.1

Chandrasen K. Sinha, Anand Pandey, and Devesh Misra

The urinary tract is a common portal of infection in childhood. Nevertheless, though symptoms may be suggestive, diagnosis is made by urine microscopy and quantitative culture of a properly collected sample of urine.

- F≫M (except in the first year of life when males predominate).
- Eight percentage of girls and 1–2% of all boys will get a urinary tract infection (UTI) during their childhood.

5.1.1
Microbiology

- *Escherichia coli* is the most common bacteria and is found in 80% of all UTIs.

Other pathogens include

- Gram −ve like *Citrobacter, Proteus, Pseudomonas*, and *Serratia*.
- Gram +ve like *Staphylococcus spp., Enterococcus spp.*, and *Hemophilus spp.*

The route of infection may be ascending (via the urethra) or hematogenous (commoner in infants).

5.1.2
Risk Factors

- Antenatally diagnosed renal anomalies
- Family history of renal disease or VUR

D. Misra (✉)
Paediatric Surgery Department, Royal London Hospital, London, UK

C. K. Sinha and M. Davenport (eds.), *Handbook of Pediatric Surgery*,
DOI: 10.1007/978-1-84882-132-3_5.1, © Springer-Verlag London Limited 2010

- Bladder outflow obstruction (i.e., urethral valves)
- Neurogenic bladder or dysfunctional voiding
- Urolithiasis
- Constipation

5.1.3
Clinical Features

Symptoms depend largely on the age of the child. Fever, dysuria, urgency, frequency, and urinary incontinence are only really seen in older children and adolescents. In infants, poor feeding, failure to thrive, temperature instability, jaundice, and vomiting may all be found.

> In general, UTI must be suspected and urine must be tested in any child with a fever above 38°C if no other cause is evident.

Examination may show renal angle, abdominal or suprapubic tenderness, an abdominal mass, or a palpable bladder. Dribbling, poor stream, or straining to void may also be noticed. Hypertension might suggest hydronephrosis or renal parenchyma disease. In severe cases, dehydration and sepsis may be evident.

Uncircumcised males have a higher incidence of UTI than circumcised ones.

5.1.4
Investigations

- Urinalysis
- *Clean-catch sample* – adhesive urobags (convenient in infants) are not ideal because of contamination. In the male, retract foreskin to expose the meatus. Catheter specimen or a suprapubic sample (under ultrasonic guidance) is needed rarely.
- *Urine dipstick* – testing for leukocyte esterase or nitrite positivity (recommended mainly for >3-year-old). The combination of both the tests increases the diagnostic accuracy. Other markers that have been evaluated albeit without any appreciable benefit are N-acetyl β-glycosaminidase (NAG), β_2 microglobulin, and interleukin-8.
- *Urine microscopy* (mainly for <3-year-old) for WBCs (>5 per high-power field), RBCs, bacteria, casts, and skin contamination (e.g., epithelial cells). Bacteriuria (preferably with pyuria) is considered positive; however, if there is pyuria without bacteriuria, then antibiotics can still be started if there is strong clinical evidence of UTI. Schistosomiasis must be suspected in children who have lived in Africa previously and who present with recurrent gross hematuria.

- *Urine culture* – sending the urine sample for culture is advisable, even if the urinalysis results are inconclusive.
  - Bacterial counts of $>10^5$ are diagnostic of UTI.
  - Bacterial counts 10^{3-5} – repeat test. A persistent pure growth of 10^{3-5} may be considered positive in the right clinical setting.
  - Bacterial count $<10^3$ – not significant. (N.B., if the sample was obtained by suprapubic puncture, then any organisms are diagnostic!).
  - If urine cannot be cultured immediately, then boric acid should be added and the sample refrigerated.

Contamination with perineal flora may mask an existing UTI. Urinary tract abnormalities may be associated with growth of multiple organisms.

5.1.5
Imaging – Proven UTI

Traditional approach

- Birth to 1 year
  - US, DMSA scan, and voiding cystourethrogram (VCUG)
- 1–5 years
  - US and DMSA only
- Five years
  - US only

In UK, the National Institute of Clinical Excellence (NICE) has suggested modification to

- Birth to 6 months
  - US only. (DMSA and VCUG are required if there is abnormality on US, or if there is evidence of severe, atypical, or recurrent UTI).
- Six months to 3 years
  - US and DMSA required if there is severe, atypical, or recurrent UTI.
  - VCUG if there are abnormalities on US, a family history of VUR, or a poor urinary stream.
- Three years
  - US and DMSA as above. No need of VCUG in most cases.
- *Renal and bladder US* – for size and shape of kidneys; presence or absence of ureter, etc. Useful in urolithiasis, hydronephrosis, hydroureter, and ureterocele. In toilet-trained children, the scan can give useful information about bladder emptying.
- *VCUG* – used to diagnose posterior urethral valves or VUR. Bladder anatomy is delineated to show bladder diverticulae or features of neurogenic bladder. In girls, a radioisotope direct isotope cystogram (DIC) is preferred, as the radiation dose is much smaller.

A DIC does not give pictures of the urethra (not required in females!). (N.B., Oral antibiotic prophylaxis should be given for 3 days, starting 1 day before the date of the cystogram).

- *Radio-isotope renal studies*
  - — DMSA[1] scan is the investigation of choice, as it shows the kidney outline and detects renal scars.
  - — MAG-3[2] renogram is preferred (to a DMSA scan) if there is hydronephrosis or if the ureters are dilated. This latter study can pick up VUR in the indirect cystogram phase in toilet-trained children.

5.1.6
Management

Parenteral antibiotics (e.g., ceftriaxone or cefotaxime) should be given to all infants (<3 month) or older patients who are sick. If acute pyelonephritis is present, then the duration of therapy should be ~10 days. Oral antibiotic (e.g., cephalexin or co-amoxiclav) can be started once the patient is afebrile.

A proposal by NICE suggests that lower UTI/cystitis in patients aged over 3 months can be treated with oral antibiotics for 3 days only, provided patients are not sick and there is a good response within 48 h. Besides cephalexin and co-amoxiclav, trimethoprim, or nitrofurantoin may be considered based on regional sensitivities. This latter is an important consideration as up to a third of community acquired UTIs in many parts of the world are nowadays resistant to trimethoprim.

Routine antibiotic prophylaxis is not recommended any more after the first UTI but may have a role to play in recurrent infections. Conditions like constipation and dysfunctional voiding are actually more common causes of recurrent UTI than diseases like VUR, and must be diligently looked for.

Asymptomatic bacteriuria does not require treatment but needs careful follow-up. If symptoms appear, then urine may need to be tested again and treatment started.

5.1.7
Outcome

Most patients with UTI are uncomplicated and respond readily to outpatient antibiotic treatment without further sequelae. Complicated UTI needs prolonged follow-up to prevent long-term sequelae like renal parenchymal scarring, hypertension, decreased renal function, and renal failure.

---

[1]Di Mercapto Succinyl Acid (DMSA) - both being attached to radioactive tracer isotope ^{99m}Technetium
[2]Mercapto Acetyl tri Glycine (MAG-3).

Further Reading

1. Goldsmith BM, Campos JM (1990) Comparison of urine dipstick, microscopy, and culture for the detection of bacteriuria in children. Clin Pediatr 29:214–218
2. Michael M, Hodson EM, Craig JC et al (2003) Short versus standard duration oral antibiotic therapy for acute urinary tract infection in children. Cochrane Database Syst Rev (1):CD003966
3. NICE recommendations. www.nice.org.uk/nicemedia/pdf/CG54quickrefguide.pdf
4. Price E, Misra D, Larcher V (2000) UTIs: accurate diagnosis and effective treatment. Prescriber 11:21–38
5. Samuel M, Misra D, Price E, Larcher V (2000) Schistosoma hematobium infection in children in Britain. Br J Urol 85:316–318

The Ureter

D. K. Gupta, Vijai D. Upadhyaya and S. P. Sharma

Anatomy

Retroperitoneal tubular structure linking kidneys to bladder; lying on psoas major, and crossing in front of bifurcating iliac artery to enter the base of the bladder in a short submucosal tunnel. The pelvic ureter is crossed by the vas in males and by the broad ligament and uterine vessels in females. Structurally, it is composed of two muscle spirals (inner "longitudinal" and outer "circular") and is lined by urothelium throughout.

Radiologically – arises at level of L1/2, descends on the tip of transverse process, crossing pelvis at ischial spine, before veering medially toward bladder.

5.2.1
Embryology

The ureteric bud branches from the caudal portion of the Wolffian (mesonephric) duct (fourth to sixth week). Cranial portion joins with the metanephric blastema and begins to induce nephron formation. The ureter is believed to be solid at this stage and recanalizes (initially in midureter). Failure of this may explain some UPJ obstructions. Caudally, the mesonephric duct (along with the ureteral bud) is incorporated into the cloaca as it forms the bladder trigone.

Alterations in bud number, position, or time of development result in ureteral anomalies; early branching may result in incomplete duplication, with a single ureteral orifice and bifid proximal ureters. An accessory ureteral bud creates a complete duplication, with the upper ureter usually protruding into the bladder more medially and inferiorly than the lower ureter. Ectopic termination of a single system or of the ureter of a duplex system is the result of the high (cranial) origin of the ureteral bud from the mesonephric duct. Because of the delayed incorporation of the ureteral bud into the bladder, the resulting position of the ureteral orifice is more caudal and medial.

D. K. Gupta (✉)
Paediatric Surgery Department, Institute of Medical Sciences, Varanasi, India

C. K. Sinha and M. Davenport (eds.), *Handbook of Pediatric Surgery*,
DOI: 10.1007/978-1-84882-132-3_5.2, © Springer-Verlag London Limited 2010

5.2.2
Ureteropelvic junction[1] (UPJ) obstruction

- Hydronephrosis ~1 in 500 pregnancies – UPJ obstruction ~50%
- M:F 2:1; L:R 3:2
- Bilateral obstruction (10–40%)
- Other urological pathology (~50%) – e.g., contralateral UPJ obstruction, VUR
- Other system pathology – uncommon, e.g., VATER association

Most UPJ obstructions are now detected by antenatal ultrasonography (U/S).

5.2.2.1
Etiology

- Intrinsic
- Usually due to the intrinsic narrowing (patent but aperistaltic). Shows ↓ muscle fibers, and replacement by fibrotic tissue with disruption of spiral orientation.
- Rarely – mucosal valves, polyps, and true ureteric strictures.
- Extrinsic
  - Aberrant or supernumerary renal vessels. ~30% of UPJ, an artery directly enters the lower pole of the kidney.

Secondary UPJ obstruction can result from severe vesicoureteral reflux (VUR).

5.2.2.2
Clinical Features

- Most infants are usually asymptomatic, having been detected through prenatal screening US.
- Older children (and adults) present episodic flank or abdominal pain (~50%), a palpable flank mass (~50%), hematuria, or recurrent UTIs (~30%).

5.2.2.3
Investigations

- Antenatal ultrasonography (definition of hydronephrosis)
- Renal pelvis AP diameter >4 mm at a gestational age of <33 weeks
- Renal pelvis AP diameter of >7 mm at a gestational age of ≥33 weeks

---

[1]For many years was pelviureteric junction (PUJ) obstruction!

Society of Fetal Urology (SFU)

Grade 0 – normal kidney

1. Grade 1 – minimal pelvic dilation
2. Grade 2 – greater pelvic dilation without caliectasis
3. Grade 3 – caliectasis without cortical thinning
4. Grade 4 – hydronephrosis with cortical thinning.

5.2.2.3.1
Postnatal Ultrasonography – Primary Investigations Tool
for Hydronephrosis

- Anechoic or hypoechoic cavity that splits the bright, central echo pattern of the renal sinus.
- AP diameter of the renal pelvis correlated with likelihood of obstruction but not degree of obstruction. Requires complementary radioisotope scans.
- False-positive, e.g., large extrarenal pelvis, peripelvic renal cyst, nonobstructive hydronephrosis, or VUR.
- Renal pyramids may look sonolucent and lead to an erroneous appearance of caliectasis because of medullary immaturity at <3 months of age.

5.2.2.3.2
Radioisotope Scan

- MAG3 (rather than DTPA[2]) is radionuclide of choice and is both filtered and secreted by the renal tubules.

  - The drainage curve of an obstructed kidney fails to decline even after the administration of diuretics – t1/2 is >20 min.
  - Reduction in differential renal function (<40%) – key sign of UPJ obstruction.

5.2.2.3.3
IVP (Uncommonly Used in Children)

- Shows dilatation of the renal calyces and pelvis, funneling down to a narrow beak end, with nonvisualization of the ipsilateral ureter.
- Delayed imaging is essential to maximize visualization of the urinary tract, because the higher volume of urine in a hydronephrotic pelvis dilutes the contrast medium and delays its passage into the ureter, even in the absence of functional obstruction.
- IV furosemide (0.5–1.0 mg/kg) may help in differentiating true UPJ obstruction from nonobstructive hydronephrosis.

---

[2]DTPA – Diethylene triamine penta-acetic acid.

5.2.2.4
Treatment

- Antenatally detected hydronephrosis – optimal management is controversial.
  - Conservative management in group with good renal function (>40%) is reasonable.
  - Pyeloplasty (needed in <50%) for group with functional deterioration and increasing dilatation.

5.2.2.5
Surgery

- Conventional pyeloplasty
  - Incision – lumbotomy, flank, or anterior extraperitoneal incision.
  - Anderson–Hynes[3] – excision of the narrowed segment, spatulation, and anastomosis to the most dependent portion of the renal pelvis.
  - Foley[4] YV-plasty for high ureteral insertion and most cases of horseshoe kidneys.
- Endourological pyeloplasty – including use of balloon dilatations, percutaneous antegrade endopyelotomy, and retrograde ureteroscopic endopyelotomy.
- Laparoscopic techniques – Laparoscopic dismembered pyeloplasty yields results that are comparable with those of the open technique.

5.2.3
Duplex Anomalies

> Ureteral duplication is the most common anomaly of the urinary tract~8% in children being evaluated for UTI.

Single renal unit with two pelvicaliceal systems, which may vary from a single ureter and a duplex collecting system, bifid ureters *(partial or incomplete duplication)*, or two ureters that empty separately into the bladder *(complete duplication)*.

- Incomplete ureteral duplication ~1 in 25.
- Complete duplication is present ~1 in 500.
- Ipsilateral complete duplication ~40% chance of a contralateral complete duplication.
- Family history ~10% of siblings.

---

[3]Jock C Anderson, Wilfred Hynes – urologist and plastic surgeon, respectively, working in Sheffield, UK.
[4]Frederic EB Foley (1891–1966) – American urologist, working in Boston, MA. More famous for his catheter, designed as a medical student in 1929.

The upper ureter is associated with ectopic insertion, ureterocele, and/or obstruction, whereas the lower ureter is frequently associated with VUR. The upper pole ureter crosses and inserts caudally and more medially in the bladder (Weigert–Meyer[5] rule).

5.2.3.1
Clinical Features

Most present with an abnormal finding on routine prenatal US. Otherwise, UTI in the first few months of life is the most common presentation, perhaps leading to life-threatening urosepsis. Infants may also exhibit failure to thrive or nonspecific gastrointestinal symptoms. Older children also present with features of UTI, but hematuria or flank pain may also occur.

5.2.3.2
Investigations

5.2.3.2.1
Ultrasound

- ↑ Renal measurements than those of the contralateral nonduplicated side.
- Disparate hydronephrosis – especially with upper pole dilation associated with an obstructed or ectopic ureter or with a ureterocele.
- ↑ Echogenicity and renal cysts suggest accompanying renal dysplasia.

IVP

May show duplicated collecting systems and their level of confluence.

- Distinct images are usually observed with single-system intravesical ureteroceles because duplicated systems generally have poorly functioning renal moieties associated with ectopia or ureteroceles.
- Delayed images are helpful in identifying poorly functioning renal units.

VCUG

Duplicated collecting systems with lower pole reflux may be visualized.

- Configuration of the kidney lacks opacification of the nonrefluxing upper pole, giving it the appearance of a *drooping lily*.
- Ectopic ureters generally do not reflux unless they are lying outside the bladder neck. In this case, the refluxing unit opacifies only during voiding, when the bladder neck is open. Occasionally, the radiologist may inadvertently pass a catheter transurethrally up the ectopic ureter. The initial films then opacify only that collecting system and not the bladder.

---

[5]Carl Weigert (1845–1904) and Robert Meyer (b1864) – German pathologist and physician, respectively.

Radioisoptope scan: usually MAG3 to evaluate relative renal function and drainage including segmental renal function (upper moiety vs. lower moiety).

5.2.3.3
Treatment

Ureteral duplication alone requires no specific intervention. Duplication anomalies with associated pathology (e.g., VUR, obstruction), however, require appropriate medical therapy and, possibly, surgical correction.

5.2.4
Ectopic Ureter

Bilateral single-system ureteral ectopia is rare and usually coexists with a multitude of other urinary tract abnormalities (e.g., VUR, renal dysplasia, rudimentary bladder development, etc.).

- Female predominant M:F 1:6.
- >80% of the ectopic ureters drain duplicated systems (usually upper pole of duplex kidney).
- Most ectopic ureters in males drain a single system (~10% bilateral).

5.2.4.1
Clinical Features

Most girls will present with constant urinary incontinence or vaginal discharge. Boys may present with recurrent epididymitis before puberty, while after puberty there may be chronic prostatitis, with painful intercourse and ejaculation.

Incontinence in males is never due to an ectopic ureter because it never inserts distal to the external urethral sphincter. Single-system ureteral ectopia reveals widespread renal dysplasia in 90% of affected kidneys. Duplicated-system ureteral ectopia reveals renal dysplasia in ~50% of affected renal moieties.

5.2.4.2
Investigations

All of the above but include cystovaginoscopy to determine the site of ectopic orifice (Table 5.2.1).

Table 5.2.1   Site of ectopic orifice

Females (%)	
Bladder neck/urethra	35
vestibule	35
Vagina	25
Uterus	<5
Males (%)	
Bladder neck/prostatic urethra	45
Seminal vesicle	40
Ejaculatory ducts	10
Vas/epididymis	<5

5.2.4.3
Surgery

Depends on symptoms, associated duplex system, and the status of kidneys.

- Nephrectomy – single system with minimally or nonfunctioning kidney.
- Heminephrectomy – duplex kidney with minimally functioning upper moiety.
- Ureteric reimplantation – single-system good functioning kidney.
- Ureteropyelostomy or ureteroureterostomy – duplex with salvageable function.

5.2.5
Megaureter

May be classified as

1. Obstructed – male predominant M:F 4:1 L>R Bilateral ~20%
    (a) Primary – due to adynamic juxtavesical segment of the ureter.
    (b) Secondary to ↑vesical pressures, e.g., PUV or a neurogenic bladder.
2. Refluxing
    (a) Primary – associated with severe VU reflux.
    (b) Megacystitis megaureter syndrome.
    (c) Secondary to ↑vesical pressures, e.g., PUV or a neurogenic bladder.
3. Obstructed/refluxing
4. Nonobstructed/nonrefluxing.

5.2.5.1
Clinical Features

Possible features include increasing hydroureteronephrosis, decrease in renal function of involved kidney, UTI, and recurrent flank pain.

5.2.5.2
Investigations

Including US (hydronephrosis and hydroureter); MAG3 scan (define degree of obstruction and assess differential renal function); IVU (delineate the anatomy), and VCUG (will show if there is associated VUR).

5.2.5.3
Management

Ureteral reimplantation – usually indicated for that associated with severe VUR or obstruction.

1. Mobilize the megaureter *via* an intravesical, extravesical, or combined approach.
2. Reduce ureteral caliber.
   (a) Hendren[6] technique – excision of distal redundant ureter.
   (b) Kalicinski[7] (plication, then folding over) or Starr (invagination) techniques.
3. Antireflux reimplant.

Occasionally, the function of the kidney drained by a megaureter is severely impaired, and nephroureterectomy may be necessary.

5.2.6
Ureteroceles

Defined as – cystic dilatations of the terminal, intravesical, and usually stenotic ureter. The opening is ectopic in ~60% cases.

- ~1 in 4,000
- Female predominant (M:F 1:4)
- ~10% bilateral

- ~80% cases are associated with duplex system
  — Usually upper pole

---

[6]W Hardy Hendren III (b 1926) American pediatric urologist working in Boston, MA.
[7]Zygmunt H Kalicinski (1927–1996) Polish pediatric urologist.

Types of Ureterocele

- Number
  - Single-system ureteroceles – single kidney, collecting system, and ureter.
  - Duplex-system ureteroceles.
- Position
  - Orthotopic ureterocele – orifice is located in a normal anatomic position. Usually arises from a single renal unit with one collecting system (more common in adults).
  - Ectopic ureterocele – orifice located in an ectopic position (e.g., bladder neck or urethra). Typically from the upper pole moiety of a duplex system (more common in children).

Stephens[8] classification – based on the features of the affected ureteral orifice:

(a) *Stenotic ureteroceles.*
(b) *Sphincteric ureterocele* – refers to those that lie distal to the internal sphincter. The ureterocele orifice may be normal or patulous, but the distal ureter leading to it becomes obstructed by the activity of the internal sphincter.
(c) *Sphincterostenotic ureteroceles* – characteristics of (i) and (ii).
(d) *Cecoureteroceles* are elongated beyond the ureterocele orifice by tunneling under the trigone and the urethra.

5.2.6.1
Clinical Features

May include UTI, urosepsis, obstructive voiding symptoms, retention, failure to thrive, hematuria, cyclic abdominal pain, and stone formation.

5.2.6.2
Investigations

- US
  - Usually seen as a well-defined cystic intravesical mass that can be proximally followed into a dilated ureter.
- IVU (not common)
  - Shows duplicated collecting systems and their level of confluence.
  - *Cobra head* or *spring onion* configuration at the bladder level.

---

[8]Frank Douglas Stephens (b 1913). One of a dynasty of Australian pediatric surgeons who worked at Royal Melbourne Childrens Hospital.

- VCUG
  - Filling defect in the bladder base. Identifying which side large ureteroceles are associated with can be difficult.
  - Reflux of the ipsilateral lower pole is observed in ~50%.
  - Contralateral reflux ~25%.
  - Reflux into the ureterocele may be observed in ~10%.

5.2.6.3
Surgery

Is aimed at relief of obstruction.

- Endoscopic decompression
  - If urgent decompression is required (e.g., urosepsis, severe compromise in renal function).
  - Better results for single-system intravesical ureterocele than for ectopic ureteroceles (10–40%).
- Reimplantation

Further Reading

1. Mears AL, Raza SA, Sinha AK, Misra D (2007) Micturating cystourethrograms are not necessary for all cases of antenatally diagnosed hydronephrosis. J Pediatr Urol 3:264–267
2. Merlini E, Lelli Chiesa P (2004) Obstructive ureterocele – an ongoing challenge. World J Urol 22:107–114
3. Ninan GK, Sinha C, Patel R, Marri R (2009) Dismembered pyeloplasty using double 'J' stent in infants and children. Pediatr Surg Int 25:191–194
4. Vemulakonda VM, Cowan CA, Lendvay TS, Joyner BD, Grady RW (2008) Surgical management of congenital ureteropelvic junction obstruction: a pediatric health information system database study. J Urol 180:1689–1692

Vesico-Ureteric Reflux

5.3

Devendra K. Gupta and Shilpa Sharma

This is rather like oesophageal reflux, common in the young and tends to improve with age.

Reflux is noted in up to 40% of fetuses.

- Female predominant
- Peak incidence at 3 years
- Familial incidence is 2–4% of all cases
- Unilateral or bilateral (60%).

5.3.1
Pathology

- Primary – presumed to occur owing to a short submucosal tunnel.
- Intravesical length:width should be about 5:1 to prevent VUR (Table 5.3.1).
- Secondary – e.g., PUV, anterior urethral valves, neurogenic bladder, ureteroceles, bladder diverticula, and ectopic ureters associated with duplex system.

5.3.2
Clinical Features

Usually with symptoms of UTI. But others include

- Renal scarring – radiologically demonstrated scarring is almost always due to reflux. Almost 30–60% of children with VUR have scars on initial evaluation. This impairs subsequent renal growth.

D. K. Gupta (✉)
Department of Pediatric Surgery, All India Institute of Medical Sciences, New Delhi, India

C. K. Sinha and M. Davenport (eds.), *Handbook of Pediatric Surgery*,
DOI: 10.1007/978-1-84882-132-3_5.3, © Springer-Verlag London Limited 2010

- Renal dysfunction – impairment of renal concentrating ability and a gradual deterioration of GFR.
- Hypertension – reflux nephropathy may lead to severe hypertension in 10–20% of children with VUR and renal scars.
- Reduced somatic growth.

5.3.2.1
Investigations

Including urine analysis for infection; US (hydroureteronephrosis); MAG 3 scan (assess differential renal function); and DMSA (for renal scars) and VCUG (once infection treated, for degree of VUR) and GFR (for baseline renal function in those likely to be poor). Direct radionuclide cystography (DRCG) is usually reserved for follow-up scans.

5.3.3
Grading

According to the severity, the reflux has been graded from 1 to 5, 1 being mild and 5 being most severe with dilatation and tortuousity of ureters (Fig. 5.3.1).

5.3.4
Management

Low-grade reflux is more likely to resolve spontaneously with age (in the absence of any malformation), but the management options include:

- Antibiotic chemoprophylaxis
  — Long-term prophylactic antibiotics (few months – 2 years).

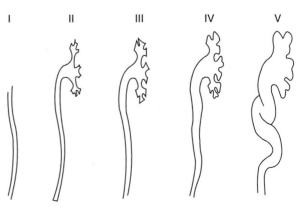

Fig. 5.3.1 Classification of ureteric reflux

Table 5.3.1   Classification of VUR

	Description
I	Lower ureter/s (without dilatation)
II	All ureter (without dilatation)
III	Dilated pelvicalyceal and ureter. Flat fornices
IV	PLUS convex ornices, dilated ureter
V	PLUS tortuosity of ureters

— Amoxycillin, co-trimoxazole, cephalexin, nitrofurantoin, and quinolones.
— Cyclic administration.
— Ensure compliance.

Better results are found in unilateral (vs. bilateral); infants (vs. >5 years), nondilated ureters (<1 cm).

- Submucosal injection therapy
  — Subureteric injection of Deflux® (dextranomer microspheres in sodium hyaluronic solution) – now used as the first choice in many centers. Teflon paste (STING) was used previously.
  — Results better for lower grades of reflux (>80% success) may be repeated to improve success rate even in higher grades.
  — Less successful in children with neurogenic bladder, etc.

5.3.5
Surgery

Surgery is indicated once the initial management with chemoprophylaxis including the submucosal injection therapy has failed. Undisputed indications for surgical therapy include:

- Secondary VUR due to anatomical anomalies such as Hutch diverticulum, ureterocele, duplex ureter, primary megaureters, PUV, and neurogenic bladder.
- Failure of conservative management despite prophylaxis therapy given for a maximum period of 2 years.
- Poor compliance to medical management.
- Persistent UTI or breakthrough infections more than twice in a year despite chemoprophylaxis.
- Appearance of new scars or enlargement of preexisting scars during medical management.
- Deterioration of renal function despite being on antibiotics at any age.
- Higher grades (IV, V) – at any age.
- Documented hypertension due to renal cause.
- Single kidney with higher grade of VUR.
- Decrease in renal growth on prophylaxis or lack of somatic growth.

- Reimplantation of ureters
- Transtrigonal ureteric (Cohen[1]) reimplantation – commonest alternative.
- Intravesical technique (Leadbetter–Politano) usually if a single-sided pathology requiring reimplantation.
- Extravesical detrusorraphy technique (Lich and Gregoir) – considered if the reflux is being treated with another operative procedure in the abdomen.
- ±Ureteric tapering or plication.

5.3.5.1
Postoperative Management

Typically, extavesical drains and a ureteric catheters are kept for 7–10 days. Continue antibiotic for ~3 months, and a follow-up VCUG or DRCG confirms the absence of reflux.

5.3.6
Complications

- Persistent reflux and ureteric obstruction due to devascularisation, kinking or torsion of the distal ureter.
- Persistent reflux – usually lower grade and it tends to improve spontaneously on continued antibiotics.
- Intravesical calculi – if nonabsorbable sutures are used.
- Ureteral obstruction due to angulation, or hiatal obstruction or temporarily due to oedema or contraction of the thickened bladder wall during spasm.
- Injury to the bowel, Fallopian tubes and vas deferens, specifically in Leadbetter–Politano technique, since there is inadequate visualization of the retrovesical structures.

5.3.7
Outcome

- Medical management, though successful in low grades of reflux, has to be continued for a long period and the outcome remains unpredictable, as it is patient-dependent.
- Surgical repair has a success rate varying from 93 to 98% with improvements in renal catch-up growth, concentration capacity and function.
- Deflux® et al. injections have reduced the number of surgical procedures performed in the recent past. However, the injection is expensive though the availability has improved worldwide.

---

[1]Joseph Cohen – South African-born pediatric urologist working in Manchester, UK.

- Severe VUR treated with medical vs. surgery
- No difference in terms of change in GFR, progression of renal scarring or recurrent UTI.

The main factor determining the outcome is the extent of renal scarring or renal parenchymal damage at the onset. Surgery does correct vesicoureteral reflux but does not significantly alter the clinical outcomes in these patients.

Further Reading

1. Birmingham Reflux Study Group (1987) Prospective trial of operative versus non-operative treatment of severe vesicoureteric reflux in children: five years' observation. Br Med J 295:237–241
2. Gupta DK (2005) Vesico-ureteric reflux. In: Willital GH, Kielly E, Gohary A, Gupta DK, Li M, Suchida YT (eds) Atlas of children's surgery, 1st edn. PABST, Germany, pp 353–356
3. International Reflux Study Committee (1981) Medical versus surgical treatment of primary vesico-ureteral reflux: a prospective international study in children. J Urol 125:272–283
4. Puri P, Chertin B, Velayudham M, Dass L, Colhoun E (2003) Treatment of vesicoureteral reflux by endoscopic injection of dextranomer/hyaluronic acid copolymer: preliminary results. J Urol 170:1541–1544; discussion 1544

Neurogenic Bladder

5.4

George Ninan

Function and ideal – the bladder should have the ability to fill to capacity while maintaining low pressures; a sensation to void when full and be under voluntary control; and to be empty at the end of voiding without residue.

5.4.1
Neurology

- Parasympathetic (predominant)
  - S2–S4 spinal segments, both afferent and efferent via the pelvic nerves to the detrusor muscle.
- Sympathetic
  - T9–L1 spinal segments via sympathetic chain and hypogastric plexus, mainly to the bladder neck.
- Somatic innervation
  - S2–S4 segments via pudendal nerve to supply the external sphincter.

5.4.2
Etiology

Congenital	Acquired
Myleomeningocele	Trauma
Spina bifida occulta (including tethered cord, lipoma of cord)	Tumors
Sacral agenesis	Infarction
	Transverse myelitis

G. Ninan
Paediatric Surgery Department, Leicester Royal Infirmary, Leicester, UK

C. K. Sinha and M. Davenport (eds.), *Handbook of Pediatric Surgery*,
DOI: 10.1007/978-1-84882-132-3_5.4, © Springer-Verlag London Limited 2010

- Neurogenic bladder in children is almost always due to spinal cord anomalies (both congenital and acquired).
- Nonneurogenic neuropathic bladder (Hinman–Allen syndrome) is a specific entity, in which there is a significant psychological overlay in addition to bladder dysfunction, and will not be considered further in this chapter.

The most common spinal cord anomaly resulting in a neurogenic bladder is myelomeningocele (see Chap. 9.1).

5.4.3
Clinical Features

- Urge incontinence (overactive detrusor).
- Stress incontinence (underactive sphincter) and giggle incontinence.

Vincent's curtsy – learned behavior in girls, whereby they squat cross-legged with the heel pressed to the perineum, to inhibit voiding.

Assess back for evidence of spina bifida occulta (a hairy patch or lumbosacral lipoma, etc.) or even sacral agenesis.

Full neurological assessment to elicit the integrity of segments S2–4. Achieved by eliciting the *anocutaneous reflex* (S1–3, pudendal nerve) or *bulbocavernous reflex* (S1–3, anal sphincter reflex from glans stimulation), and mapping perianal and lower limb sensation. The anus is usually patulus and the child soils continuously with an absent anocutaneous reflex, and this usually suggests a "safe" bladder.

Concept

- "Unsafe" bladder – inability to empty distended bladder by "Crede" maneuver.
- "Safe" bladder – leaks easily under pressure or usually empty on examination.

5.4.4
Investigations

- *Ultrasound* – looking for upper tract dilatation and postmicturition bladder residual volume.
- *Cystogram* – looking for presence of VUR, trabeculation, diverticular formation, etc.
- *Urodynamics.*

Karl Crede (1819-1892) German obstetrician

5.4.5
Basic Video Urodynamics

5.4.5.1
Essentials

- *Normal bladder capacity*
  - Infants capacity (in mL) = weight (in kg) × 7
  - 1–12 years capacity (in mL) = age (in years) × 30 + 30
  - *For example, 8-year-old child = 8 × 30 + 30 = 270 mL*
- *Detrusor hyperreflexia* – abnormal bladder contractions in a neurogenic bladder and is of significance if the pressure is >30–40 cm H_2O
- *Compliance* – relationship between volume and pressure. For example, at expected bladder capacity, detrusor pressure should be <30–40 cm H_2O
- *Sphincteric incompetence* – sphincteric mechanism opens abnormally at low pressures
- *Leak-point pressure* – point at which external sphincter opens
  - <40 cm H_2O – bladder regarded as "safe"
  - >40 cm H_2O – potential for upper tracts deterioration
- *Detrusor sphincter dyssynergia* – normally detrusor contraction and external sphincter relaxation are synergistic. The opposite may cause ↑ intravesical pressures

Technique – urethral (or suprapubic) catheter (note residual urine volume) attached to Y-connector allowing pressure measurements and filling. A rectal balloon catheter is also used to measure the intraabdominal pressure.

- *Intravesical pressure* is sum of the actual detrusor pressure and intraabdominal pressure.
- *Detrusor pressure* is intravesical pressure minus intraabdominal pressure.

Slow fill at 10–15 mL/min, depending on bladder capacity. Screen for VUR intermittently (e.g., every 50–100 mL).

5.4.6
Patterns of Neurogenic Bladder

- *Contractile bladder* – these are usually the result of suprasacral cord lesions.
  - The innervation of the detrusor and external urethral sphincter are intact and conus reflexes are positive.
  - Voiding usually occurs by detrusor hyperreflexia and is associated with detrusor sphincter dyssynergia. Intravesical pressures are usually high and may ultimately lead to secondary upper renal tract complications.
- *Acontractile bladder.*

— Innervation of both detrusor and external sphincter is destroyed, conus reflexes are negative. Detrusor contractility is absent but some degree of sphincteric incompetence is always present.

— Voiding occurs either by overflow or by raising intraabdominal pressure. A degree of detrusor noncompliance is common.

• *Intermediate bladder dysfunction.* In this bladder, a combination of anomalies is present, including various degrees of detrusor noncompliance, detrusor hyperreflexia, and sphincteric incontinence.

5.4.7
Management

Natural history is one of progressive deterioration by the age of 3 years in up to 60% of all children. This has good correlation with raised intravesical pressure.

Clean intermittent catheterization combined with an anticholinergic (oral or intravesical) is the standard therapy for neurogenic bladder.

Early institution of CIC can prevent both renal damage and secondary bladder wall changes, thereby potentially improving the long-term outcomes.

Both detrusor hyperreflexia and detrusor noncompliance can be treated medically with anticholinergics (e.g., oxybutanin and tolerodine), although surgical maneuvers to increase the capacity and outlet resistance are common.

5.4.7.1
Augmentation cystoplasty ± catheterizable conduit

A cystoplasty using ileum is most commonly performed, but alternative sources include ileocecum, sigmoid colon, and stomach.

Less common alternatives are autoaugmentation, detrusorectomy, and ureterocystoplasty.

5.4.7.1.1
Complications of Cystoplasty

1. Mucus production leading to catheter blockage, infection, and bladder stones.
2. Metabolic changes – hyperchloremic alkalosis electrolyte disturbance, systemic alkalosis (gastrocystoplasty).
3. Spontaneous perforation.
4. Metaplasia/malignancy.
5. Bowel problems, e.g., diarrhea, vitamin B12 deficiency.
6. Dysuria and hematuria (gastrocystoplasty).

5.4.8
Sphincteric Incompetence

Medical treatment remains unsatisfactory but marginal improvement may be seen with alpha-adrenergic agonists such as ephedrine.

5.4.8.1
Surgical Options

1. Periurethral bulking agents, e.g., collagen, silicone, and Deflux®.
2. Bladder neck suspension and slings, e.g., *Marshal–Marchetti bladder neck suspension* and bladder neck slings.
3. *Pippi-Salle[1] procedure* – urethral lengthening procedure suitable for girls but not for boys.
4. *Mitrofanoff[2] procedure* – involves closure of the bladder neck and using the appendix as an appendicovesicostomy. The appendix is tunneled between the bladder and the abdominal wall, which is then used as a catheterizable stoma.
5. *Artificial urinary sphincter.*
6. *Monti [3]procedure* – when the appendix is unavailable, a segment of ileum can be tubularized and used in a fashion similar to an appendicovesicostomy.

ACE procedure – most neurogenic bladders have associated bowel dysfunction due to neurogenic bowel. An appendix or Monti tube can be implanted between the cecum and the anterior abdominal wall as a catheterizable channel for antegrade continent enemas.

Further Reading

1. Bael A, Lax H, de Jong TP, Hoebeke P et al (2008) The relevance of urodynamic studies for Urge syndrome and dysfunctional voiding: a multicenter controlled trial. J Urol 180:1486–1493
2. Bauer SB (2008) Neurogenic bladder etiology and assessment. Pediatr Nephrol 23:541–551
3. Vincent SA (1966) Postural control of urinary incontinence: the curtsy sign. Lancet 2:631–634

---

[1]Joao L Pippi-Salle – Brazilian urologist, working in Porto Allegre.
[2]Paul Mitrofanoff – French urologist working in Marseilles.
[3]Paul Ricardo Monti – Brazilian urologist.

Posterior Urethral Valves

5.5

M. Gopal and A. Rajimwale

Posterior urethral valves remain the most common reasons for renal failure and renal transplantation in children.

5.5.1
Anatomy

The male urethra is divided into four segments

1. Posterior
   (a) Prostatic urethra – from the bladder neck to the site of "urogenital diaphragm."
   (b) Membranous urethra – "urogenital diaphragm".
2. Anterior
   (a) Bulbar urethra – from the distal margin of the urogenital diaphragm to penoscrotal junction.
   (b) Penile urethra – urethra that traverses the penile shaft including the glans.

5.5.2
Congenital Obstructing Posterior Urethral Membrane

This is a newer concept whereby the uninstrumented infants urethra looks more like a circumferential obstructing membrane with a small central opening, which following catheterization or instrumentation reverts to the classical "valve" appearance. Traditionally, three types of posterior urethral valve has been described (Table 5.5.1)

A. Rajimwale (✉)
Paediatric Surgery Department, Leicester Royal Infirmary, Leicester, UK

C. K. Sinha and M. Davenport (eds.), *Handbook of Pediatric Surgery*,
DOI: 10.1007/978-1-84882-132-3_5.5, © Springer-Verlag London Limited 2010

Table 5.5.1 Young's Classification[1]

	Description	Result
Type I (~95%)	Bicuspid valve from posterior edge of the verumontanum extending distally and anteriorly and fusing in the midline	Obstructive
Type II	Prominent longitudinal folds extending from verumontanum toward the bladder neck	Nonobstructive
Type III (5–10%)	Circumferential ring distal to the verumontanum at the level of the membranous urethra	Obstructive

NB, Cobb's collar[2] (or congenital urethral stricture) – distal membrane with a central opening within bulbous urethra

5.5.3
Clinical Features (Table. 5.5.1)

Antenatal (66%) – dilated posterior urethra and bladder ("key-hole" sign)±hydroureteronephrosis in male fetus on maternal US. Other key features are renal echogenicity and whether there is evidence of oligohydramnios (possible cause of hypoplastic lungs).

Postnatal (33%)

- Poor stream±palpable bladder
- UTI
- Renal failure with poor somatic growth and lethargy
- Diurnal incontinence

5.5.4
Investigation

5.5.4.1
Micturating Cystourethrogram (MCUG) (Fig. 5.5.1)

1. Wide posterior urethra and prominent bladder neck
2. Partial filling of anterior urethra
3. Posterior urethral bulging forward over the bulbous urethra
4. Valve leaflet lucencies - occasionally.

5.5.4.2
Worse Prognostic Factors

1. Antenatal factors
   (a) Gestation at detection (<24 weeks).
   (b) US appearance – cystic changes imply renal dysplasia.

---

[1]Hugh Hampton Young – Father of American urology, described classification in 1919.

Fig. 5.5.1 MCUG showing posterior urethral valves with trabeculated bladder with pseudo-diverticuli

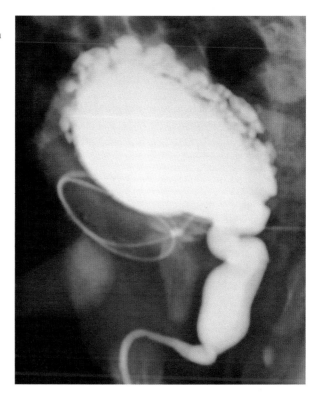

(c) Oligohydraminos.
(d) Fetal urine analysis (usually hypotonic with [Na] <100 mmol/L and [Cl] <90 mmol/L. ↑ [Na >100], [Cl >90], and [β-2-microglobulin >40], [urine osmolality >210 mOsm], and [urine output <2 mL/h] are associated with a worse prognosis).

2. Adverse postnatal factors
  (a) Nadir (i.e., lowest possible) serum creatinine >1 mg/dL (≡88 μmol/L) at 1 year of age.
  (b) US appearance: lack of corticomedullary differentiation suggests poor function.
  (c) Incontinence – inability to achieve diurnal continence signifies bladder dysfunction and this significantly worsens long-term renal function.
  (d) Lack of a protective "pop-off" mechanism such as gross unilateral reflux or urinary ascites.
  (e) Presence of severe reflux.

5.5.5
Management

The principles are

- Drain the bladder

[2]Cobb BG, Wolf JA, Ansell JS (1968) Congenital stricture of the proximal urethral bulb. J Urol; 99:629–631

— Catheterization – infant "feeding" tube is ideal, avoid Foley catheter as can stimulate bladder spasms in the already hypertrophic bladder and can cause secondary ureteric obstruction. If the urethral route is unsuccessful, use suitable suprapubic one.
- Prevent infection
  — Prophylactic antibiotics.
- Preserve renal function
  — May require intensive IV fluids and electrolyte balance.

5.5.5.1
PUV Ablation

- *Transurethral diathermy ablation* and division of the valve leaflets at the 5 and 7 o'clock. (Nd YAG laser used occasionally). Previously, access to the posterior urethra was achieved via a perineal urethrostomy or via a cystostomy. May be complicated by stricture formation or inadequate ablation.

5.5.5.2
Temporary Urinary Diversion

If ablation not feasible (small infant or lack of scopes), urinary diversion will be required. This may include vesicostomy, ureterostomy, or pelvicostomy.

- *Vesicostomy*

Dome of the bladder bought to the skin midway between the umbilicus and the symphysis pubis. This allows drainage but also cycles urine to the bladder and maintains volume. May be closed once renal function has stabilized, upper tracts have diminished, and the child is large enough for a valve ablation.

(*NB, Valve ablation should be performed at the time of vesicostomy closure to avoid urethral stricture developing in a "dry" urethra.*)

Higher levels of drainage include *the bilateral ureterostomy or pelvicostomy*. Long-term studies have shown that there is no reduction in renal failure – because of intrinsic renal dysplasia. These diversion procedures also result in a small capacity bladder. Therefore, consider only when a vesicostomy is not providing adequate drainage due to concomitant obstruction at the VUJ or in the presence of pyonephrosis.

5.5.5.2.1
Urinary Ascites (5–10%)

Usually secondary to urine leak from a renal fornix blowout, renal parenchymal rupture, or bladder perforation. Abdominal distension can be marked and cause respiratory compromise.

Peritoneal absorption of urine can lead to uremia. Paradoxically, urine leaks actually protect the kidneys from the deleterious effects of constant high back pressure from bladder.

5.5.5.2.2
Vesicoureteric Reflux (50%)

- Bilateral in 50%.
- Reflux subsides with effective valve ablation (~30%).
- Persistent reflux (~30%).

Persistent VU reflux can be treated with STING procedure or ureteric reimplantation provided that bladder function is normal on urodynamic evaluation.

(NB, Operative intervention for reflux in the "valve bladder" with PUV has a failure rate of 15–30%.)

5.5.6
VURD Syndrome (Valves Unilateral Reflux Dysplasia)

Severe unilateral reflux into a dysplastic kidney. This protects the contralateral kidney from back pressure ("pop-off" mechanism). Others "pop-off" mechanisms include large bladder diverticula, urinary ascites, and a patent urachus.

5.5.7
Bladder Dysfunction and the "Valve Bladder"

Voiding dysfunction is extremely common in children with PUV and is secondary to the long-standing obstruction and mural hypertrophy and fibrosis ("valve" bladder). Urodynamic patterns can change over time from bladder instability during infancy to myogenic failure in older boys.

Bladder dysfunction manifesting as incontinence and persistence of upper tract dilatation is being increasingly recognized as one of the factors responsible for eventual renal deterioration. The underlying mechanisms may be

1. Urine concentrating defects
   (a) Long-standing back pressure leads to the renal tubular dysfunction causing an acquired form of nephrogenic diabetes insipidus.
   (b) ↑ Urine volume exacerbates incontinence and upper tract dilatation.
2. Persistent upper tract dilation
   (a) ↑ Urine output and hold up at the VUJ – caused by ureter passing through the thick, noncompliant bladder wall.

(b) Upper tract pressure studies (Whitaker's test[3]) have shown that the VUJ obstruction is not constant but increases as the bladder fills.

Treatment is difficult and ADH treatment is not usually successful. Timed voiding in older cooperative children and overnight free drainage in children with a continent catheterisable channel (to ensure lower intravesical pressures) can protect upper tracts.

5.5.8
Urodynamic Patterns and treatment options

1. Instability – irregular contractions leading to pain and incontinence.
   (a) Anticholinergics, e.g., oxybutynin and tolterodine.
2. Hypocontractility – leading to overflow incontinence and impedance of upper tract drainage. This so-called "myogenic failure" has been attributed to long-term obstruction or prolonged use of anticholinergics.
   (a) Clean intermittent catheterization or a catheterisable stoma (e.g., Mitrofanoff).
3. Detrusor sphincter dyssynergia – bladder contracts against an unrelaxed sphincter. Historically, bladder neck hypertrophy as seen on the MCUG was thought to play a significant role. Many children went on to have bladder neck incisions. It improved voiding symptoms and upper tracts dilatation in some, but in others it also caused incontinence and retrograde ejaculation.
   (a) alpha blockers – e.g., doxazocin
4. Poor compliance/small volume bladder
   (a) bladder augmentation

5.5.9
Renal Transplantation

Up to 30% of children will ultimately require some form of renal replacement therapy culminating in a transplant. Persistent bladder dysfunction not only increases the risk of developing renal failure but has also been shown to decrease graft survival post transplant.

5.5.10
Fertility Issues

Diminished fertility possibly due to

1. ↑ Posterior urethral pressure in utero may affect prostate development.
2. ↑ Incidence of UDT.

---

[3]Mark Whitaker – British urologist at Cambridge.

3. Semen analysis has shown a much thicker ejaculate with decreased sperm motility.
4. Voiding dysfunction and retrograde ejaculation.

Further Reading

1. Dewan PA (1993) Congenital obstructing posterior urethral membrane (COPUM): further evidence of a common morphological diagnosis. Pediatr Surg Int 8:45–50
2. Elder JS, Shapiro E (2005) The valve bladder. In: Ashcraft KW, Holcomb GW III, Murphy JP (eds) Pediatric surgery, 4th edn. Elsevier Saunders, Philadelphia, pp 788–791
3. Glassberg KI, Horowitz M (2002) Urethral valve and other anomalies of the male urethra. In: Belman AB, King LR, Kramer SA (eds) Clinical pediatric urology, 4th edn. Martin Dunitz, England, pp 899–947
4. Holmdahl G, Sillen U, Bachelara M et al (1995) The changing urodynamic pattern in valve bladders during infancy. J Urol 153:463–467
5. Hoover DL, Duckett JW Jr (1982) Posterior urethral valves, unilateral reflux and renal dysplasia: a syndrome. J Urol 128:994–997
6. Young HH, Frontz WA, Baldwin JC (1919) Congenital obstruction of the posterior urethra. J Urol 3:289–354

Hypospadias

5.6

Vibhash C. Mishra and Hanif G. Motiwala

Hypospadias is a complex of an abnormal ventral meatus, chordee, and a dorsal hooded foreskin. Usually isolated, it can be part of the DSD spectrum.

- One in 300 live-births (but wide variation from 1 in 110 to 1 in 1,250)
- Rising incidence
- Associated with ↑ parity, ↑ maternal age, and ↓ birth weight
- Associated with inguinal hernia and hydrocele (~10%), undescended testes (~8%)

5.6.1
Embryology

The development of male urethra takes place between the 8th and the 15th week of gestation under the influence of testosterone.

1. Formation of posterior urethra with advancement to the developing phallus as the urethral groove.
2. Ventral fusion of urethral folds – completed distally by the in-growth of ectoderm from the tip of the glans.

5.6.2
Etiology

Multifactorial involving genetic, endocrine, and environmental factors.

- *Genetic Factors*

V. C. Mishra (✉)
Urology Department, Wexham Park Hospital, Slough, UK

C. K. Sinha and M. Davenport (eds.), *Handbook of Pediatric Surgery*,
DOI: 10.1007/978-1-84882-132-3_5.6, © Springer-Verlag London Limited 2010

The exact mode of inheritance is unknown, but is suggested by the following facts:

- Monozygotic twins – eightfold increase in the incidence of hypospadias – may be related to a net deficiency of human chorionic gonadotropin (HCG) caused by the increased demand of two fetuses.
- +ve family history – 8% of fathers and 14% of brothers.
- *Endocrine Factors*
- Deficient androgenic stimulation – which in turn may be the result of defective testosterone production, conversion (to dihydrotestosterone (DHT)), or reduced sensitivity (at target organs). Defects in testosterone biosynthesis, mutations in the 5-alpha reductase (5AR) enzyme, and androgen insensitivity syndromes have been associated with hypospadias.
- Increased maternal progesterone exposure – there is a fivefold increase in the incidence among boys conceived by IVF (progesterone is commonly administered). Progesterone is a substrate for 5AR and causes competitive inhibition of conversion of testosterone to DHT.
- *Environmental Factors*
  ↑ Incidence of hypospadias and one hypothesis suggests that there is increased maternal exposure to estrogenic substances (contained in pesticides, milk, plastic linings of metal cans, and pharmaceuticals).

5.6.3
Clinical Features

5.6.3.1
Classification (Fig. 5.6.1)

- Distal (glanular, coronal, and subcoronal) (50%)
- Middle (distal penile, midshaft, and proximal penile) (30%)
- Proximal (penoscrotal, scrotal, and perineal) (20%)

NB, True location of the meatus should be ascertained after correction of the penile curvature.

Although usually isolated, it is important to identify a disorder of sexual differentiation (DSD) – suggested by impalpable testes for instance. DSD occurs in ~15% of cases if gonad is palpable but ~50% of cases if impalpable.

Evaluate using *US, genitography, biochemical, and chromosomal analysis* before making final decisions regarding definitive management (see Chap. 5.8).

In terms of choice of surgical options, assess hypospadias by (1) location of the meatus, (2) degree of chordee, (3) penile size, (4) quality of ventral and proximal shaft skin, (5) quality of distal urethral plate, and (vi) the depth of glanular groove.

5.6.4
Surgery

5.6.4.1
Principles

A hypospadiac penis looks abnormal, may interfere with normal voiding in the standing position, and possibly affect fertility by precluding effective insemination. The goal of surgery is to create a cosmetically acceptable penis, which allows normal voiding with a forward stream and normal vaginal penetration. Therefore, some cases of glanular hypospadias can be left entirely alone.

5.6.4.2
Preoperative

- The current recommendation is to complete the repair of hypospadias before 18 months of age (minimizes psychological impact of genital surgery).
- *Hormone manipulation* – penile size can be increased by weekly intramuscular injections of testosterone or HCG or topical application of testosterone or DHT for 4–6 weeks before surgery. Concern that such prepubertal testosterone may adversely affect the ultimate penile growth has not been substantiated.
- *Orthoplasty* (correction of chordee)
    - (a) Assessment of chordee – artificial erection with intracavernosal injection of either normal saline or prostaglandin E_1.
    - (b) Straightening may be achieved by complete degloving of the penis, excision of a fibrous corpus spongiosum, and dissection of the urethral plate.
    - (c) Dorsal plication of tunica albuginea and/or ventral application of a dermal graft may sometimes be required – again assessed by erection test.
- *Urethroplasty*
    - (a) Advancement techniques (e.g., *MAGPI*[1])
    - (b) Tubularization techniques (e.g., *Snodgrass*[2]) (Fig. 5.6.2)
    - (c) Local tissue flaps (e.g., *Mathieu's perimeatal-based flap*)
    - (d) Two stages using local or extragenital free grafts (e.g., preputial skin, buccal mucosa, and postauricular skin). Two-stage procedures are particularly useful for very proximal hypospadias associated with severe chordee and a small penis. The second stage is performed 6 months or more after the first stage.

---

[1]MAGPI – Meatal Advancement GlanuloPlasty Incorporated
[2]Warren Snodgras – American urologist

Fig. 5.6.1 Types of hypospadias based on the location of meatus and include distal (glanular, coronal, and subcoronal), middle (distal penile, midshaft, and proximal penile), and proximal (penoscrotal, scrotal, and perineal) types

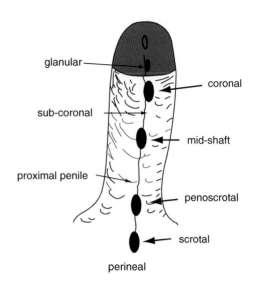

- *Meatoplasty and glanuloplasty*
    - (a) The precise technique varies according to the individual repair, but the common goal is to create a slit-like meatus and cover the distal neourethra with flaps of glans epithelium.

- *Skin coverage*
    - (a) Usually achieved by ventral transfer of preputial skin with any redundant skin trimmed away to resemble that of a circumcision. In some distal cases, a foreskin reconstruction can be contemplated (Fig. 5.6.3).

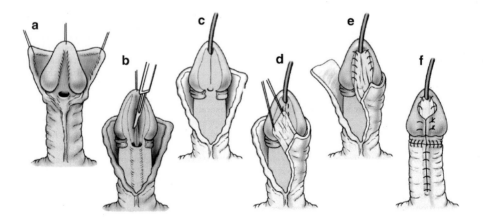

Fig. 5.6.2 Common operations for coronal hypospadias. Snodgrass repair (a-f) (Adapted from Belman et al. (Belman AB, King LR, Kramer SA (eds) (2002) Clinical pediatric urology, 4th edn. Martin Dunitz, London, p 1077, Fig. 32.16))

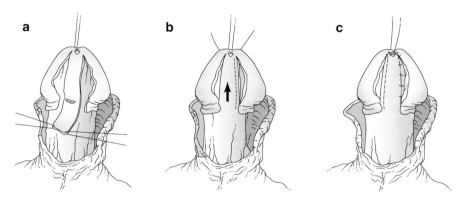

Fig. 5.6.3 Mathieu (meatal based flap) (Belman AB, King LR, Kramer SA (eds) (2002) Clinical pediatric urology, 4th edn. Martin Dunitz, London, p 1076, Fig. 32.15))

5.6.4.3
Postoperative Phase

In our practice – the bladder is drained for 1 week with a "dripping stent," an antimuscarinic agent (e.g., oxybutynin) to reduce bladder spasms, an antibiotic (e.g., trimethoprim) and a soft, pliable, foam dressing.

Early complications include bleeding, hematoma, infection, and breakdown of repair.

5.6.5
Long-Term Outcome

Most series describe a multiplicity of long-term complications such as persistent chordee, meatal stenosis, urethrocutaneous fistula, urethral stricture, and urethral diverticulum. The incidence is highly variable though. Intra-urethral hair growth used to be a complication in the past (inappropriate use of scrotal skin for instance) but should not be seen with modern techniques.

Further Reading

1. Baskin LS (2000) Hypospadias and urethral development. J Urol 163:951–956
2. Duckett JW, Coplen D, Ewalt D (1995) Buccal mucosal urethral replacement. J Urol 153:1660–1663
3. Snodgrass WT (1999) Tubularized incised plate hypospadias repair: indications, technique, and complications. Urology 54:6–11
4. Belman AB, King LR, Kramer SA (eds) (2002) Clinical pediatric urology, 4th edn. Martin Dunitz, London, pp 1076–1077

Bladder Exstrophy, Epispadias, and Cloacal Exstrophy

5.7

Bharat More and Imran Mushtaq

The exstrophy–epispadias complex is a spectrum of midline defects that includes classic bladder exstrophy, epispadias, and cloacal exstrophy.

Classic Bladder Exstrophy

- ~1 in 40,000 live births. M:F 2:1
- Recurrence risk is 1 in 100.

Cloacal Exstrophy

- ~1 in 200,000 M:F 1:1
- Associated with spinal dysraphism (~66%) and short bowel syndrome (33%)

5.7.1
Embryology

Failure of mesenchyme to migrate between the ectodermal and endodermal layers of the lower abdominal wall with subsequent premature rupture of the cloacal membrane. Rupture after complete separation of the GU and GI tracts results in classic bladder exstrophy and prior to descent of the urorectal septum results in cloacal exstrophy *Marshall and Muecke's theory*.

5.7.2
Clinical Features

Antenatal US findings suggestive of exstrophy–epispadias complex are

- Failure to visualize the bladder

B. More (✉)
Paediatric Urology Department, Great Ormond Street Hospital, London, UK

C. K. Sinha and M. Davenport (eds.), *Handbook of Pediatric Surgery*,
DOI: 10.1007/978-1-84882-132-3_5.7, © Springer-Verlag London Limited 2010

- Lower abdominal wall bulge and low-set umbilical cord
- Abnormal genitalia and abnormal widening of iliac crests

Post-natal Appearance – the bladder is open on the lower abdomen, with urothelium fully exposed. In males, the penis is short and broad with dorsal chordee. The urethral plate is short and the glans penis appears in proximity to prostatic utricle. In females, the clitoris is bifid, anterior labia are displaced laterally, and the mons pubis is absent. The vagina is anteriorly displaced relative to its usual position.

The pubic symphysis is widely separated in both sexes, with divergent recti muscles, which remain attached. The abdominal wall appears elongated because of a low-set umbilicus and the distance between the umbilicus and anus is also foreshortened.

Inguinal hernias are frequently associated with exstrophy and are typically indirect (>80% of males, >10% of females). They are the result of a wide inguinal ring and the lack of an oblique inguinal canal.

5.7.3
Management

Objectives of Management Include:

- Restoration of urinary continence.
- Preservation of renal function.
- Reconstruction of functionally and cosmetically acceptable external genitalia.
- Secondary objectives are minimization of UTIs and risk of urinary calculi, reconstruction of pelvic floor, and creation of neoumbilicus.

The infants need not be in an NICU and can be kept with the mother on the maternity ward. A piece of "cling film" should be applied to cover the exposed bladder and umbilical cord should be ligated with silk suture to avoid injury to the bladder mucosa by the cord clamp. Infants can be fed orally and there is no need for IV fluids or antibiotics initially.

The approaches used to achieve these objectives depend on institutional traditions and the experience of surgeons. It is advisable that children born with the exstrophy–epispadias complex should only be managed within a limited number of centers, having the multidisciplinary team available to manage this very complex abnormality.

There are now essentially two main approaches to management: the staged functional closure and the Kelly procedure.

5.7.3.1
Staged Functional Closure (Preferably Within 48 h of Birth)

1. *Layered bladder closure* – with indwelling ureteral stents, down to bladder neck. The pubic symphysis is recreated but the epispadias is left alone.
2. ± *Pelvic osteotomies* (if closure is delayed, if pubic diastasis is greater than 5 cm, and in redo-closures).
   Closure of pelvic ring may be important for eventual attainment of urinary continence in the functional closure approach.
3. *Postoperative care.*
   (a) Traditional – spica cast, modified Buck's traction, and mermaid bandage.
   (b) Postoperative paralysis with ventilation for 1 week.
   (c) No immobilization but good local analgesia with indwelling epidural infusion.
   (d) Ureteral stents (removed after 2 weeks), urethral catheter (removed at 3 weeks).
   (e) Prophylactic antibiotics and antifungals are prescribed in all babies due to high incidence of VUR.

- *Repair of epispadias* (e.g., Cantwell–Ransley[1] technique) with urethroplasty (12–18 months) allows an increase in bladder outlet resistance in order to increase bladder capacity.
- *Bladder neck reconstruction* (~4 years). This is normally in the form of a modified Young–Dees–Leadbetter repair. The procedure is usually delayed until bladder capacity has approached 60 mL.

5.7.3.2
Kelly Procedure[2] (Radical Soft Tissue Reconstruction)

Initial bladder closure is performed as described above.

The Kelly procedure is then performed from 6 months of age and is not dependent on the bladder achieving a predetermined capacity. It comprises the following:

1. Reopening the bladder.
2. Bilateral ureteral reimplantation.
3. Complete mobilization of the urethral plate and bladder neck from the pubic rami.
4. Division of pelvic floor muscles and identification of the pudendal vessels and nerve in Alcock's canal[3].

---

[1]FV Cantwell described repair in 1895, updated by Philip Ransley an English urologist at Great Ormond Street, London.
[2]Justin Kelly – Australian urologist.
[3]Benjamin Alcock (1801 – not known). Professor of anatomy in Dublin and Cork, Ireland.

5. Complete detachment of penis from the inferior pubic rami (preservation of the pudendal vessels and nerves).
6. Radical reconstruction of the penis and bladder neck (muscle wrap in the region of the external sphincter at the base of the urethra distal to the verumontanum).

The Kelly procedure can be combined with a Cantwell–Ransley epispadias repair as a single-stage operation. In some cases, a perineal urethostomy has to be fashioned at the time of Kelly procedure to optimize penile length. These boys would then require a two-stage hypospadias repair to complete the urethral reconstruction.

Complete Primary Repair – Mitchell Technique[4]

The Mitchell technique is an alternative but has not attained widespread popularity among surgeons. This involves primary bladder closure, urethroplasty, and genital reconstruction in a single-stage during the newborn period.

5.7.4
Complications

- Bladder dehiscence – partial/complete
- Bladder prolapse
- Upper urinary tract deterioration due to high outlet resistance and vesicoureteric reflux
- Incomplete bladder emptying

Even with successful surgery, patients may have long-term problems with

- Persistent urinary incontinence and VUR
- Recurrent urinary tract infections and urolithiasis
- Sexual dysfunction
- Malignancy (rare)

5.7.5
Outcome

Continence (daytime dry interval of 3 h) rates of 30–80% have been reported after staged reconstruction.

---

[4]ME Mitchell – American Urologist.

This is influenced by factors such as successful initial closure, bladder neck reconstruction, and experience of surgeon. Use of iliac osteotomies to reduce the tension and patient immobilization in the postoperative period helps in successful bladder closure and so further continence.

The results after complete primary repair are claimed to be promising but need further follow-up. The Kelly procedure gives a superior outcome in terms of penile length and daytime continence rates of 70% have been reported.

Although sexual function in males with bladder exstrophy is almost normal, fertility is very low owing to retrograde ejaculation or iatrogenic obstruction of the ejaculatory ducts or vas after surgical reconstruction.

Females with exstrophy report both normal sexual function and fertility. The vagina is foreshortened and as the cervix enters the vagina in the anterior wall, they are prone to uterine prolapse. Successful pregnancies have been reported and delivery by cesarean section is generally recommended to avoid injury to continence mechanism.

If continence is not achieved by above procedures by the age of 5–6 years, the available options are:

- Augmentation cystoplasty with bladder neck reconstruction and Mitrofanoff formation
- Artificial urinary sphincter
- Bladder neck sling/wrap
- Collagen injection at bladder neck
- Bladder neck closure and Mitrofanoff

In exstrophy patients with multiple failed attempts of functional reconstruction, urinary diversion can be used to provide urinary continence. Ureterosigmoidostomy was the treatment of choice until the 1970s but fell out of favor due to complications such as hyperchloremic metabolic acidosis and risk of colonic adenocarcinoma at the site of ureteral anastomosis. With the advent of CIC, continent urinary diversions like the Indiana or Mainz pouch are now the preferred options.

5.7.6
Primary Epispadias

This is usually detected in the immediate postnatal examination but in some boys may only become evident later. Boys with distal epispadias are usually continent, but in those with more proximal types the bladder neck mechanism may also be deficient.

In girls, the diagnosis is usually delayed until after the age of potty-training. Thus, they either fail or are referred with a history of constant dribbling incontinence. Although the physical findings are often missed on cursory examination, once identified it is usually very obvious.

Boys with continent epispadias and good penile length can achieve a good outcome with a Cantwell–Ransley epispadias repair. Those with a short penis and all those with incontinence are probably best managed with the Kelly procedure. As all girls with primary epispadias have a deficient bladder neck mechanism, they also would require a formal Kelly procedure. This approach would allow reconstruction of the bladder sphincter and the external genitalia.

Continence outcomes in this group of children are better than their exstrophy counterparts. This is primarily as a consequence of having an intact bladder at birth, even though the capacity is often subnormal in most epispadias patients.

5.7.7
Cloacal Exstrophy

Post-natal Appearance – bladder is open and separated into two halves by an intestinal plate. Each hemi-bladder may have a ureteric orifice. The openings on the intestinal plate are terminal ileum (which may prolapse – and looks like an elephant's trunk), hindgut (with imperforate anus), and one or two appendices. Nearly all patients have an associated exomphalos.

5.7.7.1
Surgical Principles

Closure can be performed as a one-stage procedure but more commonly is staged.

Traditionally, males with cloacal exstrophy underwent gender conversion in infancy because of small separated hemi-phalluses deemed to be inadequate for penile reconstruction. The encouraging results of the Kelly procedure now allow for even widely separated corporal bodies to be mobilized and reconstructed into a reasonable midline phallus. For this reason, gender reassignment in male cloacal exstrophy patients is now rarely necessary.

Despite these children having multiple, and sometimes, life-threatening abnormalities, many are surviving into childhood. Urinary continence can only be achieved with bladder augmentation or urinary diversion.

The sequence of reconstruction is usually as follows:

1. Closure of the omphalocele.
2. Separation of the hindgut plate from the paired separated hemibladders.
3. Formation of terminal ileostomy or colostomy incorporating the hindgut plate.
4. Bladder closure. Pelvic osteotomies are always required because of the wide pubic diastasis.

Further Reading

1. Burki T, Hamid R, Duffy P et al (2006) Long-term follow up of patients after redo bladder neck reconstruction for bladder exstrophy complex. J Urol 176:1138–1141
2. Hernandez DJ, Purves T, Gearhart JP (2008) Complication of surgical reconstruction of the exstrophy-epispadias complex. J Pediatr Urol 4:460–466
3. Ludwig M, Ching B, Reutter H, Boyadjiev SA (2009) Bladder exstrophy-epispadias complex. Birth Defects Res A Clin Mol Teratol 85(6):509–522
4. Marshal VF, Muecke EC (1962) Variations in exstrophy of the bladder. J Urol 88:766

Disorders of Sex Development

5.8

N. Patwardhan, M. Woodward, and G. Nicholls

- Rarely, genital appearance may be ambiguous or even contrary to genetic sex.
- Rightly, this should be regarded as a medical emergency to achieve the best gender outcome for the baby.

This is a complex, controversial subject with a somewhat confusing classification. Since 2006, the phrase *disorders of sexual development* (DSD) has been advocated, and appears preferable to the older terms, e.g., infants with "ambiguous genitalia," "hermaphroditism,"[1] "pseudohermaphroditism," or "intersex."

5.8.1
Embryology

From 6 weeks, early bipotential gonads develop within the genital ridge from primordial germ cells (Fig. 5.8.1).

5.8.2
Clinical Features

Although the classification of DSD is quite complex (Table 5.8.1), the presentation tends to be either that of an *undervirilized male*, or an *overvirilized female* – though there are exceptions.

The birth of an infant with ambiguous genitalia will be a cause of much anxiety for the parents and in some cases (congenital adrenal hyperplasia), the sequelae may be

---

[1]Hermaphroditos (Ερμάφρόδιτός) was the child of Aphrodite and Hermes. Although born as a boy, he was transformed by union with the nymph Salmacis.

N. Patwardhan (✉)
Paediatric Surgery Department, Bristol Children's Hospital, Bristol, UK

C. K. Sinha and M. Davenport (eds.), *Handbook of Pediatric Surgery*,
DOI: 10.1007/978-1-84882-132-3_5.8, © Springer-Verlag London Limited 2010

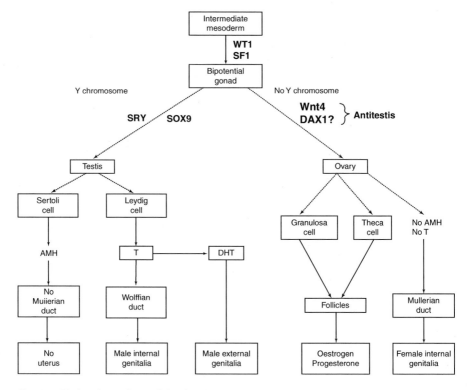

Fig. 5.8.1 Embryology of sexual development

life-threatening. This event should, therefore, be regarded as medical emergency and subsequent management should proceed in a logical and timely manner in a specialized center with multidisciplinary input. It is important to avoid guessing the sex and using pronouns such as "he" or "she." Phrases such as "your baby" are more appropriate.

Particular points to be noted when examining include:

- Presence of a palpable gonad on either side.
- Appearance of phallus including length, width, and presence of chordee.
- Appearance of scrotum/labioscrotal folds, degree of skin rugosity/pigmentation.
- Location of external urethral opening and number of orifices present on the perineum.

A proportion of children with DSD will only present later in life, such as those with Swyer syndrome who look unequivocally female (XY, complete gonadal dysgenesis), but who are unable to develop secondary sexual characteristics or menstruate.

In general, *symmetrical* genital appearance imply a *biochemical* etiology (e.g., congenital adrenal hyperplasia (CAH)), whereas *asymmetrical* appearance implies a *chromosomal* abnormality (e.g., mixed gonadal dysgenesis).

Table 5.8.1   Classification of DSD (after Lee PA, Houk CP, Hughes IA, Ahmed SF, Houk C, et al. Consensus statement on management of intersex disorders. Pediatrics 2006; 118:e488-e500)

	Variant	Notes
46XY DSD (undervirilized male)	Severe hypospadias	
	Androgen insensitivity syndromes (complete and partial)	Female phenotype, *AR* mutations
	5 α-Reductase deficiency	Failure to produce more active DHT
	Complete gonadal dysgenesis (Swyer syndrome (Swyer GI (1955) Male pseudohermaphroditism: a hitherto undescribed form. Br Med J 2:709–712); 46XY sex reversal)	Female phenotype, *SRY* mutations (~20%), usually detected at puberty
	Leydig cell hypoplasia	Autosomal recessive
	Disorders of anti-Mullerian hormone (AMH) production and receptor	*AMR* and *AMHR-II* mutations
46XX DSD (overvirilized female)	Congenital adrenal hyperplasia	*Vide infra*
	Fetoplacental aromatase deficiency	
	Exogenous androgen exposure	
	Ovotesticular DSD	
Sex chromosome DSD	45XO (Turner[2] syndrome)	Short, webbed neck, female phenotype, and aortic coarctation (60%)
	45XO/46XY (mixed gonadal dysgenesis)	
	46XX/46XY (chimeric ovotesticular DSD)	

5.8.3
Investigations

The following investigations may be required and should be tailored to each individual:

1. Genetic – karyotype and specific gene arrays
2. Endocrine – blood and urine biochemistry, hormone assays
3. Imaging – ultrasound (renal/pelvic), contrast studies (cystogram/genitogram), and MRI
4. Surgical – cystovaginoscopy, laparoscopy, and skin/gonadal biopsies

It is important that the birth is not registered until the final decision has been made, as this is extremely difficult to reverse (42 days are allowed to register a birth in the UK).

---

[2]Henry Hubert Turner (1892–1970) American physician, regarded as founder of modern endocrinology.

Wherever possible, gender is assigned according to *karyotype*, rather than being reassigned to suit the initial appearances of the external genitalia, although this may not always be possible.

5.8.4
Principles

Once a karyotype has been obtained, subsequent management should focus on

1. Hormone replacement and electrolyte balance if indicated
2. Delineation of anatomy (US, cystovaginoscopy, MRI, and laparoscopy)
3. Need for and timing of reconstruction
4. Management of gonads
    (a) ↑ Risk of malignancy, streak ovaries → gonadoblastoma
5. Genetic counseling regarding future pregnancies
6. Psychological support for family and patient

Congenital Adrenal Hyperplasia – Usually 21-Hydroxylase Deficiency

Appear as infants with ambiguous genitalia and bilateral impalpable gonads (Fig. 5.8.2). Can become life-threatening due to salt-losing nature (75%) with ↓ aldosterone.

- Urgent karyotype – XX.
- Steroid profile – ↑ 17-hydroxy progesterone ↑ androstenedione levels.

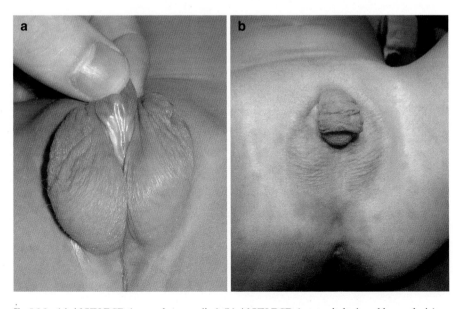

Fig. 5.8.2 (a) 46,XY DSD (severe hypospadias) (b) 46,XX DSD (congenital adrenal hyperplasia)

5.8.5
Surgery

5.8.5.1
46,XY DSD (Undervirilized Male)

The main issues for this group include:

- Hypospadias – cosmetic/functional aspects (Fig. 5.8.2 a).
- Undescended testes/impalpable gonads (?malignant potential).
- Streak gonads or intra-abdominal gonads at high risk of malignancy (e.g., mixed gonadal dysgenesis) should be removed.
- Assessment and management of persistent Müllerian structures.
    - Often asymptomatic and if so do not require excision. Recurrent infection or post-micturition dribbling may necessitate their removal.

5.8.5.2
46,XX DSD (Overvirilized Female)

The main issues are to improve the external cosmetic appearance, preserve clitoral function, and separation of the urethra and vagina. Feminizing genitoplasty may include the following:

- *Clitoroplasty* including recession, concealment, or reduction.
- *Vaginoplasty* – to separate vagina and urethra.
    - Total or partial urogenital mobilization, vaginal pull-through, or replacement.
- *Introitoplasty* to produce a more feminized appearance.

Feminizing surgery remains controversial as many adult women are unhappy with the outcome of surgery performed during their childhood, particularly with respect to cosmesis and sexual function. In recent years, there has been a move toward more conservative management, with surgery reserved for only the most virilized children, and then only when the parents have been fully counseled.

5.8.6
Long-Term Outcomes

- Data on the long-term outcome of surgery for DSD conditions are sparse.
- There are no controlled trials comparing early vs. late surgery and no data exist for the long-term outcome of newer techniques in feminizing genitoplasty, such as total or partial urogenital mobilization.
- Retrospective reviews suggest that there is much dissatisfaction with the results of surgery performed in the past with regard to cosmetic appearance and function, but this is very difficult to quantify.

By utilizing more robust classifications and better standardized recording of internal anatomy (e.g., the Rink classification for urogenital sinus anomalies), it should be possible to prospectively evaluate the results of future operations comparing like with like.

Further Reading

1. Lee PA, Houk CP, Hughes IA, Ahmed SF, Houk C et al (2006) Consensus statement on management of intersex disorders. Pediatrics 118:e488–e500
2. Rink RC, Adams MC, Misseri R (2005) A new classification for genital ambiguity and urogenital sinus disorders. BJU Int 4:638–642

Part VI

Surgery of the Liver, Pancreas and Bile Ducts

Investigation of Jaundice

6.1

Christopher J. Parsons and Mark Davenport

In most newborns, jaundice is physiological, fades within 2 weeks, and causes no harm. In a few, it can be the first sign of a deadly disease. The challenge is to find out which infant belongs to which group.

6.1.1
Metabolism of Bilirubin (Fig. 6.1.1)

Jaundice is clinically detectable when bilirubin is >50 μmol/L ($\equiv$3 mg/dL)

- Up to 60% of infants will be jaundiced in the first week of life.
- 1 in 50–100 infants will have persistence of jaundice at >2 weeks.
- 1–4/1,000 infants will have conjugated jaundice.

6.1.1.1
Physiological Jaundice

This is always unconjugated and self-limiting with a higher prevalence in the premature. It is caused by:

1. Immature liver enzymes (specifically glucuronyl transferase)
2. High red cell turnover
3. ?Exacerbated by breast feeding

C. J. Parsons (✉)
Paediatric Surgery Department, King's College Hospital, London, UK

C. K. Sinha and M. Davenport (eds.), *Handbook of Pediatric Surgery*,
DOI: 10.1007/978-1-84882-132-3_6.1, © Springer-Verlag London Limited 2010

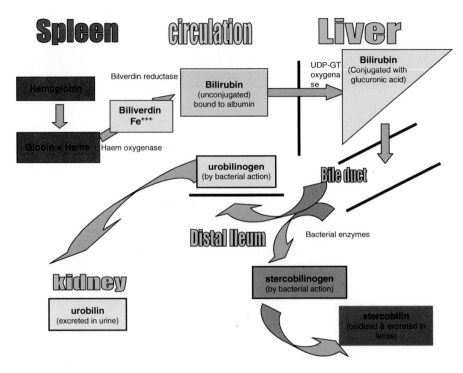

Fig. 6.1.1 Metabolism of bilirubin

6.1.2
Surgical Jaundice (always conjugated) in Infants

About 80% of such cases will be due to biliary atresia (BA) – see Chap. 6.2.
Other causes include

- Inspissated bile syndrome
- Congenital choledochal malformations (CCM) – aka choledochal cysts
- Congenital bile duct stenosis
- Spontaneous biliary perforations
- Tumors (rare)

6.1.2.1
Investigations

Ultrasonography – biliary anomalies may be evident on antenatal US.

- CCM (80%)
- Cystic BA (20%)

Prenatal differentiation is not necessary but postnatal discrimination is. Detection of an abnormality mandates early postnatal investigations (repeat US, awareness of stool color and serial split bilirubin, ±MRI).

Normal common bile duct dimensions (upper limit) (mm)	
Neonates	~1
Child up to 1 year	~2
Child over 1 year	~4
Adolescents	~7
Gallbladder (length) (cm)	
Child <1 year	1.5–3
Child >1 year	3–7
Gallbladder wall thickness (mm)	<3

US is also capable of detecting intraluminal stones, debris, and "sludge"; ascites and hepatosplenomegaly, cirrhosis of chronic liver disease, and features of BA splenic malformation (e.g., polysplenia and situs inversus).

Features suggestive of BA include

- Triangular cord sign (controversial) – represents fibrous remnants at the porta hepatis.
- Absent or atrophic gall bladder – no feeding-related changes in size.
- Cyst at the porta hepatis.

6.1.2.2
Liver Biopsy

This is used in many centers as definitive investigation for diagnosis of BA (accuracy – 85%).

Histological features of BA include

- Portal tract inflammation – mononuclear cell infiltrate
- Bile ductal plugging and proliferation
- Bridging fibrosis with overt features of cirrhosis (late findings)

Such features can also be found in nonsurgical causes of jaundice (e.g., α-1-antitryspin deficiency, giant-cell hepatitis).

Liver biopsy is invasive and carries a risk of bleeding. Interpretation requires considerable experience.

6.1.2.3
Duodenal Aspiration

Nasoduodenal tube and 24-h period measurement of aspirates for bile. Objectivity can be improved with Bilitec® 2000 device (Synectics Inc.).

6.1.2.4
Radionuclear Isotope

Technetium ^{99m}Tc-labeled iminodiacetic acid derivates can be used to assess biliary patency. It is actively taken up by the hepatocyte and excreted in bile.

- Sensitive (for BA) test (>97%), but not specific (40–70%).
- It may be improved by
    Delayed imaging (4–6 or 24 h)
    Phenobarbitol or ursodeoxycholic acid premedication (3–5 days)

Single photon emission computed tomography (SPECT)

- Performed in addition to scintigraphy
- 4–6 h after injection of isotope

The test looks for the presence of radioactivity in gastrointestinal tract.

6.1.2.5
Percutaneous Transhepatic Cholangiogam

- Only possible if US shows intrahepatic biliary dilatation (not found in BA).
- Risk of both bleeding and bile leakage.
- Most useful in inspissated bile syndrome where further saline flushing may clear obstruction.

6.1.2.6
Endoscopic Retrograde Cholangiopancreatography

Its use is limited in the diagnosis of BA, because of lack of appropriate equipment and experience. Features of BA may include

- absence of contrast in the bile duct despite filling of the pancreatic duct
- partial filling of the distal CBD and gallbladder only
- no bile in the duodenum

6.1.2.7
Magnetic Resonance Cholangiopancreatography

- Noninvasive modality but requires "breath-holding" for good-quality imaging (?GA in infants).

- T2-weighted and single-shot sequences may visualize biliary tree and the absence is regarded as diagnostic of BA (sensitivity 100% and specificity 96%) in one study.
- Key technique in the evaluation of CCM and liver cysts.

6.1.2.8
Laparoscopy ± Cholangiography

- Use of 3 mm instruments.
- Insertion of catheter into gallbladder.

6.1.3
Investigation of Surgical Jaundice in Older Child

This is virtually always associated with intrahepatic biliary dilatation and causes can be divided according to surgical tradition.

6.1.3.1
Intramural

- Calculi (choledocholithiasis)

    — Primary (uncommon) – arising in intrahepatic, common hepathic, or common bile ducts.
    — Secondary (common) – arising in the gallbladder (in children consider hemolysis, cholesterol, and metabolic (e.g. PFIC))

- Inspissated bile
- Parasites

    — Worms – nematodes (*Ascariasis lumbricoides* – Kashmir and Kenya)
    — Liver flukes – (*Clonorchis sinensis* – China, Korea, and Vietnam)

- Tumors – rhabdomyosarcoma

6.1.3.2
Mural[1]

- Congenital/acquired stenosis (ampulla and above)
- Congenital Choledochal malformation (see chapter 6.3).
- Sclerosing cholangitis
- Cystic fibrosis – cholangiopathy and inspissation of bile
- AIDS – multiple causes including opportunistic infection
- Tumors – rhabdomyosarcoma, extensive hepatoblastoma/HCC involving R and L hepatic ducts

---

[1]*Murus* (Latin) – the wall.

6.1.3.3
Extramural

- Tumors – lymphomas, head of pancreas tumors
- Mirzzi's syndrome[2] – gallbladder pathology causing secondary stenosis of adjacent CHD
- Chronic pancreatitis

Further Reading

1. Davenport M et al (2003) The spectrum of surgical jaundice in infancy. J Pediatr Surg 38(10):1471–1479
2. Hussein M, Mowat AP (1991) Jaundice at 14 days of age: exclude biliary atresia. Arch Dis Child 66:1177–1179
3. Venigalla S (2004) Neonatal cholestasis. Semin Perinatol 28:348–355
4. Woodley HE (2004) Imaging of the jaundiced child. Imaging 16:301–313

---

[2]Pablo Mirizzi (1893–1964) Argentinian. Mirizzi P (1948) Syndrome del conducto hepatico. J Int de Chir 8:731–777

Biliary Atresia

6.2

Chandrasen K. Sinha and Mark Davenport

Biliary atresia (BA) is a cholangiodestructive disease affecting all parts of biliary tract. It is invariably fatal if untreated.

6.2.1
Epidemiology

- 1 in 10,000 – Japan and China
- ↓ Incidence of BASM
- 1 in 17,000 – UK, USA, and Europe
- F > M (slight in isolated, marked in BASM)

6.2.2
Embryology

The primitive bile duct buds from the ventral pancreatic duct is engulfed by the developing liver. Bile ductules (so-called ductal plate) differentiate from hepatoblast precursors and undergo a process of selection/deletion with progressively fewer but larger remaining ducts. Critical point (5–6 weeks) is coincident with the determination of abdominal situs, spleen formation, final development of portal vein, and vena cava. Bile is secreted into the GI tract by 12 weeks.

As the etiology of BA is largely unknown, hypotheses abound. Two of them have a degree of evidential support.

- *Developmental*
  - BASM
  - Cystic BA – >50% detected on antenatal US scan

C. K. Sinha (✉)
Paediatric Surgery Department, King's College Hospital, London, UK

C. K. Sinha and M. Davenport (eds.), *Handbook of Pediatric Surgery*,
DOI: 10.1007/978-1-84882-132-3_6.2, © Springer-Verlag London Limited 2010

- *Perinatal acquired* – i.e., normal developed bile duct is damaged later, with secondary loss of luminal continuity
  - Viral insult – e.g., rotavirus, cytomegalovirus, and reovirus
- Genetic predisposition
- Immunological overreaction

6.2.3
Classification

Figure 6.2.1 illustrates classification with the most proximal level of obstruction determining the type. About 5% will have cystic change within otherwise obliterated biliary tract. These need to be differentiated from a *choledochal malformation*, which even if obstructed should connect to a smooth, progressively distended intrahepatic duct system.

6.2.4
Clinical Features

Conjugated jaundice, pale stools, dark urine, and failure to thrive. Nil specific.
    Look for situs, polysplenia, and cardiac anomalies of BASM.

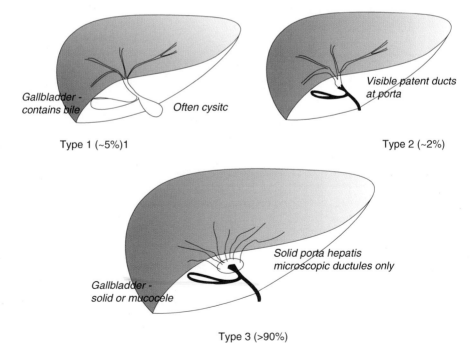

Fig. 6.2.1 Classification of biliary atresia

6.2.4.1
Investigations – see Chap. 6.1

6.2.5
Surgery

Correct coagulopathy (vitamin K).

In most cases, an attempt to preserve native liver using portoenterostomy is a better strategy than primary liver transplantation. However, latter should be considered in "old" infants (>100 days) especially those with obvious cirrhosis (ascites, portal hypertension).

6.2.5.1
Kasai Portoenterostomy[1] (Fig.6.2.2)

RUQ – muscle-cutting – extended across midline.

1. Confirm diagnosis ±cholangiogram
2. Porta hepatis dissection – facilitated by extrabdominal delivery of liver
   (a) Excision of all extrahepatic remnants to the level of liver capsule, facilitated by retraction of portal vein confluence. Clearance proceeds from bifurcation of right vascular pedicle to insertion of umbilical vein on left portal vein.
3. Roux[2] loop (~40 cm) reconstruction and portoenterostomy (6/0 PDS).

Adjuvant therapy – no real scientific evidence exists for its effectiveness.

1. Ursodeoxycholic acid
2. Steroids (2–4 mg/kg/day)

6.2.6
Complications

- Cholangitis (40%)

  — Gram −ve organisms (usually)
  — Treated with IV antibiotics (Tazocin and Gentamicin)

---

[1]Morio Kasai (1922–2008) Japanese pediatric surgeon, described concept in 1959.
[2]Cesar Roux (1857–1934) Swiss surgeon. First to successfully remove a phaeochromcytoma.

Fig. 6.2.2 Kasai portoenterostomy – close up of porta
hepatic. Transected bile
ductules are visible in this
case (unusual)

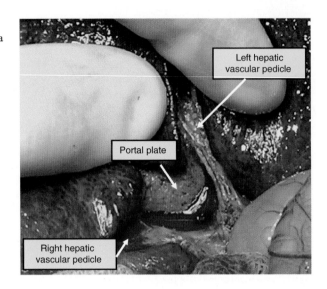

- Portal hypertension
  - Splenomegaly
  - Esophageal, gastric, and anorectal varices
- Hepatopulmonary syndrome
  - Hypoxia, cyanosis, dyspnea, and clubbing due to the development of pulmonary arteriovenous shunts.
  - ↑ Incidence with BASM, diagnosed with saturation monitoring.
  - Reversed after liver transplantation.
- Malignancy
  - HCC, hepatoblastoma, and cholangiocarcinoma (still rare).

6.2.7
Outcome

Success post-KPE can be gauged by

1. Proportion to clear jaundice (ideally <20 µmol/L)
   (a) 50–60% is achievable
2. Proportion to survive with own liver
   (a) 50% after 5 years is achievable

Prognosis post-KPE can be affected by

1. Age at surgery (explicitly with developmental variants)
2. Experience of surgeon/center
3. BASM – poor prognosis

Further Reading

1. Davenport M (2006) Biliary atresia: outcome and management. Ind J Pediatr 73:825–828
2. Davenport M, Betalli P, D'Antinga L et al (2003) The spectrum of surgical jaundice in infancy. J Pediatr Surg 38:1471–1479
3. Davenport M, Puricelli V, Farrant P et al (2004) The outcome of the older (>100 days) infant with biliary atresia. J Pediatr Surg 39:575–581
4. Hung PY, Chen CC, Chen WJ et al (2006) Long-term prognosis of patient with biliary atresia: a 25 year summary. J Pediatr Gastrol Nutr 42:190–195
5. Utterson EC, Shepherd RW, Sokol RJ et al (2005) Biliary atresia: clinical profiles, risk factors, and outcomes of 755 patients listed for liver transplantation. J Pediatr 147:180–185

Choledochal Malformations

6.3

Chandrasen K. Sinha and Mark Davenport

A choledochal cyst was first recognized by the anatomist Abraham Vater in 1723.

6.3.1
Epidemiology

- Unknown incidence
- F » M 4:1
- Chinese and Japanese > Caucasian

6.3.2
Classification

The King's College Hospital Classification is based on phenotype and is a modification of Alonso–Lej's original (Fig. 6.3.1).

- Type 1 – extrahepatic dilatation of CBD and CHD (~80%)
    - Cystic (1c) – classical type
    - Fusiform (1f) – "spindle-shaped" dilatation, no abrupt change
- Type 2 – diverticulum of the common bile duct (<2%)
- Type 3 – dilatation of the distal intramural portion of the CBD (*synonym – choledochocele*) (<2%)
- Type 4 – multiple dilatations
    - Intra- and extrahepatic (~10%)
- Type 5 – dilatation of intrahepatic ducts only (~5%)

C. K. Sinha (✉)
Paediatric Surgery Department, King's College Hospital, London, UK

C. K. Sinha and M. Davenport (eds.), *Handbook of Pediatric Surgery*,
DOI: 10.1007/978-1-84882-132-3_6.3, © Springer-Verlag London Limited 2010

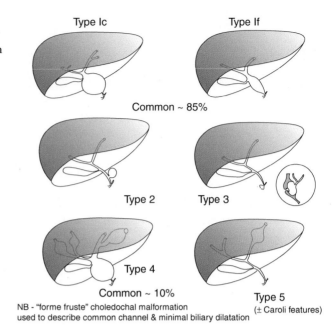

Fig. 6.3.1 King's College Hospital Classification of choledochal malformation

Type Ic

Type If

Common ~ 85%

Type 2

Type 3

Type 4

Common ~ 10%

Type 5
(± Caroli features)

NB - "forme fruste" choledochal malformation used to describe common channel & minimal biliary dilatation

With possible exception of duodenal atresia, the above are usually found as isolated lesions.

Caroli's[1] *disease* – distinct anomaly with multiple intrahepatic cysts and duct ectasia (left > right) and intrinsic liver fibrosis. Caroli's syndrome (usually autosomal dominant) refers to the association with polycystic kidney disease and usually renal failure.

6.3.3
Pathogenesis

The exact etiology is unknown. Two hypotheses
- 2° to congenital bile duct segmental stenosis (can be detected on antenatal US – Type 1c).
- Reflux of activated pancreatic enzymes via the common channel causes mural weakness and 2° dilatation (Babbitt[2] hypothesis).

The wall of the typical choledochal cyst (Type 1c) is usually thick, vascular, and has an incomplete mucosal lining (this will vary with the age of the child and length of symptoms). Large cystic malformations tend to displace adjacent viscera such as duodenum and colon and expand into head of pancreas.

[1]Jacques Caroli (1902–1979) – French physician, worked at Saint Antoine Hospital, Paris.
[2]Donald P. Babbitt (1923–2005) – American radiologist, working at Milwaukee, WI.

6.3.4
Clinical Features

Classic triad of presentation (jaundice, pain, and abdominal mass) (~15% of most series)

- Jaundice and acholic stool (usually infants – differential with cystic biliary atresia).
- Abdominal pain and pancreatitis (usually older children ± jaundice).
- Cholangitis ± stones.
- Intra- or extraperitoneal rupture.
- Biliary cirrhosis – portal hypertension, ascites, and liver failure.
- Malignant epithelial change (e.g., cholangiocarcinoma) – usually during adulthood.

Laboratory: conjugated jaundice, ↑GGT, ↑alkaline phosphatase, and ↑transaminases. Coagulation profile may be deranged in those with long-standing biliary obstruction due to vitamin K malabsorption.

- *US* – degree (CBD size); intrahepatic dilatation; intralumenal stones.
- *MRCP* – excellent anatomical imaging.
- *ERCP* – currently only indicated if there is doubt about diagnosis (minimal biliary dilatation) or if definitive pancreatic ductal anatomy is required.

6.3.5
Surgery – Type 1c (Cystic Malformation)

Aim – excision of the dilated extrahepatic biliary tract together with proximal biliary reconstruction to achieve perfect bile drainage.

Incision – RUQ (laparoscopic reconstruction is possible but requires considerable dexterity).

1. Cholangiography – define proximal and distal common channel anatomy.
2. Cholecystectomy and mobilization of cyst from adjacent viscera, hepatic artery, and portal vein. Proximal division at the level of CHD allows separation of distal cyst from within head of pancreas. Identify distal, nondilated CBD. Transfix after probing, and clearing common channel. Transduodenal sphincteroplasty may be required for those with dilated common channels.
3. A long Roux loop (~45 cm) is the recommended reconstruction technique (hepaticoduodenostomy is possible but not widely advocated)
4. Hepaticojejunostomy (after choledochoscopy, if possible, to define areas of intrahepatic stenosis/stones, etc.). Usually straightforward anastomosis but may require variation due to local anatomy.

(NB, If dissection is difficult with marked with infection and inflammation, then removal of the cyst wall can be treacherous – simple removal of mucosa from the inner lining may be a safer pragmatic approach (Lilly's[3] procedure). Also, in sick infants with

------

[3]John R. Lilly (1929–1995) American pediatric surgeon, Denver, CO.

perforated cysts, for instance, a two-stage procedure, i.e., preliminary external drainage using a T-tube may be safer).

- For localized, symptomatic Type V cysts typically containing stones, liver resection should be considered.

6.3.6
Outcome

It tends to be related to what's left behind

- Intrahepatic ducts (residual stones/strictures – cholangitis).
- Common channel (residual stones/debris – pancreatitis).
- Biliary mucosa – possible long-term risk of malignancy (limited data).

Further Reading

1. Dabbas N, Davenport M (2009) Congenital choledochal malformation. Ann R Coll Surg Eng 91:100–105
2. Davenport M, Basu R (2005) Choledochal malformation manometry – under pressure. J Pediatr Surg 40:331–335
3. Hong L, Wu Y, Yan Z, Xu M, Chu J, Chen QM (2008) Laparoscopic surgery for choledochal cyst in children: a case review of 31 patients. Eur J Pediatr Surg 18:67–71
4. Todani T, Watanabe Y, Urushihara N et al (1995) Biliary complications after excisional procedure for choledochal cyst. J Pediatr Surg 30:478–481

Gallbladder Disease

6.4

Chandrasen K. Sinha, Masih A. Kadar, and Mark Davenport

Even children can get gallstones!

There are a number of true congenital anomalies of gallbladder; most are rare and usually asymptomatic. They are:

- Duplication, triplication, etc.
- Agenesis – can have otherwise normal biliary tract; associated with some chromosomal anomalies.
- Multiseptate – separate nonbile-containing spaces within gallbladder.
  Some are acquired.
- "Porcelain" calcification, associated with gallstones. Rare in children.
- Cystic fibrosis – micro-gallbladders, webs, and mucus-filled epithelial cysts

6.4.1
Gallstone Disease

Unknown incidence

- ~30% of adolescents with sickle cell disease (↑ homozygous SCD)
  — <10% symptomatic

Gallstones are predominantly of three types:

- Cholesterol (50%) – yellowish, often solitary
  — Usually adolescent girls

- Bilirubin pigment (45%) – pigmented, multiple, and sludge
  — Sickle Cell Disease (SCD), thalasemia, spherocytosis, and progressive familial cholestasis (PFIC)

C. K. Sinha (✉)
Paediatric Surgery Department, King's College Hospital, London, UK

C. K. Sinha and M. Davenport (eds.), *Handbook of Pediatric Surgery*,
DOI: 10.1007/978-1-84882-132-3_6.4, © Springer-Verlag London Limited 2010

- Calcium carbonate ($\uparrow$ in children)
  - Postinfection/dehydration/TPN, etc. in infancy
    NB: mixed stones with differing proportions of above also occur commonly.

6.4.2
Clinical Features

Gallstones may cause

1. Biliary colic – postprandial pain, >4 h duration
2. Acute and chronic cholecystitis – $\uparrow$ temperature $\uparrow$ duration $\uparrow$ tenderness (+ve Murphy's sign[1])
3. Empyema – palpable RUQ mass and pyrexia
4. Mucocele – stone impacted in Hartmann's[2] pouch preventing ingress of bile, but with mucus build-up
5. Choledocholithiasis – $\uparrow$ conjugated jaundice
   (a) Cholangitis – pyrexia (~40°C). Charcot's triad[3]
6. Acute pancreatitis – $\uparrow$ amylase
   (a) Stone impacted in ampulla

6.4.2.1
Investigations

1. *US* – sensitive, may show thickened wall, sludge, and $\uparrow$CBD
2. *MRCP* – sensitive to CBD stones, choledochal malformation, etc.
3. *Underlying cause*
   (a) Evidence of hemolyis ($\uparrow$ reticulocytes)
   (b) Cholesterol and triglyceride (fasting) level
   (c) $\downarrow$ GGT and cholestasis may indicate PFIC

6.4.3
Management

- Asymptomatic stones – probably best left alone, certainly those detected incidentally without obvious underlying cause
- Advise cholecystectomy in SCD during adolescence (better elective than emergency, $\uparrow$ deposition with age).

---

[1]J.B. Murphy – involuntary gasp when examining hand touches inflamed gallbladder during inspiration.

[2]Henri Albert Hartmann (1860–1952) French surgeon, working at Hotel Dieu in Paris.

[3]Jean Martin Charcot (1825–1893) French physician. Triad is rigors, jaundice, and RUQ tenderness.

- Cholangitis/cholecystitis
  (a) IV Antibiotics (Gram –ve predominantly)
  (b) Intervention – 2–4 weeks
- Choledocholithiasis (stone in duct) – elective ERCP±sphincterotomy

6.4.4
Surgery

6.4.4.1
Laparoscopic Cholecystectomy

- Undoubted benefit compared to open surgery
- Three working ports (5 mm) and umbilical camera port (10 mm/5 mm)
- Calot triangle[4] dissection – identify and clip cystic duct/artery
- On-table cholangiogram – (not routine) indicated if ?CBD stones, i.e., history of jaundice±pancreatitis
- Mobilize gallbladder. Remove intact in purse-string bag

6.4.4.1.1
Complications

- Bleeding (from GB bed or artery)
- Bile leak (from cystic duct or less commonly damage to CBD)
- Subphrenic or subhepatic collection±abscess
- Sepsis
- Biliary stricture – from bile duct damage (diathermy/laceration)
- Missed stone in CBD

6.4.5
Acalculous Cholecystitis

Usually associated with sepsis (particularly *Salmonella* spp.), trauma, diabetes, and burn injury.

6.4.6
Hydrops

Features include distended but normal GB and ducts and absence of gall stones. This condition is commonly seen in association with Kawasaki syndrome. Hydrops may lead to necrosis of GB, perforation, and bile peritionitis.

---

[4]Jean-Francois Calot (1861–1944) French surgeon. He actually described cystic artery, duct, and common hepatic duct as the triangle (i.e., pretty small) – now considered to be cystic duct, CHD, and liver.

6.4.7
Biliary Dyskinesia

Poorly defined condition, typically in adult women but children may also be susceptible. Sometimes, true sphincter of Oddi-invoked pressure changes can be shown by biliary manometry (ERCP), or provocation by cholecystokinin.

Some children may get symptomatic relief after cholecystectomy.

Further Reading

1. Durakbasa CU, Balik E, Yamaner S et al (2008) Diagnostic and therapeutic endoscopic retrograde cholangiopancreatography (ERCP) in children and adolescents: experience in a single institution. Eur J Pediatr Surg 18:241–244
2. St Peter SD, Keckler SJ, Nair A et al (2008) Laparoscopic cholecystectomy in the pediatric population. J Laparoendosc Adv Surg Tech A 18:127–130
3. Stringer MD, Soloway RD, Taylor DR et al (2007) Calcium carbonate gallstones in children. J Pediatr Surg 42:1677–1682
4. Ure BM, Jesch NK, Nustede R (2004) Postcholecystectomy syndrome with special regard to children – a review. Eur J Pediatr Surg 14:221–225

Portal Hypertension

6.5

Chandrasen K. Sinha and Mark Davenport

Significant portal hypertension tends to present with precipitant variceal bleeding.

6.5.1
Incidence

- Not known
- Normal portal pressure ~5 mmHg
  - Portal hypertension >10 mmHg
- Commonest single cause is *portal vein thrombosis* (PVT) (long-standing)

6.5.2
Anatomy

Portal vein is formed by confluence of superior mesenteric and splenic vein, behind neck of pancreas ascending as the posterior component of the portal triad (CBD and hepatic artery). It divides into right and left portal veins at porta hepatic and these branch within liver to empty into the sinusoids. Direction of blood flow is determined entirely by the pressure gradient.

Portosystemic collaterals open up around the esophagus, distal rectum, retroperitoneum, and anterior abdominal wall (*caput medusae*[1]).

- Portal vein ~75% of liver blood flow.
- Hepatic artery ~25% (has ability to ↑ to compensate).

---

[1]*Caput medusae* (Latin) head of the medusa – mythical being with a bunch of snakes for hair – capable of turning a man to stone.

C. K. Sinha (✉)
Paediatric Surgery Department, King's College Hospital, London, UK

C. K. Sinha and M. Davenport (eds.), *Handbook of Pediatric Surgery*,
DOI: 10.1007/978-1-84882-132-3_6.5, © Springer-Verlag London Limited 2010

6.5.3
Causes of Portal Hypertension

- Extrahepatic (prehepatic)
  - Portal vein thrombosis
- Intrahepatic
  - Cirrhotic
    - (Post-Kasai) Biliary atresia
    - Cystic fibrosis
    - Alpha-1 antitrypsin deficiency
    - Posthepatitis (viral, autoimmune)
    - Congenital hepatic fibrosis
  - Schistosomiasis

- Posthepatic
  - Budd–Chiari syndrome – hepatic vein occlusion
  - Idiopathic, congenital web, and posttransplant
  - Veno-occlusive disease
  - Drugs (typically postleukemia)

6.5.4
Portal Vein Thrombosis

Initial thrombus formation is asymptomatic (and probably occurs in neonatal period), but gradually collateral veins develop and can be recognized as a "cavernoma" on US. Overall "portal" blood flow may be maintained but at higher pressure, but slow flow is the norm. The liver is usually smaller than normal, arterialized but biochemically and histologically normal.

6.5.4.1
Etiology

- *Idiopathic* (50%)
- *Congenital* (20%) – assumed as occurs with other malformations, e.g., radial, craniofacial, and vertebral deformities.
- *Neonatal-acquired* (30%) – either directly due to umbilical vein catheter abuse, or indirectly related to omphalitis, sepsis, dehydration, etc.

Thrombogenic coagulopathy is an uncommon cause of both hepatic and PVT in children (cf. adults).

6.5.5
Clinical Features

Children present with

- Bleeding
- Palpable splenomagaly

Even the initial bleed (hematemesis and/or melena) can be life-threatening and torrential due to PHT. A history of liver disease (and visible jaundice) makes the diagnosis obvious (although still requiring endoscopic confirmation), though there is a lag time to develop varices (months). If the only abnormal sign is a palpable spleen, then PVT is the likeliest cause.

Varices develop in a predictable sequence (esophageal, gastric, and anorectal), again over time, and the latter variants will not be a cause of de novo bleeding.

Rarely, PHT causes secondary biliary obstruction (bilopathy) and hepatopulmonary syndrome.

6.5.5.1
Investigations

1. Laboratory
   (a) Liver biochemistry (normal in PVT) including PT.
   (b) Full blood count ($\downarrow$Hb, $\downarrow$ WBC, and $\downarrow$ platelet count – due to hypersplenism).
   (c) Viral serology, Cu and Fe estimation, and autoantibodies (underlying cirrhosis).
2. US – looking for cavernoma formation, portal blood flow, and liver parenchymal appearance.
3. MRV – to define porto-mesenteric venous anatomy (if shunt is considered).
4. Upper GI endoscopy – diagnostic and therapeutic.

6.5.6
Management

6.5.6.1
Management of Acute Bleed

If after hemodynamic resuscitation (±blood transfusion), then PHT appears the likeliest cause of the bleeding, then use octreotide infusion (dose) to reduce PHT, and proceed to urgent endoscopy (±definitive therapy).

- Endoscopic variceal therapy
  — Band ligation (older child) or sclerotherapy (infant)

— Usually requires course of treatment for eradications (three to four sessions)
— Superglue injection for gastric varices
- Sengstaken tube[2] – device with gastric and esophageal balloons (only former is usually needed in children), applied under GA and tension for 24 h. Confirm correct positioning radiologically. Use in conjunction with endoscopy.
- Transjugular intrahepatic portosystemic shunt
  — Little use in children – only indicated as short-term "bridge" in cirrhotic livers on way to transplantation.

6.5.6.2
Secondary Prophylaxis

Few studies in children but possible use of

- Propranolol
- Depot somatostatin analog
- Shunt surgery – for PVT (good liver function)
- Transplantation – for cirrhotic disease (poor liver function)

6.5.7
Surgery

6.5.7.1
Shunt Surgery

For PVT and (rarely) cirrhotic liver disease with good liver function.
Indications include

- Persistent bleeding uncontrolled by endoscopic treatment
- Massive splenomegaly

6.5.7.1.1
Options

- *Meso-Rex shunt*
  — Native (internal jugular vein) conduit between left portal vein (in Rex fossa) and superior mesenteric vein.
  — Only type with no risk of encephalopathy.

---

[2]Robert Sengstaken, Arthur Blakemore. New York surgeons who described custom-made tube with esophageal and gastric balloons in 1950. First patient was 15-year-old girl with portal vein thrombosis.

- *Portosystemic shunt*
  - Mesocaval shunt – conduit between IVC and SMV.
  - Lienorenal shunt ± splenectomy – anastomosis between lienorenal vein and splenic vein.

6.5.7.2
Transplantation – see chapter 6.7

Further Reading

1. Abd El-Hamid N, Taylor RM, Marinello D et al (2008) Aetiology and management of extrahepatic portal vein obstruction in children: King's College Hospital experience. J Pediatr Gastroenterol Nutr 47:630–634
2. Celinska-Cedro D, Teisseyre M, Woynarowski M et al (2003) Endoscopic ligation of esophageal varices for prophylaxis of first bleeding in children and adolescents with portal hypertension: preliminary results of a prospective study. J Pediatr Surg 38:1008–1011
3. de Ville de Goyet J, Alberti D et al (1999) Treatment of extrahepatic portal hypertension in children by mesenteric-to-left portal vein bypass: a new physiological procedure. Eur J Surg 165(8):777–781
4. Zargar SA, Yattoo GN, Javid G et al (2004) Fifteen-year follow up of endoscopic injection sclerotherapy in children with extrahepatic portal venous obstruction. J Gastroenterol Hepatol 19:139–145

Pancreatic Disease

6.6

Chandrasen K. Sinha and Mark Davenport

Recognized as separate organ and named pancreas ("All Flesh") by Ruphos, Greek physician working in Ephesus.

Embryology (Fig. 6.6.1)

- Ventral anlage[1] (appears ~5th week of gestation), arises from biliary diverticulum. Rotates around behind duodenum and sandwiches superior mesenteric vessels.
- Coalesces with dorsal anlage (~7 weeks).
- Exchange of duct systems – original ventral duct becomes the draining duct for dorsal (majority) pancreas (duct of Wirsung[2]). Original dorsal duct becomes more proximal duct of Santorini[3].
- Final stage is absorption of ventral duct (and attached bile duct) into wall of duodenum.

This complex process results in three key pathologies:

- *Annular pancreas*

Persistence or anterior rotation of the ventral anlage, leading to a ring (*Latin annulus*) of normal pancreatic tissue around duodenum.

---

[1]*Anlage* (sing.) *anlagen (pl.)* – Middle German for "plan or arrangement" used in context as cluster of embryonic cells.
[2]Johann Georg Wirsung (1589–1643) – German anatomist working in Padua (Italy), who identified duct in 1642 when dissecting the corpse of a convicted murderer.
[3]Giovani Domenico Santorini (1681–1737) Italian anatomist.

C. K. Sinha (✉)
Paediatric Surgery Department, King's College Hospital, London, UK

C. K. Sinha and M. Davenport (eds.), *Handbook of Pediatric Surgery*,
DOI: 10.1007/978-1-84882-132-3_6.6, © Springer-Verlag London Limited 2010

May cause

— Duodenal obstruction – probably due to associated anomalies such as malrotation and duodenal atresia/stenosis.
— Susceptibility to acute pancreatitis.

If obstructive features are present, then duodenoduodenostomy is a better option that attempts to divide the ring.

• *Pancreas divisum*

It is due to the failure of duct exchange leaving the dominant dorsal duct to drain via the accessory duct alone. Present in up to 10% of normal population. This is relatively inefficient as a physiological system and predisposes to pancreatitis (acute or chronic). Diagnosed by ERCP (only), MRCP insensitive.

Surgical options include

1. Endoscopic sphincterotomy
2. Transduodenal sphincterotomy
3. Retrograde duct drainage (e.g., longitudinal pancreato-jejunostomy – Puestow[1] procedure)

• *Common channel*

The ampulla of Vater[4] results from absorption of ventral duct and attached bile duct into the duodenal wall and results in a mechanism keeping bile and pancreatic juices apart. There is an additional sphincter mechanism (of Oddi[5]) controlling the flow. A common channel (defined as 5 mm in child) results from failure of this absorptive process and allows free interchange of secretions.

Associated with

— Choledochal malformation

Predisposes to

— Acute pancreatitis

The most effective surgical treatment is biliary diversion (even if bile duct is of relatively normal diameter). Consider additional sphincteroplasty if there is marked common channel dilatation.

---

[4]Abraham Vater (1684–1751) German anatomist, described this in 1720.
[5]Ruggero Oddi (1864–1913) Italian physician who described this while still a medical student.

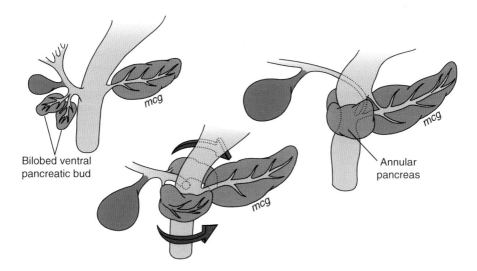

Fig. 6.6.1   Rotation of ventral and dorsal pancreatic anlagen. (Adapted from Shoenwolf et al.)

6.6.1
Acute Pancreatitis

It is an acute inflammation of the pancreas with variable severity, which may range from mild inflammation to severe necrotizing pancreatitis.

6.6.1.1
Surgical Etiology

- Choledochal malformation
- Gallstones (Sickle cell anemia, spherocytosis)
- Congenital ductal anomalies (pancreas divisum, common channel, annular pancreas, and congenital strictures)
- Cysts (e.g., duplication)
- Blunt abdominal trauma (~25%) (See chapter 8.2)

6.6.1.2
Medical Etiology

- Multisystem disease

  — Reye's[6] syndrome – acute onset encephalopathy and fatty liver associated with aspirin use in children.

---

[6]R. Douglas Reye. Australian paediatrician who published this in 1963.

— Hemolytic uremic syndrome – severe diarrheal illness (often bloody) usually associated with *Escherichia coli* (serotype O157:H7).
— Cystic fibrosis (<2% of CF population) occasionally presenting feature.

- Viral infections (e.g., mumps, rubella, cytomegalovirus, HIV) (~10%).
- Ascariasis (helminthic infection – India and China) adults >children – although prevalence of infection ↑children.
- Drugs (e.g., sodium valproate, steroids, azathioprine, and L-asparaginase (~10%).
- Metabolic diseases (e.g., hypercalcemia (hyperparathyroidism), familial hypertriglyceridemia) (~2%).

Hereditary pancreatitis – autosomal dominant mutation in cationic trypsinogen gene (PRSS1, on Chromosome 7) (~2%). Premalignant.

6.6.1.3
Pathology

↑ Pancreatic duct pressure or premature enzyme activation within acinar cells may lead to autodigestion, inflammatory reaction and initiation of SIRS, and even MODS (see chapter 2.2). Leakage of secretions (from trauma or duct necrosis) into surrounding tissue may lead to acute fluid collections (if early, <4 weeks)) or with creation of actual nonepithelial lined cavity (>4 weeks, pseuodcyst).

6.6.1.4
Clinical Features

Often misdiagnosed initially, but usual features are sudden-onset abdominal pain (often radiating to back, relived by leaning forward) and vomiting. On examination, there may be low-grade fever±signs of shock (↑ pulse ↓BP) depending on severity. Examination will reveal tenderness in upper abdomen. Late signs include bruised appearance of umbilicus (Cullen's sign) or loins (Grey–Turner's sign).

Acute necrotizing pancreatitis (potential for mortality) is uncommon in children, but will show shock, disseminated intravascular coagulation, GI bleeding, respiratory, and renal failure (i.e., MODS).

6.6.1.5
Investigation

1. Laboratory tests:
   (a) ↑↑ Amylase and ↑ lipase – no correlation of level with severity
   (b) ↑ White cell count
   (c) ↓ Calcium, ↓ glucose
   (d) Blood gas analysis (evidence of ↓pH)
   (e) ↑ Bilirubin, ↑ GGT
   (f) ↑ INR
   (g) Urinary TAP (trypsin activation peptide) level – may predict severity

2. *USS* – showing retroperitoneal and pancreatic edema and looking for evidence of gall-stones, biliary dilatation, etc.
3. *CT/MRI* – defines extent of disease process and able to detect pancreatic necrosis
4. *ERCP* – indicated in acute gallstone pancreatitis

6.6.1.6
Management

(a) Supportive – including fluid resuscitation, NG tube (if vomiting) with analgesia, and H₂ blockers (↓ gastric acidity). Few need ventilation and blood gas support. Parenteral nutrition important from >48 h. Antibiotics if evidence of systemic infection or sepsis

(b) *Surgery*
   Early – consider necrosectomy (open or laparoscopic) (<5%) if CT evidence of necrosis and severe systemic illness
   Late

   - *Pseudocyst formation*
     - Supportive (~30% will spontaneously diminish)
     - Aspiration – US- or CT-guided±pigtail drain
     - Cystgastrostomy
       — Endoscopic – feasible
       — Open – classical approach
       — If cyst not near stomach, then a Roux loop will achieve drainage

---

Characterized by recurrent episodes of symptomatic pancreatic inflammation together with gradual decline of exocrine and endocrine function.

- *Pancreatic ascites* – duct open to peritoneal cavity with free flow
  — *ERCP* (diagnosis), treated by stent
  — *Open* – identify leak and oversew/resect or Roux loop to drain

---

6.6.2
Chronic Pancreatitis

6.6.2.1
Etiology

Previous list still applies but congenital anatomical duct anomalies, HP, and cystic fibrosis are leading causes.

6.6.2.2
Clinical Features

Intermittent epigastric pain (as before), with pain-free intervals (varying duration). Anorexia and weight loss may be features, exacerbated by exocrine failure (e.g., steatorrhoea). Endocrine failure (i.e., diabetes) is a late sign, whatever the cause.

6.6.2.3
Investigations (List as Before in Acute Episodes)

- *Specific laboratory studies* – fecal elastase (<200 µg/g of stool); Fecal fat estimation.
- Secretin-cholecystokinin provocation test.
- *AXR* – may show calcification.
- *US* – biliary and pancreatic duct dilatation; pseudocysts, calculi, or ascites.
- *CT/MR scan.*
- *ERCP* – defines ductal anatomy and is key to determine the role of surgery.

6.6.2.4
Surgery

Indicated if persistent pain (despite standard therapy of fat restriction enzymes and adequate analgesia), complications (e.g., pseudocyst).
Options include

- *ERCP and stent* (*e.g., Sherman stent*) – only short-term but if successful predicts success of open surgery.
- *Sphincteroplasty* (*endoscopic or open*) – for localized ampullary stenosis or common channel only.

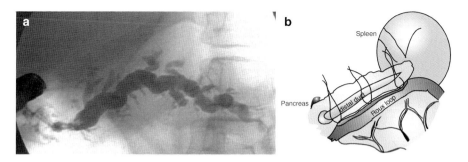

Fig. 6.6.2 (**a**) ERCP showing dilated main pancreatic duct, secondary to chronic pancreatitis. (**b**) Treated effectively with Puestow[8] procedure

- *Internal open retrograde duct drainage.*
    - Puestow[8] procedure – longitudinal pancreatojejunostomy – usually to left of mesenteric vessels.
    - Frey[7] procedure – extension of duct open into head of pancreas (Fig. 6.6.2).

Pseudocyst formation (management uses same principles as for acute pancreatitis).

Further Reading

1. Chiu B, Lopoo J, Superina RA (2006) Longitudinal pancreaticojejunostomy and selective biliary diversion for chronic pancreatitis in children. J Pediatr Surg 41:946–949
2. Houben C, Ade-Ajayi N, Patel S et al (2007) Traumatic pancreatic duct injury in children: minimally invasive approach to management. J Pediatr Surg 42:629–635
3. Iqbal CW, Moir CR, Ishitani MB (2009) Management of chronic pancreatitis in the pediatric patient: endoscopic retrograde cholangiopancreatography vs operative therapy. J Pediatr Surg 44:139–143
4. Kandula L, Lowe ME (2008) Etiology and outcome of acute pancreatitis in infants and toddlers. J Pediatr 152:106–110
5. Lowe ME, Greer JB (2008) Pancreatitis in children and adolescents. Curr Gastroenterol Rep 10:128–135
6. Molinari I, Souare K, Lamireau T et al (2004) Fecal chymotrypsin and elastase-1 determination on one single stool collected at random: diagnostic value for exocrine pancreatic status. Clin Biochem 37:758–763
7. Schoenwolf GC, Bleyl SB, Brauer PR, Francis-West PH (2009) Larsen's human embryology, 4th edn. Churchill Livingstone, Philadelphia, p 452
8. Terui K, Yoshida H, Kouchi K et al (2008) Endoscopic sphincterotomy is a useful preoperative management for refractory pancreatitis associated with pancreaticobiliary maljunction. J Pediatr Surg 43:495–499

[7]Charles F. Frey – American surgeon.
[8]Charles Bernard Puestow (1902–1973) American surgeon.

Liver Transplantation

6.7

Jonathan S. Karpelowsky and Alastair J. W. Millar

The first attempt at human liver transplantation occurred in Denver, USA, in 1963, in a child with biliary atresia (Thomas Starzl).

6.7.1
Indications and Contraindications

The most common indications for LT in children are: (Table 6.7.1)

- Biliary atresia (~40%)
- Metabolic diseases (~15%) – e.g., alpha-1-antitrypsin deficiency, tyrosinosis, cystic fibrosis, and hyperoxaluria
- Acute liver failure (~11%)

Chronic liver disease indicators would include

1. Ascites
2. Esophageal varices – bleeding not controlled by endoscopic methods
3. Poor response to nutritional resuscitation
4. Evidence of impaired synthetic function, including prolonged prothrombin time, reduced serum cholesterol levels, and low serum albumin

In acute hepatic failure, clinical indicators would include encephalopathy, hypoglycemia, and prothrombin time of >50 s, though early treatment of paracetemol overdose with acetyl cysteine may prevent irreversible liver failure.

Timing of liver transplantation not only affects survival rate, but may influence neurodevelopmental outcome. Timely referral for assessment is important as the debilitating effects of liver disease impact negatively on surgical morbidity and mortality.

Alastair J. W. Millar (✉)
Department of Paediatric Surgery, Red Cross War Memorial Children's Hospital, Health Sciences Faculty, University of Cape Town, Cape Town, South Africa

C. K. Sinha and M. Davenport (eds.), *Handbook of Pediatric Surgery*,
DOI: 10.1007/978-1-84882-132-3_6.7, © Springer-Verlag London Limited 2010

Table 6.7.1 Indications for which liver transplantation has been performed in children

Obstructive biliary tract disease
Biliary atresia
Choledochal cyst with cirrhosis
Metabolic (inborn errors of metabolism)
Alpha-1-antitrypsin
Tyrosinemia
Glycogen storage disease type III and IV
Wilson's disease
Neonatal hemochromatosis
Hypercholesterolemia
Cystic fibrosis
Hyperoxaluria (+renal transplant)
Hemophilia A + B
Protein C deficiency
Crigler–Najjar syndrome
Acute and chronic hepatitis
Fulminant hepatic failure (viral, toxin, or drug-induced).
Chronic hepatitis (B, C, etc. toxin, autoimmune, idiopathic)
Intrahepatic cholestasis
Neonatal hepatitis
Alagille syndrome
Biliary hypoplasia
Familial cholestasis syndromes
Neoplasia
Hepatoblastoma
Hepatocellular carcinoma
Sarcoma
Hemangioendothelioma
Miscellaneous
Cryptogenic cirrhosis
Congenital hepatic fibrosis
Caroli's disease
Budd–Chiari syndrome
Cirrhosis from prolonged parenteral nutrition

There are few contraindications. Irreversible major cardiorespiratory or neurological disease, which would be incompatible with quality of life and long-term survival, malignancy outside the liver, and uncontrolled systemic sepsis are absolute contraindications. Relative contraindications include cyanotic pulmonary arteriovenous shunting with portal hypertension, chronic hepatitis B, HIV/AIDS, psychosocial factors, and inadequate vascular supply.

6.7.2
Assessment

- *Child assessment*

All children require initial confirmation of the diagnosis, intensive medical investigation (cardiovascular, respiratory, and renal), and nutritional resuscitation to treat the complications of the liver disease, portal hypertension, and nutritional deprivation. Disease assessment includes identification of risk factors and contraindications. Viral screening and immunization should be complete.

- *Family assessment*

Transplant candidacy inevitably results in enormous emotional stress for parents while waiting for the appropriate donor. Family life may become disrupted especially for those who live afar. This provides opportunity to assess the family's commitment to sustain long-term compliance after transplantation and to put in place supportive strategies to ensure adherence to treatment regimens, which need to be lifelong.

Compliance is more difficult to predict in children with acute hepatic failure.

Living related transplant requires extensive evaluation of the potential donors including both physical and psychological assessment.

6.7.3
Surgery

6.7.3.1
Donor Operation

Age limits for suitable donors are being extended due to shortage of organs. Pediatric or neonatal donors can be accepted while livers procured from older children and adults can be transplanted into small children after ex vivo reduction of the size of the graft.

Splitting the donor liver into two functioning units for two recipients is now routine in good donors (Fig. 6.7.1).

Ideal donors fulfil the following criteria.

1. Stable cardiorespiratory function
2. Age <45 years with a short intensive care unit stay (<3 days)
3. Little requirement for inotrope support
4. Normal or near normal liver function

This should be associated with a <5% incidence of primary nonfunction.

Liver biopsy is useful if steatosis is suspected. Viral screening of the donors is essential (Hepatitis A, B, and C; CMV; EBV and HIV). Core HBV antibody and HCV +ve donors would only be considered in selected viral-infected recipients.

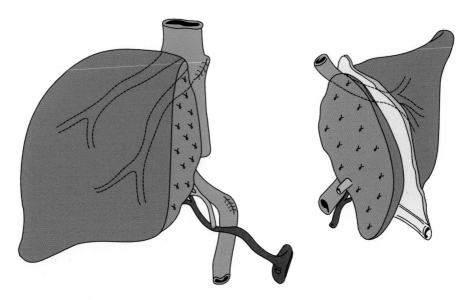

Fig. 6.7.1 Donor liver split into two functioning grafts; the right liver split graft consists of segments 4–8 for an adult recipient and the left lateral segment (segments 2 and 3) for a pediatric recipient. The latter is the usual graft taken from an adult living related donor for an infant or child. The arterial division as depicted here is obligatory in the living donor but in a cadaver split liver the common hepatic artery/coeliac axis can be left with the smaller graft and the right hepatic artery is designated to the right liver graft

The majority of donor livers are removed as part of a multiorgan procurement procedure, which would include various combinations of kidneys, liver, heart, or heart and lungs, small bowel, and pancreas. The organs are perfused with cold preservation solution, placed in a plastic bag also filled with the same solution and stored in ice at 4°C. Cold ischemic times should preferably be kept to <12 h.

6.7.3.2
Recipient Operation

The recipient procedure is often a complex operation taking several hours and is approached in four stages.

1. Removal of the native diseased liver (usually with preservation of the IVC).
2. Anhepatic phase – hepatic vein, portal vein, and hepatic artery anastomoses are performed enabling reperfusion of the new liver. In most cases, the liver is first perfused after portal vein reconstitution and the artery is done later.
3. Bile duct reconstruction – Roux-en-y loop in most cases.
4. Wound closure with drainage to the suprahepatic and infrahepatic spaces.
   (a) If there is any tension at sheath closure due to bowel edema or graft size, it is wise to insert a temporary patch of nonadherent material as a "tight" abdominal closure is associated with an increased incidence of vascular thrombosis and graft

dysfunction. Tension-free definitive closure is usually possible a few days after the initial procedure.

6.7.4
Living-Related Donors

Left lateral segment donation from living donors has become widely accepted as a method of acquiring a liver graft in the face of severe donor shortages, particularly in countries with cultural or religious reticence to accept brain death in a ventilated heart-beating donor (e.g., Japan). Advantages may include

1. Elective procedure preferably before end-stage liver disease in the recipient
2. Excellent graft quality and short ischemic time
3. ↑ Availability of donor organs for other patients on the waiting list

The donor should first undergo a thorough screening both clinical and psychological without coercion and be given an option to withdraw from the procedure at any time before the transplant. Parents usually approach living-related liver transplantation with enthusiasm. They should be advised of the high chance of their own possible unsuitability, including the finding of significant pathology and complications, including death.

> Donor morbidity of ~10% (wound sepsis, hernia, bile leak, and adhesive bowel obstruction). Donor mortality of ~0.2%.

6.7.4.1
Postoperative Care

Meticulous postoperative care is essential with close monitoring of the graft and patient.

- Ventilation – usually 24–48 h (often affected by preoperative health condition).
- Hypertension – almost universal but can be initially managed with appropriate treatment.
- Nutritional and vitamin supplementation – after 72 h by enteral feeding or parenteral nutrition if there is a delay in restoration of bowel function.
- Immunosuppression naturally leads to susceptibility to bacterial, fungal, and viral infections and vigilant monitoring for infections must be undertaken by culture of blood and secretions for bacterial and fungal infections and PCR monitoring of CMV and EBV.
- Prophylaxis is provided against fungal infection (mycostatin), *Pneumocystis jiroveci* (formerly *Pneumocystis carinii*) (trimethoprin-sulfamethoxazole), and viral infection (e.g., CMV and Epstein–Barr virus) (gancyclovir/valganciclovir).

The graft is monitored for

- Vascular patency – daily Doppler US. Patency may be augmented by
  - Hematocrit at <30%
  - Anticoagulants – aspirin and/or dipyrimadole and (high-risk cases) heparin

Technical complications of vascular thrombosis, venous outflow obstruction, bile leak, or abdominal compartment syndrome tend to occur early on and require immediate corrective surgical or radiological intervention.

- Immunological rejection, with liver function tests and biopsy.
  - Anti-CD25 monoclonal antibodies (diclazumab or basiliximab),
  - Steroids (methylprednisolone),
  - Calcineurin 2 inhibitor (tacrolimus), and
  - Antimetabolite (azathiaprine or mycophenolate mofetil)

Steroids are weaned to a low maintenance of 0.25 mg prednisolone/kg over 3 months and tacrolimus levels of 10–12 ng/mL initially can be reduced to maintenance of 5–8 ng/mL in the early period and reduced even further later on depending on host response.

6.7.4.1.1
Complications

Surgical complications include

1. *Biliary (10–20%)*
   (a) Associated with split liver and living-related left lateral segment grafts. Include bile leak, anastomotic strictures, and nonanastomotic strictures of the donor bile duct with sludge formation. Most biliary complications occur in the first few weeks.
   (b) US and MRCP are the principle imaging modalities. It is also imperative with all suspected biliary complications to ensure that the hepatic artery is patent.
2. *Graft ischemia*
   (a) Either from hepatic artery thrombosis (~5%) or portal vein thrombosis (uncommon) and can be devastating. A significant rise in liver enzyme activity, particularly in the first few days after transplant, may be the first indication.
   (b) Arterial thrombosis may lead to graft necrosis, intrahepatic abscess, biliary necrosis, and bile leakage.
   (c) Portal vein thrombosis usually presents with a degree of liver dysfunction, poor clotting function, and portal hypertension, which may be heralded by gastrointestinal bleeding from esophageal varices. Immediate thrombectomy may be successful.
3. *Bowel perforation (~5%)*
   (a) Contributory factors included previous operation with multiple adhesions and the use of diathermy for dissection, steroid therapy, and viral infection. Diagnosis may be difficult and a high index of suspicion is needed.
4. *Inferior vena cava thrombosis (rare)*
   (a) Usually presents early with ascites and lower body edema or later due to regeneration of the graft and twisting of the caval anastomosis.

5. *Hepatic venous outflow obstruction*

   (a) Can be due to kinking of the hepatic vein in reconstruction of a partial graft. Suspect if there is persistence of ascites after the early posttransplant period. Confirmation of the diagnosis may require liver biopsy, which indicates perivenular congestion and hepatic venogram. Most respond well to dilatation.

6. *Diaphragmatic paresis and hernia (rare)*

   (a) Diaphragmatic paresis and hernia may result from excessive use of diathermy and crushing of the phrenic nerve in the caval clamp.

   (b) Plication or repair of the diaphragm is required.

Medical complications include

1. *Infections* (~1.4 infections/patient).

2. *Acute rejection*

   (a) Diagnosis of rejection can be made on the basis of clinical, biochemical, and histological changes and usually presents in the first few weeks after transplant with fever, malaise, a tender graft, and loose stools usually associated with a low calcineurin inhibitor serum level.

   (b) Treated with methyl prednisolone and adjusted baseline immunosuppression.

3. *Late acute cellular rejection* (>3 months)

   (a) Usually due to ↓ immunosuppression from nonadherence and is associated with long-term complications.

4. *Chronic rejection*

   (a) Irreversible phenomenon, which is chiefly intrahepatic and ductular rather than a vascular phenomenon (in contrast to other organ transplants).

   (b) ↓ Intrahepatic bile ducts and ↑ cholestasis. Accompanying CMV infection is frequent.

5. *Chronic graft hepatitis* (20–30%)

   (a) Cause is often not known. Serum liver-associated autoantibodies are often positive. It is most frequently seen in children transplanted for cryptogenic cirrhosis (~70%). Management is with reintroduction or ↑ in steroids.

6. *Cytomegalovirus (CMV) infection*

   (a) CMV infection (seroconversion or virus isolation)

   (b) CMV disease (infection plus clinical signs and symptoms)

   (c) Viral naive recipients receiving a CMV +ve graft are most at risk and should receive antiviral prophylaxis. These patients are treated with a combination of antiviral agents, ↓ immunosuppression, and supportive therapy.

7. *Epstein–Barr virus (EBV) and posttransplant lymphoproliferative disease (PTLD)*.

   (a) PTLD is a spectrum of EBV-driven B-lymphocyte-driven proliferation and may present as a polymorphic B-cell hyperplasia, polymorphic lymphoma, or lymphomatous PTLD.

   (b) Histology must demonstrate lymphoproliferation that disrupts the architecture of the tissue, oligoclonal or monoclonal cell lines, and the presence of EBV in the tissue.

   (c) First manifestations – adenoidal and/or tonsillar involvement. Often widespread and GI and CNS involvement is common. Management strategies include prevention with close PCR monitoring of viral load and reduction of immunosuppression, which may require complete withdrawal, rituximab (anti-CD 20 monoclonal antibody) along with standard antilymphoma chemotherapy, particularly with the monoclonal type.

8. *Renal impairment*

   (a) Is almost inevitable in those patients suffering from chronic liver disease and exacerbated by nephrotoxic immunosuppressive drugs such as cyclosporin and tacrolimus. Renal sparing protocols of immune suppression may include sirolimus (rapamycin), which is nonnephrotoxic.

9. *Drug toxicity*

   (a) Nephrotoxicity and posterior reversible encephalopathy syndrome (PRES) are the most frequently seen in association with calcineurin 2 inhibitor use. Long-term adverse effects of steroids mandate their minimal use. Peptic ulceration from aspirin and steroids is common and requires antacid therapy prophylaxis.

6.7.4.1.2
Retransplantation

Approximately 10–15% of patients may suffer graft failure at some time and need retransplantation. Early indications may be primary nonfunction, early hepatic arterial thrombosis, severe drug-resistant acute rejection, and established chronic rejection. The outcome largely depends on the indication for retransplantation and is good for technical causes but less satisfactory for rejection and infection.

6.7.5
Outcome

- One-year survival of >95% is being achieved in the best centers.

   — Predicted 10-year survivals of 80–85%.
   — Acute liver failure is less successful with a ↑ early death rate usually associated with cerebral complications and multiorgan failure.

- Excellent quality of life can be achieved and most children are fully rehabilitated.
- Liver transplantation is a lifelong commitment from the transplant medical/surgical team and the patient.

Further Reading

1. Baker A, Dhawan A, Heaton N (1998) Who needs a liver transplant? (new disease specific indications). Arch Dis Child 79:460–464
2. Cox KL, Berquist WE, Castillo RO (1999) Paediatric liver transplantation: indications, timing and medical complications. J Gastroenterol Hepatol 14 suppl:S61–S66
3. Muiesan P, Vergani D, Mieli-Vergani G (2007) Liver transplantation in children. J Hepatol 46:340–348
4. Otte JB (2002) History of pediatric liver transplantation. Where are we coming from? Where do we stand? Pediatr Transplant 6:378–387
5. Otte JB (2004) Paediatric liver transplantation – a review based on 20 years of personal experience. Transpl Int 17:562–573
6. Shneider BL (2002) Pediatric liver transplantation in metabolic disease: clinical decision making. Pediatr Transplant 6:25–29
7. Vilca-Melendez H, Heaton ND (2004) Paediatric liver transplantation: the surgical view. Postgrad Med J 80:571–576

Part VII

Principles of Surgical Oncology

Wilms' Tumor

7.1

Ramnik V. Patel, Chandrasen K. Sinha, Shawqui Nour,
and Jenny Walker

Wilms' tumor is a highly malignant renal tumor, derived from embryonic tissue; at present, it has reasonable prognosis due to successful application of multimodal therapy.

7.1.1
Epidemiology

Wilms'[1] tumor *(nephroblastoma)* is the most common pediatric renal tumor and second most common intra-abdominal malignancy (after neuroblastoma).

- Incidence – 10 per million children (~100 cases each year in the UK)
- Ten percent of all pediatric malignancies
- Median age of onset – 3.5 years (unilateral ~36 months; bilateral ~25 months)
- M:F ratio=0.9:1 (unilateral); 0.6:1 (bilateral)
- Nearly all renal, occasional extra-renal WTs described
- Solitary 88%; multicentric 12%
- Unilateral 93%; bilateral 7% (synchronous 85%; metachronous 15%)
- *Geography* – Africans>Caucasians>East Asians

---

[1]Max Wilms (1867–1918) – German surgeon working in Basel and Heidleberg described cases in 1899. He died on the Western Front of diphtheria.

R. V. Patel (✉)
Department of Paediatric Surgery, Sheffield Children's Hospital, London, UK

C. K. Sinha and M. Davenport (eds.), *Handbook of Pediatric Surgery*,
DOI: 10.1007/978-1-84882-132-3_7.1, © Springer-Verlag London Limited 2010

7.1.1.1
Clinical Patterns

There are four clinical patterns/settings:

- *Sporadic* (*>90%*) – no other association, otherwise healthy
- *Recognized associations with congenital anomalies (~5%)*
  — GU anomalies

- *Familial/hereditary* (*1–2%*)
  — Multiple, bilateral, earlier age of onset
  — AD, specific cytogenetic mutations in one of at least three genes

- *Syndromic* (*rare, <1%*)
  — *Overgrowth phenotypic syndromes* – excessive pre and postnatal somatic growth resulting and hemi-hypertrophy
    — Beckwith[2]–Wiedemann[3] Syndrome (BWS) (macroglossia, exomphalos, organomegaly)
    — Isolated hemi-hypertrophy
    — Perlman syndrome (fetal overgrowth, renal hamartomas, nephroblastomatosis)
    — Sotos syndrome (cerebral gigantism)
    — Simpson – Golabi – Behemel Syndrome (similar phenotype to BWS, gene [Xq26] mutations)

- *Nonovergrowth phenotypes*
  — Wilms' Aniridia GU anomalies (sometimes gonadoblastoma) retardation syndrome (*WAGR*) – 11p deletion syndrome.
  — Denys – Drash syndrome (gonadal dysgenesis, nephropathy, mutation in WT-1 gene). Also, Frasier Syndrome (similar phenotype).
  — Bloom syndrome (AR, short stature, distinct facies, hypogonadism, widespread cancer risk).
  — Isolated anorexia, Trisomy 18, etc.

WT-1 gene – Wilms' tumor suppressor gene on Ch 11 (11p13).

---

[2]John Bruce Beckwith (1933) – American pathologist, describing key features in abstract format in 1963.

[3]Hans Rudolf Wiedemann (1915) – German pediatrician in Kiel, independent report in 1964.

7.1.2
Pathology

WT arises from fetal undifferentiated metanephric blastema tissue via nephrogenic rests (incidence 1%, but only 1% progress to WT).

- *Favorable histology* (*90%*) – classic histologic pattern is *triphasic* (i.e., tubular epithelial, blastemal, and stromal elements). Occasionally, in teratoid WT, foci of cartilaginous, adipose, or muscle tissue may appear.
- *Unfavorable histology* (*10%*) – anaplasia seen in higher clinical stage and characterized by focal (<10% of specimens) or diffuse (>10% of specimens) nuclear enlargement, nuclear hyperchromasia, and abnormal mitoses.

7.1.3
Clinical Features

Usual presentation is a small child with an asymptomatic abdominal mass (80%), sometimes abdominal pain (~20%) or hematuria (~20%) may be seen.
Rarer features include

- Urinary tract infection
- Fever from tumor necrosis
- Hypertension and anemia
- Varicocele
- Acute abdomen with tumor hemorrhage or rupture (uncommon)

Differential – Xanthogranulomatous pyelonephritis, mesoblastic nephroma, renal cell carcinoma, renal rhabdoid tumor, and neuroblastoma.

7.1.3.1
Investigations

Specific laboratory studies – βFGF, renin, erythropoietin, cytogenetics studies.

- *US* – heterogenous mass
- *CT Scan/MRI* – accurate staging, including any extension into renal veins and cava (~40%)
- Bone and brain scan – to identify metastatic spread
- *Echocardiogram* – assess right atrial involvement
- *Arteriography* – for preoperative planning/embolization in large tumors, solitary kidney, bilateral tumors, or tumor in a horseshoe kidney
- *DMSA* – bilateral WT to assess individual renal function

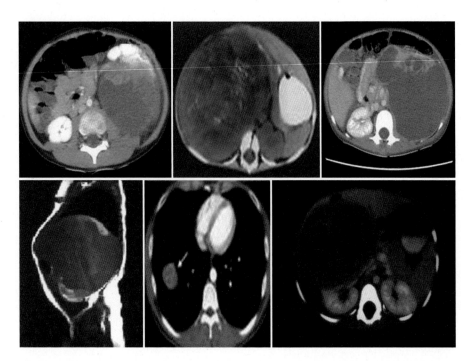

Fig. 7.1.1 Wilms' tumor. *Top row*: Stage I, II, III. *Bottom row*: metastatic WT Stage IV, bilateral WT Stage V

Histology – US-guided spring-loaded 14–16G cutting-core needle biopsy. *Essential* as 1% have benign disease and 5% have non-WT variants (Fig. 7.1.1 and Table 7.1.1).

Table 7.1.1 Staging of WT (UK): preoperative biopsy and chemotherapy

WT has been divided into five stages (with some national differences)
Stage I – confined to kidney and completely excised
Stage II – extending beyond kidney but completely resected
Stage III – incompletely resected, +ve abdominal lymph nodes, peritoneal spread, rupture (pre or intraoperative), open biopsy
Stage IV – distant metastasis (lungs, liver, bone, or brain)
Stage V – bilateral synchronous

In NWTS, the staging is at presentation and stage V can be subdivided into Stage I–III for both sides. SIOP do not advocate a pre-operative biopsy

7.1.3.2
Histological Risk Stratification for Prenephrectomy Chemotherapy-Treated WT

Based on these, three groups of tumors have been classified:

- *Low-risk*: Mesoblastic nephromas, cystic partially differentiated WT, and completely necrotic WT.

- *Intermediate-risk*: Nephroblastoma: (epithelial, stromal, mixed type); regressive type with more than two-thirds tumor being necrotic; and focal anaplasia.
- *High-risk*: Nephroblastoma: blastemal type and diffuse anaplasia; clear-cell sarcoma of kidney; and Rhabdoid tumor of kidney.

7.1.4
Management

There are clear differences in the philosophy of treatment across the world. In European centers, the aim has been to give chemotherapy initially to downstage the tumor (advantage – ↓ operative morbidity). In North America, surgery is still the preferred initial treatment.

7.1.4.1
Routine Preoperative Chemotherapy (UK Practice)

- *UKW3 trial* gave preoperative chemotherapy (Vincristine and Actinomycin D) for 6 weeks.
- *SIOP 2001* management as above but limited to 4 weeks (except for stages IV and V tumors).

7.1.5
Surgery

- Transverse supraumbilical.
- Mobilize colon and duodenum (on right) to expose tumor and vascular pedicle.
- Evaluate nodal spread and palpate opposite kidney.
- *Nephrectomy including perinephric fascia* and *regional lymph nodes* – ligation of ureter, then renal artery, and lastly vein. The adrenal may also need to be excised.
- *Partial Nephrectomy.*

    — Bilateral WT contralateral pre-existing abnormality of kidney
    — WT in single kidney
    — WT with nephroblastomatosis

- *Venous extension* – infrahepatic extension can be removed by venotomy after caval control. Suprahepatic and atrial involvement may require cardiopulmonary bypass.
- Hepatic or pulmonary resection for persistent metastases (if necessary).

Bilateral Wilms' Tumor (Stage V)

A range of procedures have been used including local enucleation of small tumors, partial nephrectomy and contralateral excision biopsy, bilateral partial nephrectomy, unilateral nephrectomy and contralateral partial nephrectomy, bilateral nephrectomy + dialysis + renal transplant, and finally removal, "bench surgery," intra-operative radiotherapy + auto-transplant.

7.1.5.1
Postoperative Chemotherapy

Based on the stage and histological risk group as follows:

	Low	Intermediate	High
Stage I	None	A, V (4 weeks)	A, V, D (4 months)
Stage II	A, V (2–4 months)	2 (A, V) or 3 (A, V, D) drugs (4 months) (randomized)	2 (A, V) or 3 (A, V, D) drugs (4 months) (randomized) + RT
Stage III	A, V, D (4 months)	VP-16, Carbo, Cyclo, D (6 months)	VP-16, Carbo, Cyclo, D (6 months) + RT

V vincristine; *A* Actinomycin-D; *D* Doxorubicin; *VP-16* etoposide; *Carbo* carboplatin; *Cyclo* cyclophosphamide; *RT* radiotherapy

7.1.5.2
Prognosis

Overall, long-term survival rates of >90% can be achieved with Stage I–III tumors; even with metastatic disease, ~70% can still achieve long-term survival. *Stage and tumor histology* and, to a lesser extent, *age at diagnosis* (↓ survival in infants) are the most important prognostic factors.

Further Reading

1. Green DM (2007) Controversies in the management of Wilms' tumour – immediate nephrectomy or delayed nephrectomy? Eur J Cancer 43:2453–2456
2. Malogolowkin M, Cotton CA, Green DM et al (2008) Treatment of Wilms' tumor relapsing after initial treatment with vincristine, actinomycin D, and doxorubicin. A report from the NWTS group. Pediatr Blood Cancer 50:236–241
3. Mitchell C, Pritchard-Jones K, Shannon R et al (2006) Immediate nephrectomy versus preoperative chemotherapy in the management of non-metastatic Wilms' tumour: results of a randomised trial (UKW3) by the UK Children's Cancer Study Group. Eur J Cancer 42:2554–2562

4. Spicer RD (2005) Wilms' tumour. In: Burge DM, Griffiths DM, Steinbrecher HA, Wheeler RA (eds) Paediatric surgery, 2nd edn. Hodder Arnold, London, pp 367–374

5. Van den Heuvel-Eibrink MM, Grundy P, Graf N et al (2008) Characteristics and survival of 750 children diagnosed with a renal tumor in the first seven months of life: A collaborative study by the SIOP/GPOH/SFOP, NWTSG, and UKCCSG Wilms' tumor study groups. Pediatr Blood Cancer 50:1130–1134

Liver Tumors

7.2

Chandrasen K. Sinha and Mark Davenport

The treatment of hepatoblastoma has been revolutionized by effective chemotherapy and judicious surgery with an overall survival of ~90%.

- Third commonest intra-abdominal malignancy in children.
- Two real malignant variants – *hepatoblastoma* (typical embryonic tumor) and *hepatocellular* carcinoma (HCC) (end result of chronic liver disease).
  - Rarely, *rhabdomyosarcoma* – botryoid[1] tumor from bile ducts causes early-onset jaundice.
- Three benign variants – *hemangiomas* (ubiquitous, mono or bilobar), *mesenchymal hamartomas* (adolescent girls), and *adenomas*.
- M>F (Hepatoblastoma).
- Geographical variation.
  - ↑ HCC in East Asia, China, Japan (↑ Hepatitis B)

7.2.1
Associations:

- Hepatoblastoma
  - Beckwith–Wiedeman syndrome
  - Hemihypertrophy
  - Low birth weight
    Fetal alcohol syndrome

- HCC
  - Cirrhotic liver disease (e.g., biliary atresia, tyrosinemia, etc.)

---

[1]*Botryoid* (Greek) *grape-like.*

C. K. Sinha (✉)
Paediatric Surgery Department, King's College Hospital, London, UK

C. K. Sinha and M. Davenport (eds.), *Handbook of Pediatric Surgery*,
DOI: 10.1007/978-1-84882-132-3_7.2, © Springer-Verlag London Limited 2010

7.2.2
Pathology: Malignant Tumors

Hepatoblastoma – usually unifocal and commoner in the right lobe. Two types recognized:

1. Epithelial type
   (a) Fetal, embryonal, or small cell undifferentiated pattern

2. Mixed epithelial and mesenchymal type
   (b) Teratoid or nonteratoid features

7.2.3
Clinical Features

Both tumors present with a combination of a palpable mass and usually signs of anemia, etc. Hepatoblastoma tends to occur in young (1–3 years), while HCC occurs usually in adolescence. Metastases at presentation are more common with HCC (~30%). Rarely, the tumor (more characteristic of embryonal sarcoma) may rupture and present acutely.

7.2.3.1
Investigations

- *Specific Laboratory studies* – ↑↑α-fetoprotein (AFP) and β human chorionic gonado-tropin (hCG) levels.
  - AFP – normal (~10% HB (implies anaplastic variant) vs. 40% HCC).
  - AFP – initial level has no prognostic significance, although degree of fall postchemo may do.
- *US/Doppler* – confirms cystic vs. solid; site; ?multicentric and evidence of portal vein involvement.
- *CT/MRI (±angiography) scans* – evidence of metastases (other lobe/chest/brain). Resectability and involvement of portal and hepatic veins.
- *Percutaneous biopsy.*

7.2.4
Staging

There are two staging systems in use; the older is derived from largely American practice (what was left after the surgeons had had a go at resection) and the more recent based on the concept of PRETEXT (PRETreatment EXtent of disease), which has found favor in

Europe and the UK. Table 7.2.1 illustrates the former and Fig. 7.2.1 the latter. The advantage of the American approach is that some children with favorable histology with complete resection may not require chemotherapy. The advantage of the SIOPEL approach is that large unresectable tumors become resectable and diminish the complications of untoward surgical adventure.

Table 7.2.1   Children's oncology group (COG) staging

Stage	Features	
I	Complete resection	30%
II	Resection with microscopic residual disease	30%
III	Resection with gross residual tumor/tumor spillage/positive lymph nodes/incomplete resection	30%
IV	Distant metastases	10%

7.2.5
Management

The current trend is for preoperative chemotherapy followed by complete surgical resection unless the imaging shows a small peripheral, usually exophytic, tumor suitable for straightforward excision or there is histological doubt.

1. Chemotherapy.
   (a) Cisplatin, carboplatin – trialed currently as monotherapy.
   (b) Doxorubicin
   (c) Vincristine
   (d) Cyclophosphamide
   (e) Paclitaxel and etoposide.
Usually six cycles of chemotherapy are administered every 2–4 weeks. AFP levels are used as a guide to determine response to therapy.

2. Radiotherapy – may be used when microscopic disease is seen at the resection margins and in chemoresistant pulmonary metastases. Dose (usually 1,200–2,000 centiGray).

7.2.6
Surgery

The aim is complete surgical resection of all disease. This may be accomplished by

- *Liver resection* (see Chap. 10.2)

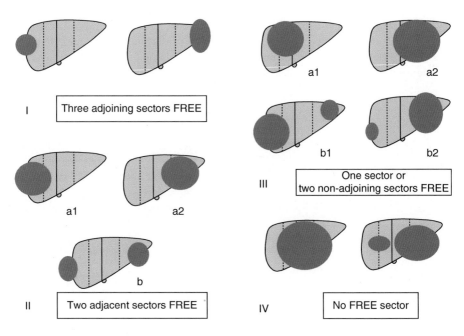

Fig. 7.2.1 PRETEXT classification of hepatoblastoma

- — Segmentectomy
- — R or L hemihepatectomy (V, VI, VII, VIII) or (II, III, IV)
- — R or L extended hemihepatectomy (plus IV) or (plus V, VIII)
- • ± Caudate (I) – unusual to completely resect this.
- • *Liver transplantation*
- — Indications include unresectable primary, multifocal, or central tumors or when diaphragmatic extension precludes complete resection.

Resection of pulmonary metastases may also be needed in some children with long-term disease-free survival, where primary tumor has been already eradicated.

7.2.7
Outcome

Patients who undergo complete resection of the tumor and adjuvant chemotherapy approach 100% survival.

- • Five-year survival (overall) in hepatoblastoma 57–69% (COG)
- • Five-year event-free survival rates

- — Stage I with UH → 91%
- — Stage II → 100%
- — Stage III → 64%
- — Stage IV → 25%
- Five-year survival (overall) ~ 90% (SIOPEL)
  - — event-free survival rates ≤ 80%
- Two-year event-free survival (HCC) ~40%

7.2.8
Hepatic Metastases

Possible sites include

- Neuroblastoma
- Wilms' tumor
- Rhabdomyosarcoma
- Non-Hodgkin's lymphoma
- Osteogenic sarcoma

The criteria for resection of these metastases are reasonable expectations of life with control of the primary tumor and limited number of metastases.

7.2.9
Benign Liver Tumors

7.2.9.1
Hemangiomas (Hemangioendotheliomas)

Common if looked for, with the majority remaining clinically silent. Some may present in infants with hepatomegaly, high-output cardiac output, and thombocytopenia.

- Other hemangiomas – usually skin, intestinal, pulmonary (up to 40% of severe examples)
- Female predominant

7.2.9.1.1
Pathology

Endothelial-lined vascular spaces with variable size. Hemangioendothelioma is used to describe typical lesions of infancy. Some merge with angiosarcoma-like lesions and are best treated as malignant.

7.2.9.1.2
Clinical Features

Symptoms may include abdominal distension and hepatomegaly within 1 month of birth. Platelet sequestration and consumptive coagulopathy (Kasabach–Merritt syndrome) may occur (especially if bilobar).

7.2.9.1.3
Investigations

- Specific laboratory studies – FBC (anemia and ↓ platelets), thyroid function tests (both hypo and hyperthyroidism have been reported).
- US and Doppler – mono or bilobar high, flow through hepatic artery
- CT/MRI ± angiogram – will delineate anatomy, respectability, and degree of vascular function (Fig. 7.2.2).

7.2.9.1.4
Management

There is a potential for spontaneous regression in the first few years of life. However, active treatment is required for all symptomatic lesions. All those with high-output cardiac failure require support with diuretics and digoxin.

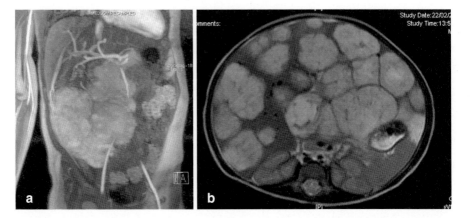

Fig. 7.2.2 MRI scans showing (a) angiogram phase – large heterogeneous right lobe tumor (biopsy – hepatoblastoma). (b) T2-weighted – multiple bilobar vascular tumors in a 1-month-old infant – hemangioendothelioma

1. Chemotherapy
   (a) Steroids
   (b) Propranolol
   (c) Vincristine
   (d) α-Interferon

2. Surgery

   (a) Isolated lesions are best treated with surgical excision.
   (b) Hepatic artery embolization/ligation indicated for multifocal or extensive lesions.
   (c) Liver transplantation for multifocal lesions (typically low-flow) and those poorly responsive to HAE/L.

7.2.9.2
Mesenchymal Hamartomas

These are multicystic heterogeneous lesions, which can be massive. They have been associated with placental pathology and show no evidence of spontaneous regression. Controversial as to whether they have a malignant potential.

Liver resection is usually preferred.

7.2.9.3
Focal Nodular Hyperplasia and Hepatic Adenomas

FNH and hepatic adenomas are benign tumors seen in children. There is some evidence of a relationship with estrogen exposure (e.g., contraceptive pill), and most do occur in adolescent girls.

7.2.9.3.1
Investigations

- *CT/MR scans* – appearance of a central scar is a pathognominic feature of FNH.
- Tc-sulfur colloid radioisotope scan.
- Percutaneous biopsy may be needed for definitive diagnosis.

Indications for resection in both lesions are symptoms and diagnostic doubt.

Further Reading

1. Ortega JA et al (2000) Randomized comparison of cisplatin/vincristine/fluorouracil and cisplatin/continuous infusion doxorubicin for treatment of pediatric hepatoblastoma: A report from the Children's Cancer Group and the Pediatric Oncology Group. J Clin Oncol 18:2665–2667

2. Aronson DC et al (2005) Predictive value of the pretreatment extent of disease system in hepatoblastoma: results from the International Society of Pediatric Oncology Liver Tumor Study Group SIOPEL-1 study. J Clin Oncol 20(23):1245–1252
3. Roebuck D et al (2007) 2005 PRETEXT: a revised staging system for primary malignant liver tumours of childhood developed by the SIOPEL group. Pediatr Radiol 37:123–132
4. Litten JB et al (2008) Liver tumors in children. Oncologist 13:812–820

Neuroblastoma

Nadeem Haider and Roly Squire

Enigmatic embryonal tumor arising from neuroblasts with somewhat unpredictable behavior.

5–10% of all childhood cancers
- Age of onset
  Infancy ~30%
  1–4 years ~50%
  10–14 years ~5%
- M>F (slight)

7.3.1
Sites of Origin

- Adrenal medulla (~50%)
- Abdominal sympathetic ganglia (~25%)
- Posterior mediastinum (~20%)
- Pelvis (~3%)
- Neck (~3%)

7.3.2
Pathology

Tumor appears as soft with areas of hemorrhage and necrosis. More mature areas tend to be firm. Histological appearance is as sheets of dark blue round cells with scanty cytoplasm, embedded in a delicate vascular stroma. Tends to spread with local extension and

N. Haider (✉)
Paediatric Surgery Department, Leeds General Infirmary, Leeds, UK

C. K. Sinha and M. Davenport (eds.), *Handbook of Pediatric Surgery*,
DOI: 10.1007/978-1-84882-132-3_7.3, © Springer-Verlag London Limited 2010

encasement of major vessels. May metastasize to lymph nodes, bones, bone marrow, liver and skin. Secondary spread is usually associated with large primaries (except stage 4S tumors).

- Characteristic ring of neuroblasts around a neurofibrillary core (rosette formation) differentiate from other blue, round cell tumors (e.g., Ewing's sarcoma, lymphoma and rhabdomyosarcoma).

7.3.3
Shimada[1] System Classification

Based on the

1. Mitosis karyorrhexis index (MKI)
2. Age of child
3. Degree of differentiation (towards ganglioneuroma)
4. Stroma-rich or stroma-poor

Favorable prognosis includes infants, low MKI, stroma-rich tumors, well differentiated tumors or tumors with intermixed degrees of differentiation.

7.3.4
Cytogenetics and Prognostic Factors

A large number of molecular abnormalities have been identified in the neuroblastoma cells. These include

- *MYCN* amplification
  - Gene on Ch 2p.
  - Leads to activation of angiogenesis pathways and ↑tumor growth
  - Advanced vs. low-stage disease stage (amplification present ~40% vs. ~10%)
  - 90% of patients with MYCN amplification will die of disease progression irrespective of treatment modality used

- Ch 17q gain, Ch 1p deletion
- Expression of the H-*ras* oncogene – associated with low-stage disease

---

[1]Hiroyuki Shimada – Japanese pathologist, latterly working in Los Angeles, USA.

- DNA ploidy and index – diploid DNA associated with *MYCN* amplification
- CD44 expression – ↑expression associated with good prognosis
- TRKA expression – ↑expression associated with good prognosis
- Multidrug resistance-associated protein (MRP) – ↑ levels associated with poor prognosis

7.3.5
Clinical Features

Palpable abdominal mass. Unlike other tumors (e.g., Wilms') children often appear sick, lethargic with fatigue, bone pain, weight loss, fever, sweating and anemia.

7.3.5.1
Unusual But Characteristic

- Periorbital ecchymosis or proptosis (racoon eyes) – retro-orbital secondaries.
- Horner's[2] syndrome – apical thoracic tumors.
- Progressive cerebellar ataxia and trunk opsomyoclonus.
- Dancing eye syndrome – rapid but chaotic, conjugate eye movements.
- Progressive paraplegia – from extradural cord compression.
- Hypertension (~25%) due to catecholamine production or renal artery compression.
- Skin nodules – stage 4S disease.
- Diarrhea – due to vasoactive intestinal polypeptide (VIP) release – more typical of ganglioneuromas and ganglioneuroblastomas.

7.3.5.2
Investigations

7.3.5.2.1
Specific Laboratory Studies

- ↑↑ Vanillylmandelic acid (VMA) and homovanillic acid (HVA) – urinary metabolites of catecholamines.
- ↑ ferritin, ↑ lactate dehydrogenase (LDH), and ↑ Neuron specific enolase (NSE).
- AXR – tumor calcification (~50%).

---

[2]Johann F. Horner (1831–1886) – Swiss ophthalmologist named triad as meiosis, ptosis and enopthalmos, but can have ↓ facial sweating and iris color change. Described many times before Horner's case in 1869.

- *US* – solid vs. cystic, may suggest renal vein and caval involvement.
- *CT/MRI scans* – anatomy of tumor search for metastases. Possible intraspinal extension ("dumb-bell" tumor).
- Radio-isotopes.
  - — MIBG (meta-iodobenzylguanidine) scan – for abnormal medullary tissue.
  - — Tecnetium
- *Biopsy* – percutaneous or open.
- *Bone marrow*

7.3.6
Staging: Complex and Evolving

- Evans classification (1971) – site of origin and behavior
- TNM (tumor-node-metastasis)

7.3.6.1
International Neuroblastoma Staging System (INSS) 1989

Simple

1. Stage 1 – completely resectable localized tumor.
2. Stage 2 – incompletely resected tumor and/ or presence of +ve I/L nodes.
3. Stage 3 – primary tumor crossing the midline or unilateral tumor with +ve C/L nodes. Also midline tumor with bilateral +ve nodes.
4. Stage 4 – tumor with spread to other organs, bone or lymph nodes.
   (a) Stage 4S – infants. Skin, liver and bone marrow (Table 7.3.1)

There is a new staging system for tumor stratification that has been proposed by the International Neuroblastoma Risk Group (INRG). This will define the risk group by the pretreatment grade as opposed to postsurgery staging in the INSS system, as well as age, tumor biology, histology and MYCN status.

7.3.6.2
Infantile Neuroblastoma

Infants (<1 year) carry a much better prognosis and is true for all stages. For example, 5 year survival in stage 4: 75% vs. 10%.

Table 7.3.1   International neuroblastoma staging system (INSS) 1989

Stage 1	Localized tumor with complete gross excision, ±microscopic residual disease; representative I/L nodes –ve for tumor microscopically (nodes attached to and removed with the primary tumor may be +ve)
Stage 2A	Localized tumor with incomplete gross excision; representative I/L no adherent lymph nodes negative for tumor microscopically
Stage 2B	Localized tumor ± complete gross excision, with I/L nonadherent lymph nodes +ve for tumor. Enlarged contralateral lymph nodes must be negative microscopically
Stage 3	Unresectable unilateral tumor infiltrating across the midline, ±regional node involvement; or localized unilateral tumor with C/L regional node involvement; or midline tumor with bilateral extension by infiltration (unresectable) or by node involvement
Stage 4	Any primary tumor with dissemination to distant lymph nodes, bone, bone marrow, liver, skin, and/or other organs (except as defined for stage 4S)
Stage 4S	Localized primary tumor (as defined for stage 1, 2A, or 2B), with dissemination limited to skin, liver, and/or bone marrow (limited to infants <1 year). Marrow involvement should be minimal (i.e., <10% of total nucleated cells identified as malignant by bone biopsy or by bone marrow aspirate). More extensive bone marrow involvement would be considered to be stage IV disease. The results of the MIBG scan (if performed) should be –ve for disease in the bone marrow

7.3.6.3
Stage 4S Neuroblastoma

- ~30% of infantile neuroblastoma
- Spontaneous regression possible

Features include hepatosplenomegaly (may cause respiratory failure), subcutaneous nodules, and a positive bone marrow.

Life-threatening hepatomegaly can be treated with low dose radiotherapy (effect may be slow in onset) or cyclophosphamide (5 mg/kg/day). Aggressive chemotherapy may be required in cases with >10 copies of *NMYC*, serum ferritin levels of >142 mg/mL and other adverse biological markers.

- More than 80% of these infants with 4S disease will survive without any specific treatment.

7.3.6.4
Risk Groups

Patients are assigned into one of three groups	(Predicted 3 year survival rates)
Low risk	>90%
Intermediate risk	70–90%
High risk	<30%

The North American COG base their risk groups on overall survival rates of >90%, 70–90%, and <30% three years after diagnosis. Patients risk grouping is based on INSS stage, age, MYCN status, Shimada classification and DNA ploidy.

7.3.7
Management

- *Immediate resection* – current practice suggests that this is reserved for tumors in the absence of *image defined risk factors* (IDRF) i.e., (INRG "L1 TUMORS"). If there are IDRF's preresection, then neoadjuvant chemotherapy should be given.
- *Tumor biopsy* – treatment of metastatic and localized tumors with IDRF's (INRG "L2 Tumors") can be influenced by their *MYCN* status.
  - The risk groups are then defined by a combination of stage, age, histology and cytogenetics.
- Stage 2 – Surgical excision.
  - Not always feasible especially those with intraspinal extension or apical thoracic tumors. In these cases, chemotherapy prior to surgery is advisable.
- *Stage 3 and 4* – chemotherapy followed by attempt at surgical resection.
  - tumors are less vascular and are downstaged postchemotherapy.

7.3.7.1
Low Risk Group

- Stage 1 (i.e., localized resectable neuroblastoma)
- Stage 2 in those <1 year (regardless of *MYCN* status or histology)
- Stage 4S disease

Adjuvant chemotherapy is generally not needed for this group of patients except in very few life-threatening cases of 4S disease.

7.3.7.2
Intermediate Risk Group

- Stage 3/4/4S disease in those <1 year of age and favorable biology irrespective of histology.
- Stage 3 in those >1 year with non-*MYCN* and favorable histology.

Four agent chemotherapy (Cyclophosphamide, Doxorubicin, Carboplatin, Etoposide) for 4 or 8 cycles depending on the histology.

Surgery is performed after chemotherapy. If residual disease is present, radiotherapy can be considered (controversial).

7.3.7.3
High Risk Group

- Stage 2A/2B disease who are >1 year and have *MYCN* amplified unfavorable histology tumors.
- Stage 3/4/4S who are <1 year and *MYCN* amplified tumors.
- Stage 3 in children >1 year with *MYCN*-amplified or non-*MYCN*–amplified tumors, and unfavorable histology.
- Stage 4 in children >1 year.

Multiagent induction chemotherapy to induce tumor remission, and improve chance of resection. If response is poor, then second line chemotherapy is used.

Surgery to excise the tumor is then carried out.

Further high-dose chemotherapy and peripheral stem cell rescue for reconstitution of patient's bone marrow ± retinoic acid ± radiotherapy.

Spinal Cord Compression

Spinal cord compression by dumb-bell type tumors may cause paralysis, paresthesia, or bladder dysfunction. Immediate treatment is mandatory. Treament options include surgical decompression of spinal cord, chemotherapy or radiotherapy. Since most patients will require chemotherapy, hence chemotherapy is used most commonly with the surgical option reserved for the nonresponders.

7.3.8
Fetal Tumors

Increasingly frequent clinical scenario. Most have favorable biologic markers with no *MYCN* amplification (i.e., Low Risk with excellent survival following surgery alone). Some advocate observation only in the early management expecting regression and small (<5 cm) tumors appear to be good candidates for this approach. About 60% of infants can avoid surgery following spontaneous tumor regression.

7.3.9
Surgery

- Aim of surgery postchemotherapy is to achieve complete resection.
- Complete resection has demonstrated to be an advantage in advanced disease.
- Aim of second-look procedure is to achieve as complete a debulking as possible without sacrificing major organ function.

Possible role for laparoscopic and thoracoscopic surgery is diagnostic and excision biopsies of smaller tumors.

7.3.10
New Treatments

- I^{131} labeled MIBG.
- New chemotherapy agents – topotecan, irinotecan, etoposide, oral topoisomerase II inhibitor.
- Immunologic therapies include monoclonal antibodies, cytokine therapies and vaccines.
- Antiangiogenic factors.
- Other experimental agents include, tyrosine kinase inhibitors, direct targeting of *MYCN* amplified cells and creation of chimeric antibodies to deliver cytotoxic drugs.

Further Reading

1. De Bernardi B et al (1992) Disseminated neuroblastoma (Stage IV and IV S) in the first year of life. Cancer 70:1625–1629
2. Iwanaka T, Kawashima H, Uchida H (2007) The laparoscopic approach of neuroblastoma. Semin Pediatr Surg 16:259–265
3. Lacreuse I, Valla JS, de Lagausie P et al (2007) Thoracoscopic resection of neurogenic tumors in children. J Pediatr Surg 42:1725–1728
4. Paul SR et al (1991) Stage IV neuroblastoma in infants: long term survival. Cancer 67:1493–1498
5. Titilope AI, Dai H et al (2007) Neuroblastoma. Surg Oncol 16:149–156

Teratomas

7.4

Erica Makin and Mark Davenport

Teratomas are germ-cell tumors (GCTs) that contain all three embryonic layers (endoderm, mesoderm, and ectoderm) and most of them (~80%) are benign.

Teratomas[1] are germ-cell tumors arising from the gonads or (usually midline) extragonadal sites. Sacrococcygeal teratoma (SCT) is the commonest variety and the commonest of all solid neonatal tumors. This chapter focuses on extragonadal GCTs.

7.4.1
Incidence

- Teratomas (overall) → *teratoma (overall)*
  — 4 per million children under the age of 15 years
- Sacrococcygeal teratoma → *SCT*
  — 1 in 30,000, M:F 2:1

7.4.2
Embryology

GCTs arise from primordial cells derived from the embryonic yolk sac endoderm at around 24 days of gestation. During the fifth and sixth week, these cells migrate along the mesentry of the hindgut toward the genital ridge. Premature migration arrest is thought to result in the formation of extragonadal GCT arising in or near the midline (Table 7.4.1).

---

[1]*Teratoma* is derived from the Greek *teratos* meaning monster and *onkoma* meaning swelling.

M. Davenport (✉)
Paediatric Surgery Department, Kings College Hospital, London, UK

C. K. Sinha and M. Davenport (eds.), *Handbook of Pediatric Surgery*,
DOI: 10.1007/978-1-84882-132-3_7.4, © Springer-Verlag London Limited 2010

Table 7.4.1 Distribution of extragonadal GCT

Site	%	Notes
Sacrococcygeal	70	
Intracranial	10	Usually pineal gland
Mediastinal	5	Commoner in male adolescents. (NB Testicular examination essential as mediastinal mass could be a secondary)
Other (cervical, retroperitoneum, omentum, pancreas, stomach, and vagina)	15	*Retroperitoneum* – usually benign *Vaginal* – malignant ESTs at presentation *Gastric* – benign

7.4.3
Pathology and Classification (Fig. 7.4.1)

- *Immature teratomas* are not strictly benign and usually contain one or more of the somatic tissues (most commonly neuroepithelial cells). Metastases usually arise from undiagnosed malignant cells within the teratomas at the time of resection.
- *Endodermal sinus tumors (ESTs)* are the commonest malignant GCT.
- *Choriocarcinomas* arise from placental tissue (gestational) or extraplacental tissue in the mediastinum or gonad (nongestational) in an adolescent or via transplacental spread in a newborn.
- *Embryonal carcinomas* are capable of differentiating into embryonic or extraembryonic tumors. They are poorly differentiated, anaplastic, and are highly malignant with the worst prognosis.

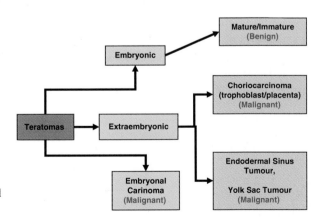

Fig. 7.4.1 A schematic demonstrating the pathological classification of teratomas

Table 7.4.2   Staging of extragonadal GCT

Stage		Overall survival (%)
I	Complete resection. Negative tumor margins. Coccygectomy for sacrococcygeal site;	90
II	Microscopic residual disease, lymph nodes normal;	90
III	Gross residual disease or biopsy only; retroperitoneal nodes either normal or showing evidence of malignancy;	75
IV	Distant metastases, including liver	75

7.4.3.1
Staging

The Pediatric Oncology Group/Children's Cancer Group (POC/CCG) staging system for malignant extragonadal GCTs is outlined in Table 7.4.2.

7.4.3.2
Tumor Markers

1. *α-feto protein (α-FP)* – protein produced by embryonic liver, yolk sac, and gastrointestinal tract
   — Very sensitive to the presence of malignant EST.
   — Normally elevated in the neonatal period and reaches normal levels by 9 months of age (Fig. 7.4.2). It is routinely measured postoperatively as screening for recurrence. *(NB. Also elevated in benign and malignant liver disease).*
2. *Human chorionic gonadotropin (HCG)* – released by syncytiotrophoblasts
   — Sensitive marker for choriocarcinoma.

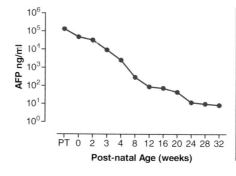

Fig. 7.4.2   Serum α-FP levels in normal infants. (Adapted from Wu JT, Book L, Sudar K (1981) Serum Alpha Fetoprotein (AFP) levels in normal infants. Pediatr Res 15:50–52)

PT	135000
0	48500
2	33000
3	9500
4	2600
8	300
12	90
16	75
20	45
24	12
28	10
32	9

7.4.4
Management

7.4.4.1
Principle

- Most GCTs are treated with a combination of surgery and chemotherapy (e.g., UKCCSG GC II protocol (carboplatin ("JM8"), etoposide, and bleomycin – JEB regimen)), which has increased the 5-year survival to ~90%. A more toxic regimen (cisplatin, etoposide, and bleomycin – PEB) is reserved for recurrence.
- Radiotherapy is the mainstay for intracranial GCTs.

7.4.5
Sacrococcygeal Teratomas (SCT)

Antenatally diagnosed in >90% cases at 20-week anomaly scan.
Antenatal complications include

- Polyhydramnios and premature delivery.
- Fetal hydrops (placentomegaly, ascites, pleural effusions) and the development of *"maternal mirror" syndrome*.

The need for antenatal intervention (exception amnioreduction) is associated with a poor prognosis.

7.4.5.1
Delivery

Ideally should be via C-section (particularly if tumor is >5 cm), to minimize the risks of rupture, hemorrhage, or dystocia during birth. Once stabilized, the extent of the tumor should be ascertained by USS±MRI and classified according to the Altman[2] criteria (Table 7.4.3).

Table 7.4.3 Altman classification (1974)

Type	Description	%
I	Predominantly external	45
II	External with intrapelvic extension	35
III	Externally visible, mainly pelvic with intra-abdominal extension	10
IV	Entirely intrapelvic/intra-abdominal, no external findings	10

[2]R. Peter Altman – American pediatric surgeon at Columbia University, New York.

7.4.5.2
Surgery

Preoperative imaging (MR/US) should define upper extent of tumor. If upper extent is below sacral promentary, then sacral-only approach should be possible. Very vascular tumors may benefit from initial laparotomy and preliminary ligation of median sacral vessels.

1. Position – "skydiver" with urethral catheter and rectal pack.
2. Incision - "chevron," "Mercedes-Benz," or "pi."
3. Create skin flaps, and dissect from stretched gluteal and anorectal muscle groups. Define plane between rectum and tumor working toward pelvis.
4. Define and divide sacro-coccygeal joint (always remove coccyx with tumor).
5. Once tumor is mobile enough, the median vascular pedicle can be defined, transfixed, and divided.

(NB – although early vascular control via the sacrum is often advocated, this can be difficult with large, bulky tumors within the pelvis.)

6. Reconstruction – important stage but often hurried after long period of dissection. Ensure re-alignment of anorectal and levator muscle complex, adequate buttock volume (consider de-epithelializing excess skin flaps), median sacral cleft, and "normal" distance between anus and sacrum.

Histology – presence of yolk-sac elements (~5%) or "immature" tumors (50%) has little prognostic significance if tumor is completely resected.

All patients should be followed-up for at least 3 years and screening should include a rectal examination and αFP at regular intervals (e.g., every 2 months for first 6 month, then every 3 months for 18 months).

Potential long-term morbidity related largely to neurological involvement (tumor/iatrogenic).

- Urological – ↓ sphincter function (incontinence) (5–30%)
- Anorectal – ↓ sphincter function (incontinence or constipation) (10–30%)
- Lower limb impairment (rare)
- Cosmetic - leave secondary surgery until primary school years

7.4.7
Outcome

- Antenatally diagnosed SCT – overall survival of ~75%.
- If live born – >90% survival.
- Recurrence occurs in 10–20% of benign SCTs and in ~30% of malignant stage 1 SCTs (often late presenters).

Further Reading

1. Altman RP, Randolph JG, Lilly JR (1974) Sacrococcygeal teratoma: American Academy of Pediatrics Surgical section survey - 1973. J Pediatr Surg 9:389–398
2. Derikx JP, De Backer A, van de Schoot L et al (2007) Long-term functional sequelae of sacrococcygeal teratoma: a national study in The Netherlands. J Pediatr Surg 42:1122–6
3. Makin EC, Hyett J, Ade-Ajayi N et al (2006) Outcome of antenatally diagnosed sacrococcygeal teratomas: single-center experience (1993–2004). J Pediatr Surg 41:388–93

Miscellaneous Tumors

7.5

Anindya Niyogi, Chandrasen K. Sinha, and Robert Carachi

7.5.1
Lymphomas

Lymphomas can be divided into

- *Hodgkin's lymphoma* (HL) (45%)
  — *All B cell origin*
- *Non-Hodgkin's lymphoma* (NHL) (55%)
  — *Both B- and T-cell origin*

7.5.1.1
Hodgkin's[1] Lymphoma

- ~45% of all childhood lymphomas.

7.5.1.1.1
Etiology

- Unclear.
- Genetic immunosupression.
- Delayed exposure to infection.
- Epstein–Barr virus (EBV) infections were identified as predisposing factors.
- HLA-DP alleles are more common in Hodgkin disease.

HL is characterized by the presence of pathognomonic Reed–Sternberg[2] cells.

---

[1]Thomas Hodgkin (1798–1866), English physician at Guy's Hospital, London described this in 1832.
[2]Dorothy Reed (1874–1964) and Carl Sternberg (1872–1935), American and German pathologists who distinguished these cells independently.

A. Niyogi (✉)
Paediatric Surgery Department, Chelsea and Westminster Hospital, London, UK

C. K. Sinha and M. Davenport (eds.), *Handbook of Pediatric Surgery*,
DOI: 10.1007/978-1-84882-132-3_7.5, © Springer-Verlag London Limited 2010

7.5.1.1.2
Clinical Features

Rye[3] classification divides classical HL into four histological subgroups:

1. Nodular sclerosing (70%) best prognosis
2. Mixed cellularity (20%) associated with HIV
3. Lymphocyte predominant (<10%)
4. Lymphocyte depleted (<2%) worst prognosis

NB, WHO classification also includes a fifth nonclassical type, the nodular lymphocyte-predominant HL.

Painless, rubbery, typically fixed, lymphadenopathy (usually cervical), with later involvement of mediastinal lymph nodes causing dyspnea, cough, or stridor. Sometimes, spread is extralymphatic, for instance, with liver and spleen involvement.

Constitutional (so-called B) symptoms are also seen (e.g., weight loss, fever (Pel-Ebstein; ~40°C every 7–10 days), night sweats, pruritus, fatigue, and anorexia).

Investigations

- Specific laboratory studies.
  - ↑ESR, ↑ serum copper, and ↑ ferritin (worse prognosis).
  - ↑ Lactate dehydrogenase (LDH) may correlate with tumor bulk.
- CT scan (chest, abdomen, and pelvis).
- Positron emission tomography (PET) ↑ sensitivity (cf. CT scan).
- Surgical biopsy (histology and immunohistochemistry).

Table 7.5.1 illustrates the commonest staging system for HL.

7.5.1.1.3
Management

Combined-modality therapy (typically radiation and chemotherapy) is the preferred approach for most patients. The goal is to induce a complete remission, defined as the "disappearance of all evidence of disease" as evaluated by PET/CT, physical examination, and bone marrow examination (if appropriate).

Currently, the following are used:

- *ABVD* (adriamycin, bleomycin, vinblastine, and dacarbazine) regimen.

---

[3]Rye – After conference held in Rye, New York state in 1966.

Table 7.5.1 Ann Arbor[4] classification

Stage	Definition
I	Involvement of a single lymph node region (I) or single extralymphatic site (Ie)
II	Involvement of two or more lymph node regions on the same side of the diaphragm (II) or of one lymph node region and a contiguous extralymphatic site (IIe)
III	Involvement of lymph node regions on both sides of the diaphragm, which may include the spleen (IIIs) and/or limited contiguous extralymphatic organ or site (IIIe, IIIes)
IV	Disseminated involvement of one or more extralymphatic organs

N.B. Spleen is considered as a lymph node area. Involvement of the spleen is denoted with the S suffix (i.e., IIB$_S$). A or B designations denote the absence or presence of B symptoms, respectively

- *BEACOPP* (bleomycin, etoposide, adriamycin, cyclophosphamide, vincristine, procarbazine, and prednisone).
  - — ↑ Cure rate but more toxic.

For disease recurrence after an initial chemotherapy-induced remission, then high-dose chemotherapy and autologous bone marrow transplantation or peripheral stem cells treatment may be used.

7.5.1.1.4
Outcome

- 5-year survival rate ~90%.

Most acute and late complications are due to treatment-related toxicities. One-third of patients who survive pediatric HL may develop a secondary malignancy, which includes lung (most common), thyroid, breast, skin, leukemia, and (second) lymphoma.

NHL has the greatest chance of acute complications due to rapid tumor growth.

7.5.1.2
Non-Hodgkin's Lymphoma

- NHL accounts for ~4% of all pediatric cancers.

7.5.1.3
Etiology (unknown)

- HLA – specific includes HLA-A*02
- HIV infection

---

[4]Ann Arbor – Site of conference in Michigan, USA in 1971.

Common link is probably Epstein–Barr[5] virus in most lymphomas.

- Secondary NHL after previously treated HL.

Most childhood NHLs can be classified into three types:

- *Lymphoblastic lymphomas (LBL)* (most often T cell)
- *Small noncleaved cell lymphomas (SNCCL)* (B cell)
  - (Burkitt[6] lymphomas or Burkitt-like/non-Burkitt lymphomas)
- *Large Cell Lymphomas (LCL)* (T cell, B cell, and anaplastic)

7.5.1.3.1
Pathology

Many of the molecular alterations that contribute to the malignant phenotype are chromosomal translocations involving genes for immunoglobulin or T-cell receptor (TCR) molecules. Some characteristic chromosomal translocations associated with NHL are highlighted below.

- Burkitt's lymphoma: t(8;14)(q24;q32) translocation → aberrant c-MYC
- LBL: t(11;14)(p13;q11) translocation → enhanced LMO2 expression
- LBL: deletion in a regulatory region of the gene TAL1
- LBL: Inactivation of the multiple tumor suppressor gene 1 (MTS-1/p16INK4 alpha/CDKN2)
- LCL (B cell): t(8;14)(q24;q32) translocation (same as Burkitt's Lymphoma)
- LCL (9T cell): t(2;5)(p23;q35) translocation → nucleophosmin (NPM)/anaplastic lymphoma kinase (ALK) fusion protein p80 (expression may have survival advantage)

7.5.1.3.2
Clinical Features

Typically presents as extranodal disease with rapid growth (<1 month).

- Abdomen (~30%) especially SNCCL
  - E.g., "appendicitis," intussusception
- Head and neck (~30%)

---

[5]Michael Epstein and Yvonne Barr –Virologists (English and Australian), who identified this at Middlesex Hospital, London in 1964.
[6]Denis Parsons Burkitt (1911–1993) – British (N Irish) surgeon, famously one-eyed, who identified the tumor in Uganda and showed a marked geographical relationship with endemic malaria.

- Mediastinum (~25%), especially LBL
  - SVC syndrome or airway compromise
- Peripheral nodes or bones, typically LCL

Investigations

Diagnostic and staging evaluation

- Bloods: Blood count, Hepatic and renal function tests, ESR, LDH
- Chest x-ray
- CT scan
- Bone scan
- Gallium 67 scan / PET scan
- Excisional biopsy: histopathology, cytogenetics, molecular genetics
- Bone marrow aspirate
- CSF analysis
- HIV and other viral serology
- Echocardiography (To check cardiac function before administering cardiotoxic chemotherapeutic agents)

NHL is staged according to the St Jude (Murphy) classification (Table 7.5.2).

7.5.1.3.3
Management

- Childhood NHLs are extremely chemosensitive.

Table 7.5.2   St Jude (Murphy) System

Stage	Definition
I	Single extranodal tumor or single anatomic area (nodal), excluding the mediastinum or abdomen
II	Single extranodal tumor with regional node involvement, or
	Primary GI tumor±mesenteric nodes, with gross total resection, or
	On same side of diaphragm, 2 or more nodal areas or 2 single (extranodal) tumors±regional node involvement
III	Any primary mediastinal, pleural, or thymic intrathoracic tumor, or
	Any extensive and unresectable abdominal tumor, or
	Any primary paraspinous or epidural tumor regardless of other sites, or
	On both sides of the diaphragm, 2 or more nodal areas or 2 single (extranodal) tumors±regional node involvement
IV	Any of the above with initial central nervous system or marrow (<25%) involvement

- *Tumor lysis syndrome* – metabolic derangements caused by a highly proliferative and/
  or bulky malignancy.

Several chemotherapeutic regimes stratified for biologic subtypes and stage has been recommended. Debulking surgery is rarely indicated even for patients with bulky disease.

7.5.1.3.4
Outcome

- Complete remission achieved in >90% patients.
- Survival rate for patients with advanced disease.
  - ~70% for T-cell (lymphoblastic) lymphomas
  - ~85% for B-cell lymphomas
- Long-term sequelae include cardiomyopathy from anthracyclines, infertility from alka-
  lyting agents, and secondary leukemias due to epipodophyllotoxins used in the treatment of NHL.

7.5.2
Rhabdomyosarcoma

Rhabdomyosarcoma is the most common soft tissue sarcoma in children.

Tumor arising from immature mesenchymal cells

There are four main histological   of RMS:

1. Embryonal RMS (ERMS)   (~55%) intermediate prognosis
   (a) Botryoid variant   (~5%) best prognosis
2. Alveolar RMS (ARMS)   (~20%) poor prognosis
3. Undifferentiated sarcoma (UDS)   (~20%) poor prognosis

7.5.2.1
Etiology (unknown)

- Genetic associations
  - Embryonal variant – Loss of heterozygosity at Ch 11p15.5 (IGFII gene)
  - Alveolar variant
    - t(2;13) or t(1;13) translocations
    - PAX3 (Ch 2, poor prognosis) or PAX7 (Ch 1, better prognosis) and FKHR (Ch
      13) genes

- RMS has been associated with
  - p53 mutations (50% of patients).
  - Li-Fraumeni syndrome, Neurofibromatosis, Rubinstein–Taybi syndrome, Gorlin basal cell nevus syndrome, Beckwith–Wiedemann syndrome, Costello syndrome.

7.5.2.2
Pathology

RMS is one of the small, round blue-cell tumors of childhood showing variable differentiation along the myogenesis pathway. Diagnosis is confirmed by cytogenetics or reverse transcriptase polymerase chain reaction (RT-PCR) to identify specific chromosomal abnormalities. The protein myo D1 is a protein normally found in developing skeletal muscle cells, which serves as a useful immunohistochemical marker of RMS.

7.5.2.2.1
Investigations (as above)

- MRI scan – assess degree of local invasion
- CT scan – predominantly for distal metastasis

The current staging system is the *Lawrence/Gehan Staging System for Intergroup Rhabdomyosarcoma Study (IRS) IV*, which is initiated preoperatively and then completed after resection (Tables 7.5.3 and 7.5.4).

7.5.2.3
Clinical Features

Most children with RMS present with a painless swelling, which varies by site of presentation. The most common sites are

Table 7.5.3 TNM Lawrence/Gehan pretreatment staging for IRS IV

Stage	Site	Tumor	Node	Metastasis
I	Orbit, head, and neck (not parameningeal), genitourinary (not bladder/prostate)	<5 cm or >5 cm	N0,1,X	M0
II	Bladder/prostate, extremity, trunk, parameningeal, others	<5 cm	N0,X	M0
III	Bladder/prostate, extremity, trunk, parameningeal, others	<5 cm	N1	M0
		>5 cm	N0,1,X	
IV	All	<5 cm or >5 cm	N0,1,X	M1

Notes

N0 no nodal metastasis; *N1* regional nodal metastasis; *NX* unknown nodal status; *M0* no distant metastasis; *M1* distant metastasis

Table 7.5.4 Clinical grouping classification

Group	Extent of disease
I	Localized tumors, completely resected, no microscopic residual
IIa	As above PLUS microscopically +ve resection margin
IIb	As above PLUS +ve regional lymph nodes
IIc	As above PLUS +ve regional lymph nodes and margins of resection
III	Localized or locally invasive tumor, gross residual disease after attempted resection or biopsy only
IV	Distant metastatic tumor

- Head and neck (~30%)
- Extremities (~25%)
- GU tract (~20%).

7.5.2.4
Management

- *Primary resection* with no microscopic residual disease, if feasible, without causing unacceptable disfigurement or loss of function offers the best chance of cure.
  - *Primary re-excision* is frequently attempted for microscopically positive margins before the initiation of any other form of therapy.
  - *Regional LN evaluation* is recommended in extremity and trunk tumors.
  - *Lymphatic mapping and sentinel node biopsy* may allow adequate staging while limiting the operative morbidity.

Medical therapy depends on the staging.

- *ERMS (completely excised).*
  - Vincristine and dactinomycin (also known as Actinomycin-D) (VA regimen)
- *ARMS and Gp II and III RMS.*
  - *VAC regimen* – addition of cyclophosphamide.
  - Irinotecan or topotecan may be added to this combination for high-grade tumors.
- *Radiation therapy (XRT)* – residual localized disease.
- *Second-look operation* to remove residual tumor after chemotherapy with or without radiotherapy has also shown to improve survival.

7.5.2.5
Outcome

- Five-year survival rate
  - >90% (localized disease) <20% (metastatic disease).

About 30% of RMS patients will relapse, and between 50% and 95% of these will die of progressive disease.

7.5.3
Malignant Melanoma

Melanoma is the most common tumor to involve the fetus by transplacental spread.

- Melanoma is a malignancy of primarily skin pigment-producing cells (melanocytes) with a clear relationship to with sunlight exposure.
- 0.3–0.4% of melanomas appear in prepubertal children.
- Half of melanomas occur in previous pigmented lesions.
- Owing to poor prognosis of metastatic melanoma, early diagnosis is essential to reduce mortality.

7.5.3.1
Clinical Features

The mnemonic ABCDE (asymmetry, border irregularity, color variegation, diameter, evolving) is useful to remember the features of melanoma development.

7.5.3.2
Management

- Excisional biopsy, lymphatic mapping and sentinel node biopsy, and regional lymphadenectomy in sentinel node positive patients are the management methods of choice.

Tumor thickness and skin penetration and sentinel node status are the most important prognostic factors. This is described by

1. Clark's level (progressive involvement of skin structures)
2. Breslow's depth (measured in millimeters)

The narrowest efficacious margins for cutaneous melanoma have yet to be determined. *American Joint Commission on Cancer (AJCC) staging* is most widely accepted.

Prognosis for distant metastatic disease is extremely poor. Systemic chemotherapy is the mainstay of treatment for metastatic disease. Biochemotherapy, using standard chemotherapeutic agents with biologic response modifiers such as IL-2, IFN-alfa, or granulocyte macrophage colony-stimulating factor, has shown some promise.

7.5.4
Pancreatic Tumors

7.5.4.1
Pancreatoblastoma

This is the embryonal equivalent for this organ although <100 cases have been reported.

- The majority of these tumors are of an embryonal type, which develops at an early stage of pancreatic differentiation, thus contains both exocrine and endocrine cell types.
- They are usually present as an asymptomatic mass in the upper abdomen.
- Tumor markers (e.g., α-1-fetoprotein, LDH) may be elevated.
- Complete excisional surgery is the mainstay of treatment (usually pancreaticoduodenectomy).
- Prognosis is poor in metastatic disease, primarily inoperable disease, or local recurrence.

7.5.4.2
Adenocarcinoma

Islet cell and papillary (Frantz's tumor[7]) cystic tumors, etc. are rare in children. The latter appears characteristically in teenage girls, and 50% are of African origin.

7.5.4.3
Islet cell hyperplasia

This is a diffuse increase of pancreatic islet cell tissue, which may result in hyperinsulinism and hypoglycemia leading to seizures, cerebral damage, and even death. In persistent hypoglycemia, placement of a central venous catheter for 20% glucose infusion is advisable to maintain an adequate blood glucose level. Operative excision is required if it fails to respond to diazoxide. If no localized adenoma is found, a 95% pancreatectomy is recommended.

7.5.5
Thyroid Tumors

Carcinoma accounts for

- ~1% of all childhood malignancies.
- ~5% of cancers arising in the head and neck.

---

[7]VK Frantz – American pathologist described in 1959.

- Is identified in ~30% of children, who undergo surgical resection for cold nodules.
- F>M 2:1 ↑incidence with age (peak at adolescence).

7.5.5.1
Etiological Factors

- Previous irradiation and chemotherapy for other malignancies (e.g., HL, leukemia, and other head and neck malignancies).
- Iodine deficiency (↑risk of follicular ca.).
- Genetic (e.g., mutations in the RET proto-oncogene identified in the *multiple endocrine neoplasia [MEN2] syndromes*).
- ~40% of medullary thyroid carcinomas (MTC) are related to autosomal dominant familial syndromes.

Histologic types include:

- *Papillary* (~75%) – epithelial cells arranged as papillae disseminated throughout the gland. Lymphocytic infiltrates and psammoma[8] bodies are common.
- *Follicular* (~20%) – malignant cells are adenomatous with follicle formation and are distinguished from benign adenomas only by the presence of nuclear atypia, capsular invasion, or vascular invasion.
- *Medullary* (~5%).
  1. Arises from the parafollicular C cells, derived from neural crest cells.
  2. Appear as solid islets of regular, undifferentiated cells with abundant granular cytoplasm. The stroma contains fibrotic tissue, amyloids, and calcifications.
- *Anaplastic* (rare).

7.5.5.2
Clinical Features

Painless thyroid mass with or without cervical adenopathy. Advanced cases may present with dysphagia, features of tracheal/esophageal compression (e.g., hoarseness), or metastasis.

7.5.5.2.1
Investigation

- Thyroid function tests (normal in most cases)
- Plasma calcitonin (↑ MTC), thyroglobulin (↑ differentiated TC)
- Genetic testing for MTC (e.g., *RET* proto oncogene mutations)
- US – differentiate between solid and cystic lesion
- Thyroid scan – Tc 99m-pertechnetate shows functioning thyroid tissue
- Fine-needle aspiration cytology (FNAC) – role poorly defined in children
- >13 years → FNAC, <13 years → excision

---

[8]*Psammoma* (Greek) – sand.

Benign nodules can be followed safely with serial physical examination and US scans but are resected if growth is shown. Surgical resection is indicated for malignant or suspicious nodules. An aspirated cyst that collapses completely can be observed, but should be removed, if recurs.

7.5.5.3
Surgery

Total or subtotal thyroidectomy is indicated for differentiated carcinoma. Tumor involving the recurrent laryngeal nerve should be shaved off, preserving the nerve with the parathyroid glands. If viability of the parathyroid glands is questionable, they should be autotransplanted into the sternomastoid muscle of the nondominant forearm.

Further Reading

1. Arya LS, Dinand V (2005) Current strategies in the treatment of childhood Hodgkin's disease. Indian Pediatr 42:1115–1128
2. Harris NL (1999) Hodgkin's disease: classification and differential diagnosis. Modern Pathol 12:159–175
3. Murphy SB (1980) Classification, staging and end results of treatment of childhood non-Hodgkin's lymphomas: dissimilarities from lymphomas in adults. Semin Oncol 7:332–339
4. Crist WM, Anderson JR, Meza JL et al (2001) Intergroup rhabdomyosarcoma study-IV: results for patients with nonmetastatic disease. J Clin Oncol 19:3091–3102
5. Robison LL (2009) Treatment-associated subsequent neoplasms among long-term survivors of childhood cancer: the experience of the Childhood Cancer Survivor Study. Pediatr Radiol 39(Suppl 1):S32–S37

Part VIII

Principles of Trauma

General Principles

8.1

Shailesh B. Patel

Trauma continues to be the commonest cause of death, by a long way, in children in developed countries (>350 deaths/year in UK). Most have multiple injuries, and presence or absence of significant head injury is the usual determinant of outcome.

One-third of childhood deaths occur at home, with burns and falls being the most common. Most accidental childhood deaths could be considered avoidable if proper safety measures had been followed.

Prevention strategies are of major importance to reduce mortality and morbidity which can have long-term financial and economic implications. After targets were set in 2000, the number of children killed or seriously injured in motor vehicle accidents in 2007 in UK was reduced to 55% below the 1994–1998 average baseline.

8.1.1
Basic Approach to Trauma

8.1.1.1
Important Differences Between Children and Adults

- *Weight*

Drugs and fluids are given as dose per kilogram of body weight. Weighing on scales is most accurate, but may have to be estimated prior to the arrival of the patient.

S. B. Patel
Department of Paediatric Surgery, King's College Hospital, London, UK

C. K. Sinha and M. Davenport (eds.), *Handbook of Pediatric Surgery*,
DOI: 10.1007/978-1-84882-132-3_8.1, © Springer-Verlag London Limited 2010

- *Anatomical*
- *Psychological*
- Fear is a common response. Gentle reassurance, explanation, and honesty are vital in order to let the child develop trust in the carer and allow repeated assessments.
- Presence of parents may be helpful.
  - *Airway*
- Large head and short neck allows neck flexion and airway narrowing
- Large tongue may obstruct airway
- Floor of mouth is soft. Airway is easily obstructed during chin lift maneuvers
- Narrowest part of airway is cricoid (larynx in adults)
  - *Breathing*
- Ribs are more horizontal in young children
- Compliant chest wall – serious parenchymal damage can occur without rib fractures. Rib fractures denote very large compression forces
- Abdominal organs are more exposed due to flatter diaphragm
  - *Circulation*
- Circulating blood volume per kilogram of body weight is high, but actual volume is low. Small amounts of blood loss can be critical
- Body surface area (BSA) to weight ratio falls with increasing age. Small children lose heat more rapidly and are prone to hypothermia

Estimated weight (kgs) for age 1–10 years $= 2 \times (\text{age in years} + 4)$

8.1.2
Management Plan

Treatment is based on a structured approach:

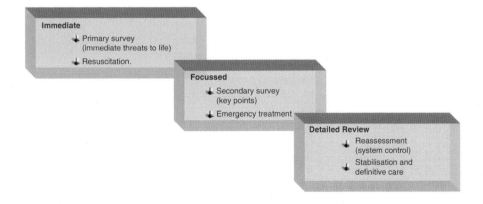

8.1.3
Primary Survey and Resuscitation

Assessment begins with SAFE approach

Shout for help
Approach with care
Free from danger
Evaluate ABC

Primary survey identifies life-threatening problems and is completed within 1–2 min. Each problem is corrected before moving on to the next step, with reassessment after each intervention. Any deterioration at any stage requires A, B, and C to be rechecked.

Basic life support measures are initiated.

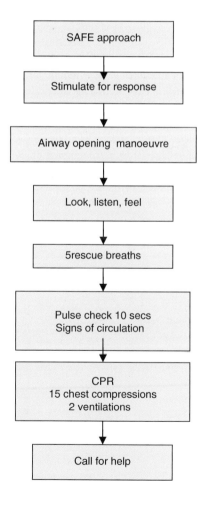

- Airway with cervical spine control
- Breathing with ventilatory support
- Circulation with hemorrhage control
- Disability with prevention of secondary insult
- Exposure with temperature control

8.1.4
Airway and Cervical spine

Airway assessment has top priority and starts with placing the cheek over the child's mouth and

Looking   for chest and/or abdominal movement
Listening   for breath sounds
Feeling   for breath

Airway compromise may be due to material *in lumen* (blood, vomit, teeth or foreign body), or damage or loss of control of structures *in wall* (mouth, tongue, pharynx, larynx, and trachea), or *outside wall* (prevertebral haematoma, maxillary fracture). Soot traces, erythema, and blisters around mouth/nostrils may indicate smoke or heat inhalational injury requiring early intubation. Commonest cause is a floppy tongue in an unconscious child and is corrected by an appropriately sized Guedel airway. Blind finger sweep is *contraindicated*.

Spinal precautions must be taken from the beginning unless the mechanism of trauma clearly excludes the possibility of cervical injury. Child must be *either* immobilized on a firm surface with appropriately sized hard neck collar and side supports with blocks and straps, *or* head held in *manual in-line immobilization* by a competent assistant. A combative child may be safer if left alone with only a hard collar.

Airway management sequence

- Jaw thrust (no head tilt/chin lift)
- Suction/removal of foreign body under direct vision
- Oro/nasopharyngeal airways (beware basal skull fracture)
- Tracheal intubation
- Surgical airway

8.1.5
Breathing

Assessment of the adequacy of breathing is the next priority after airway. *Look, listen,* and *feel* approach is used, but also *percuss* chest for dullness/hyperresonance.

Examination includes signs of obvious chest injury, e.g., bruising, tyre marks, crepitus, open wounds, and flail chest (see chapter 8.3). High flow O_2 by non-rebreathing face mask and reservoir bag should be routinely applied to all patients. If breathing is inadequate, assisted bag-mask ventilation must be started, and subsequent endotracheal intubation and ventilation may be required.

Causes of unequal breath sounds may include aspiration of vomit/blood, pneumothorax, haemo-pneumothorax, misplaced/dislodged tracheal tube, blocked main bronchus, diaphragmatic rupture, and pulmonary contusion.

Effort of breathing

- Recession
- Respiratory rate
- Inspiratory/expiratory noises
- Grunting
- Accessory muscle use
- Flaring of nasal alae

Efficacy of breathing

- Breath sounds
- Chest expansion
- Abdominal movement

Effects of inadequate respiration

- Heart rate
- Skin color
- Mental status

Indications for Intubation and Ventilation

- Persistent airway obstruction
- Likelihood of airway loss, e.g., inhalational burn
- No airway reflexes
- Inadequate ventilatory effort/fatigue
- Severe flail chest
- Persistent hypoxia with supplemental oxygen
- Head injury requiring controlled hyperventilation

8.1.6
Circulation

Rapid assessment of heart rate and rhythm, central and peripheral pulse volume and peripheral perfusion (color, temperature, and capillary return) is performed. Capillary return is assessed by pressing on a warm area of the body for 5 s and counting the number of seconds for return of capillary flush (normal value is <2 s).

Signs of circulation include movement, coughing, or normal breathing. Failure of circulation is indicated by the absence of central pulse for 10 s.

A quick check for signs of external haemorrhage is made, and pressure applied if appropriate. Tourniquets should not be used.

Pulse oximetry, BP cuff, and ECG leads should be attached at the earliest opportunity.

Systolic pressure is usually raised in injured children, and hypotension is therefore a dangerous sign.

Two large bore peripheral intravenous cannulae must be inserted urgently. If any difficulty is encountered, intraosseous cannulation of the tibia or femur is the quickest option in the seriously injured child, avoiding limbs with proximal fractures. More secure access can be obtained once stabilized.

Fluids in hypovolaemic shock due to trauma:

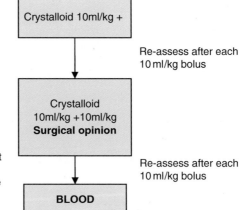

If rapid transfusion is required, O-negative or type-specific blood may be necessary.

Circulating blood volume = 70–80 ml/kg

Chest compressions must be started if

- No pulse
- Slow pulse (less than 60 beats/min with poor perfusion)
- No signs of circulation

8.1.7
Disability

Rapid assessment of conscious level using AVPU, pupil size and reactivity, and posture is performed.

Level P or U indicates the need to protect the airway and equates to Glasgow coma scale 8 or less. Neurological resuscitation must be initiated to prevent secondary brain insult. Unequal pupils mean that immediate intervention is required.

(See Chap. 8.3).

A	Alert
V	Responds to Voice
P	Responds only to **P**ain
U	Unresponsive to all stimuli

8.1.8
Exposure

Proper assessment requires clothes to be removed, but heat loss and embarrassment should be prevented by covering with a blanket.

8.1.9
Life-Threatening Conditions

- Airway obstruction
- Tension pneumothorax
- Open pneumothorax
- Massive haemothorax
- Flail chest
- Cardiac tamponade
- Shock (haemorrhage or otherwise)
- Decompensating head injury

These conditions should have been diagnosed on clinical findings alone and treated as soon as they are found.

8.1.10
Other Procedures During Resuscitation

- Chest and pelvic X-ray
- Blood tests – Cross-match, full blood count, clotting, amylase, urea, and electrolytes, **D**on't **E**ver **F**orget **G**lucose

- Nasogastric tube – acute gastric dilatation is common; use oral route if basal skull fracture is suspected
- Urinary catheter – only if the child is unable to void spontaneously or accurate monitoring is required
- Analgesia – morphine (0.1–0.2 mg/kg IV) in small boluses, reduce if hypotensive or in case of altered conscious level

8.1.11
Secondary Survey

A thorough top-to-bottom examination is performed once all life-threatening conditions have been identified and stabilized. Secondary survey may have to wait until life-saving surgery is performed, but must be subsequently carried out and fully documented. Relevant investigations, e.g., cervical spine imaging, head, chest or abdominal CT or ultrasound may be indicated at this stage.

- Surface (head to toe, front, and back – will require log roll)
- All orifices (mouth, nose, ears, eyes rectum, and perineum
- All body cavities (chest, abdomen, pelvis, retroperitoneum)
- All extremities and joints

An **AMPLE** history should be taken from paramedics or carers at the first opportunity:

Allergies.
Medications.
Past history of any major illness. Pregnancy.
Last meal (if the patient needs surgery).
Environment surrounding injury (e.g., other casualties/fatalities, speed of impact, use of restraints, height of fall, cold/hot environment, drowning).

8.1.11.1
Emergency treatment

Treatment plans for key findings from secondary survey are started promptly to minimize the risk of deterioration or increased morbidity, e.g. limb-threatening injury.

8.1.11.2
Reassessment and System Control

Detailed attention is now paid to maintaining and normalizing all physiological systems:

- Respiratory
- Circulatory
- Central nervous system
- Metabolism
- Host defenses

8.1.12
Continuing Stabilization and Definitive Care

These represent the last stage of trauma resuscitation:

- Note taking
- Referral
- Transfer

Useful Formulae During Resuscitation (WETFLAG)

Weight	$2 \times (age+4)$ kg
Electricity	2 J/kg DC for defibrillation shock
Tube	$4+(age/4)$ mm internal diameter tracheal tube
FLuids	10 mL/s/kg + 10 mls/kg
Adrenaline	10 μg/kg = 0.1 mls/kg of 1:10,000 solution
Glucose	5 mls/kg 10% dextrose

8.1.13
Supplemental Data

- *Physiological*

Respiratory rate, heart rate, and systolic blood pressure all change with age.

Age (years)	Respiratory rate (breaths per minute)	Heart rate (beats per minute)	Systolic pressure (mmHg)
<1	30–40	110–160	70–90
1–2	25–35	100–150	80–95
2–5	25–30	95–140	80–100
5–12	20–25	80–120	90–110
>12	15–20	60–100	100–120

- *Typical laboratory cross-match time*
- *Typical notes template*

Cross-match times		
Blood type	Cross-match	Time (min)
O-negative	No	0
Type-specific	ABO	10–15
Full cross-match	Full	45–60

History

- Mechanism of injury
- AMPLE

Primary survey and resuscitation

- A
- B
- C
- D

Secondary survey and emergency treatment

- Head
- Face
- Neck
- Chest
- Abdomen
- Pelvis
- Spine
- Extremities

Continuing stabilization

- Respiration
- Circulation

Based on courses and with permission of APLS (Advanced Paediatric Life Support).

ALSG Centre for Training and Development 29–31, Ellesmere Street, Swinton, Manchester, M27 0LA, UK. Tel.: +(44) 161 794 1999. www.alsg.org

Abdominal Trauma

8.2

Ramnik V. Patel, Emmanuel M. L. Endeley, Mark Davenport, and Jenny Walker

8.2.1
Epidemiology

- M ≫ F

Ethnic factors

- Bimodal age distribution (toddlers and teenagers)
- Summer > winter

8.2.2
Mechanism of Injury

- Blunt (90%) – falls, RTA, bicycle related
  — Kidney (25%), spleen (25%), and liver (15%)
- Penetrating (10%) – knives, gunshot, and impalement injuries
  — Small bowel (20%), colon (15%), and stomach (10%)
- Combined

8.2.2.1
Factors predisposing to abdominal injury in the child

- Shape – square becoming more rectangular with age
- Thinner abdominal wall musculature. Lower abdominal fat content
- Flexible ribs

R.V. Patel (✉)
Department of Paediatric Surgery, Sheffield Children's Hospital, London, UK

C. K. Sinha and M. Davenport (eds.), *Handbook of Pediatric Surgery*,
DOI: 10.1007/978-1-84882-132-3_8.2, © Springer-Verlag London Limited 2010

- Solid organs are anterior and comparatively larger in the child (more surface area is exposed)
- The bladder is intraabdominal
- Lap belt injury – causes peculiar flexion-distraction injury to the lumbar spine (Chance[1] fracture) as it acts as a fulcrum

8.2.3
Clinical Features

The key element in the history is the precise nature and circumstances of the traumatic episode and the degree and type of force which caused it. This should lead to a raised index of suspicion if there is no external evidence of injury.

Various signs of injury include abrasions and contusions, tenderness, distention, (associated with bleeding or intraperitoneal air) and a scaphoid abdomen (e.g., traumatic diaphragmatic hernia). Intraperitoneal blood may be evident after 24 h as bruising in the loins (Grey-Turner's sign[2]) or around the umbilicus (Cullen's sign[3]). Abrasions from the lapstrap may be evident in seat-belt injury. Rarely, the scrotum may act as a repository for air, blood, or fluid from intraperitoneal injury.

8.2.4
Management (See Part VIII, Chap 8.1, PP 418–428)

1. *Primary survey* – assessment of
   (a) Airway
   (b) Breathing
   (c) Circulation
2. *Secondary survey* – head-to-toe physical examination
3. *Tertiary survey* – usually performed >24 h after admission and aims to identify missed or hidden injuries

8.2.4.1
Investigations

FBC, hematocrit, urinalysis, liver function tests, and amylase (occasionally lipase).

---

[1]G.Q. Chance – British radiologist who described three cases in 1948, later associated with seat-belt injury in 1965.

[2]George Grey-Turner (1877–1951) – English surgeon, who reported this as late sign of hemorrhagic pancreatitis.

[3]Thomas Stephen Cullen (1868–1953) – Canadian gynecologist, who mentioned sign in connection with ectopic pregnancy.

8.2.4.2
Trauma Imaging

- *X-ray* – commonly performed as a part of secondary survey including spine series, AP chest, and pelvis series. Specific abdominal X-ray may show free air.
- *CT scanning* (double contrast, i.e., IV for solid organ injury and oral selectively for stomach, duodenum, and proximal bowel). This is currently the standard tool for the assessment of significant abdominal injury in the hemodynamically stable child.
- *Ultrasound* (*Focused Assessment by Sonography in Trauma – FAST*) FAST is mainly used and evaluated in adults and those who are hemodynamically unstable. Its aim is to detect free fluid, and is highly sensitive in this role. It is also operator-dependent, and lacks specificity providing no real information on the grade of organ injury. Currently it cannot be recommended to replace CT scanning in children.
- *Diagnostic peritoneal lavage* – limited role in children because positive result doesn't necessarily require laparotomy. May be considered if
  - CT scanning is not available.
  - In a hemodynamically unstable child with suspected bleeding from an intraabdominal injury or in the ICU.
  - Other injuries (e.g., head or orthopedic injuries) requiring immediate surgical intervention and with no time for CT scanning.
- *Emergent laparoscopy* – role is yet to be defined, but should be considered in suitable patients. Should reduce the incidence of negative laparotomies. Indicated in blunt abdominal trauma with suspicious examination findings (e.g., abdominal wall contusions, peritonitis, falling hematocrit with free intraperitoneal fluid but no radiographic solid organ injury). In penetrating injury, accompanied by local wound exploration; then laparoscopic survey may replace the need for formal laparotomy.
- *Interventional radiology.*
  - Diagnostic angiography and therapeutic embolization may be considered in on-going liver/spleen bleeding.
- *ERCP* – specific role in the determination of bile and pancreatic duct injury.
- *Exploratory laparotomy* – indicated as a diagnostic procedure in.
  - Hemodynamically unstable with unequivocal abdominal signs.
  - Penetrating injuries.

Hemodynamically "unstable" vs. "stable"?

This concept underlies a key principle in the management of abdominal trauma but definition tends to be imprecise.

Initial volume resuscitation should begin with a bolus of 10 mL/kg of crystalloid solution, and may be repeated with a blood transfusion to follow (e.g., 10 mL/kg of packed RBC).

8.2.5
Nonoperative Management of Blunt Abdominal Trauma (~95%)

This concept was introduced in the late 1970s, initially for splenic injury, and is currently accepted as the standard for most solid organ injury. It includes

- Bed rest and hemodynamic monitoring (for at least 24 h)
- Serial haematocrit
- Frequent physical examinations

There should be restriction on sporting activities after discharge from hospital for up to 4 weeks (depends on the grade of injury).

8.2.5.1
Interventional Radiology

Minimally invasive techniques now play a larger role in stopping bleeding or drainage of collections. Examples would include embolization of hepatic arterial pseudoaneurysms following liver injury and percutaneous drainage of urinomas and pseuodcysts following renal and pancreatic injury respectively. Pelviureteric stents may be placed cystoscopically or percutaneously; pancreatic duct stents via an ERCP may be used to improve organ function.

8.2.6
Laparotomy for Abdominal Trauma (~5%)

Indications include

- Unstable/shocked cases
- A transfusion requirement of ≥40 mL/kg within a 24-h period *probably* mandates laparotomy and intervention.

Principles

- Midline incision.
- Four quadrants packing and inspection for injury of each in turn.
- *Damage control surgery* – extensive, prolonged surgery in multitrauma patients is associated with a potentially lethal combination of metabolic acidosis, coagulopathy, and hypothermia. A multistage approach is therefore preferable.
  - Phase I – short primary operation to control bleeding and prevent contamination (stapling/oversew of intestinal lacerations, etc.)
  - Phase II – ICU resuscitation.
  - Phase III – reoperation (>24 h) and definitive repair of specific injury.

- Penetrating injuries (see later)
- Specific organ injury (e.g., hollow viscus injury – stomach, small and large bowel, bladder, and diaphragm laceration)

8.2.7
Penetrating Injuries

While exposure to motor vehicles and falls from a height are fairly ubiquitous scenarios for children in the developed world; exposure to guns, knives, etc. is highly variable. Mostly, this is seen as an urban problem and confined to specific areas.

The at-risk population is 10–24 year old males, and in the USA, gun-related (usually) homicides (~17%) are second only to motor vehicle crashes (~40%) in terms of cause of death.

- Black > white
- Adolescents
- Males ≫ females

Most penetrating abdominal injuries involve violence, but at least in children, gunshots tend to be accidental while knife injuries are all too deliberate.

The degree of injury with most gunshots is related to the kinetic energy of the missile fired, and therefore, a product of the projectile mass and the square of its velocity. Thus, it can be divided into:

- Low velocity (<250 m/s) – most civilian handguns, shotguns, etc.
  - Track injury, little cavitation effect.
- High-velocity (750–1,000 m/s) – military rifles.
  - Track injury and ↑ cavitation (increased potential for massive soft-tissue injury perpendicular to track).

8.2.7.1
Management of Penetrating Abdominal Injuries

According to the principles above with the addition of mandatory definition of the trajectory of blade or bullet. What starts off in the chest may well end up in the abdomen – transiting the diaphragm in the process.

- Plain radiographic films (radiopaque markers at entry and exit wounds)
  - ?Pneumoperitoneum
- CT scan (ideally triple contrast) for solid and hollow organ injury

Poor prognostic features include, arrival measurements of:

- Initial core temperature of <34°C
- Systolic blood pressure of <90 mmHg

In general, formal laparotomy is still the usual surgical option in (definitely) penetrating injuries. In certain areas with a high prevalence of such injuries (e.g., South Africa), a policy of "wait and watch" has been adopted for those who are otherwise stable and have no obvious signs of peritonism.

Laparoscopy may be used in selected cases (e.g., diaphragmatic injury, tangential gunshot wound in hemodynamically stable cases).

8.2.7.2
Laparotomy

- Small bowel injury.
  - >50% of circumference involved – aim for resection.
  - <50% – aim for repair.
- Colon injury
  - Depends on the time to laparotomy (≥24 h), associated injuries, and degree of fecal contamination. For most cases, primary repair without covering colostomy is practical.

> Impalement injuries are uncommon, but the recommendation is to leave them in place until they can be removed in the operating theater because of the potential for bleeding.

8.2.8
Specific Organ Injury

8.2.8.1
Splenic Injury

Commonly injured in blunt abdominal trauma. In case of an apparently innocuous injury, suspect the underlying splenic pathology (e.g., malaria). Most injuries can be treated conservatively, but usually the reason for failure is continued bleeding (Table 8.2.1).

8.2.8.1.1
Surgical Options

- *Splenectomy (e.g., Grade IV/V) total or partial*
- *Splenorrhaphy (e.g., Grades II/III/IV)*
  - Direct suture/Argon Beam coagulator
  - Topical agents (e.g., Surgicel®, fibrin glue)
  - Absorbable mesh (e.g., Dexon®, Vicryl®)
- *Splenic autotransplantation (omental pocket, etc.)*

Table 8.2.1   Spleen injury scale

Grade	Descriptors
I	Subcapsular hematoma (<10% surface area)
	Capsular laceration (<1-cm deep)
II	Subcapsular hematoma (10–50% surface area)
	Laceration (1–3 cm deep)
III	Subcapsular hematoma (>50%), ruptured
	Parenchymal hematoma(>5 cm)
IV	Hilar or segmental vessel injury ± major (>25%) devascularization
V	Hilar injury + devascularization
	Shattered spleen

Notes – if multiple lacerations, advance one grade
Adapted from American Association for Surgery of Trauma

8.2.8.2
Liver Injury

Common organ (because of size) to be the target of blunt force trauma, and typically involves the posterior segments of the right lobe. CT scans tend to overestimate the degree of injury, and again, most (>90%) can be treated nonoperatively (Table 8.2.2).

Table 8.2.2   Liver injury scale

Grade	Descriptors
I	Subcapsular hematoma (<10% surface area)
	Capsular laceration (<1-cm deep)
II	Subcapsular hematoma (10–50% surface area)
	Laceration (1–3 cm deep)
III	Subcapsular hematoma (>50%), ruptured parenchymal hematoma (>10 cm)
	Laceration (>3 cm)
IV	Laceration – disruption of <75% of lobe or up to three segments
V	Laceration – disruption >75% of lobe, or more than three segments
	Juxta-venous injury (hepatic veins/IVC)
VI	Avulsed liver

Notes – if multiple lacerations, advance one grade

Adapted from American Association for the Surgery of Trauma, Chicago, USA

8.2.8.2.1
Surgical Options

- *Temporary vascular control (Pringle's[4] maneuver)* – sling or finger around the portal triad, through the lesser omentum. Stops portal venous and arterial inflow.
  - In case of significant bleeding from injury site, suspect caval or hepatic vein laceration/avulsion.
  - *Topical agents (as above)*/Argon beam coagulator/fibrin glue
- *Perihepatic packing* – large operative gauze packs compressing RUQ. Close abdomen, and remove after 24 h.
- Embolization – may complement the above in acute stage, or as definitive treatment for pseuodaneurysm.

NB – partial hepatectomy, etc. is unwise outside of specialist centers
Late complications include

- Biliary leak (5%) (second week postinjury).
- Pseudoaneurysm formation and delayed hemorrhage.
- Hemobilia (bleeding into the biliary tract).
- Bilhemia (bile leaking into the bloodstream).
- Abscess formation.

8.2.8.3
Renal Injury

Relative lack of perirenal fat may predispose to injury in children. This usually involves parenchymal contusions, but injury to the ureteropelvic junction or the vascular pedicle may occur.

- Blunt (90%) ≫ penetrating – although latter, much more likely to be serious.
- Haematuria (microscopic or frank) and flank mass.

Most (>95%) can be treated conservatively, but the indications for intervention (surgical or radiological) include:

- Expanding retroperitoneal hematoma
- Vascular pedicle injury (nonfunction on contrast CT scan)
- Urinoma

Nephrectomy is the usual outcome of surgical exploration for major vascular injury. Partial nephrectomy should be possible for parenchymal lacerations/devascularizations, etc.

---

[4]James Hogarth Pringle (1863–1941) Glasgow surgeon describing this in 8 patients in 1908.

8.2.8.4
Pancreatic Injury

The usual mechanism of injury is a sharp blow to the epigastrium (bicycle, horse kick, etc.) which compresses the neck of the pancreas onto the underlying vertebral column. This splits the parenchyma and lacerates the duct. Presentation is usually delayed, as bleeding is not a problem. Presence of duct injury is the single most important prognostic feature (CT scan suggestive, ERCP definitive), and leads to pancreatitis and pseudocyst formation.

Possible interventions include

- Distal pancreatectomy (if duct injury is recognized early enough)
- ERCP and stenting
- Allow pseudocyst to form and then intervene.
    - Aspiration (percutaneous ± drain)
    - Cystgastrostomy

Further Reading

1. Tinkoff G, Esposito T, Reed J, Kilgo P, Fildes J, Pasquale M, Meredith J: 2008 American Association for the Surgery of Trauma Organ Injury Scale I: Spleen, Liver, and Kidney, Validation based on the National Trauma Data bank Journal of the American College of Surgeons, 207(5): 646–655.
2. Advanced Life Support Group (2005) Advanced paediatric life support: the practical approach, 3rd edn. BMJ Publishing Group, London
3. Walker J (2005) Abdominal trauma. In: Burge DM, Griffith DM, Steinbrecher HA, Wheeler RA (eds) Paediatric surgery, 2nd edn. Hodder Arnold, London
4. Coley BD, Mutabagani KH, Martin LC et al (2000) Focused abdominal sonography for trauma (FAST) in children with blunt abdominal trauma. J Trauma 48:902–906
5. Feliz A, Shultz B, McKenna C, Gaines BA (2006) Diagnostic and therapeutic laparoscopy in pediatric abdominal trauma. J Pediatr Surg 41:72–77
6. Upadhyaya P (2003) Conservative management of splenic trauma: history and current trends. Pediatr Surg Int 19:617–627
7. Houben CH, Ade-Ajayi N, Patel S et al (2007) Traumatic pancreatic duct injury in children: minimally invasive approach to management. J Pediatr Surg 42:629–635
8. Rogers CG, Knight V, MacUra KJ, Ziegfeld S, Paidas CN, Mathews RI (2004) High-grade renal injuries in children – is conservative management possible? Urology 64:574–579

Thoracic Trauma

8.3

Mark Davenport

After the head, chest injuries are the most lethal of childhood accidents.

8.3.1
Mechanisms of Injury

- Blunt (85%)
  - MVA
  - Bicycle-related, horse-related
  - Falls from height
  - Blast injury
- Penetrating (15%)
  - Knives, gunshot
  - Railings, fence-posts

Nonaccidental injury
  Rib fractures
  Toddlers and infants
  Variable ages (healing etc)
  Other injuries
High index of suspicion

8.3.2
Anatomy

Evolution has dictated that the vital cardiopulmonary organs are protected from injury by providing a significant composite structure of bone and muscle allowing just enough flexibility to breathe but resistant to all but the most severe crushing or penetrating force.

M. Davenport
Paediatric Surgery Department, Kings College Hospital, London, UK

C. K. Sinha and M. Davenport (eds.), *Handbook of Pediatric Surgery*,
DOI: 10.1007/978-1-84882-132-3_8.3, © Springer-Verlag London Limited 2010

8.3.2.1
Surface Landmarks

- Manubrio-sternal Angle of Louis[1] – insertion of the 2nd rib (T4/5 level)
- Vertebral prominens – spine of C7
- Nipple line – overlies the fourth intercostal space
- Diaphragm – Right dome higher than left. Up to the level of T 9/10

8.3.3
Ribcage Injury

These range from contusion, through actual rib fracture (commonest 4th – 9th) to multiple segmental involvement and a flail chest. All increase the work of breathing, either through inhibition and pain or by rendering the actual mechanics of breathing impossible. There is elasticity in the structure (AP rather than lateral), which is commonly observed in children. Sometimes, this results in severe lung parenchymal crush injury, yet, the shell remains intact.

Flail Chest – (≥3 ribs broken twice) – paradoxical movement (inwards on inspiration). Treatment depends on the severity, but ET intubation and IPPV, which removes the mechanical element of lung dysfunction should remain a possibility.

8.3.3.1
Investigation

1. CXR (AP and lateral) – essentially cartilaginous ribs in young may lead to false –ve films
2. CT scan

8.3.3.2
Atypical (Hence Suspicious) Injury

- 1st and 2nd rib fracture – should be well-protected, and implies significant blunt force trauma. Beware of the injury to subclavian vessels.
- *Sternal fracture* – seen in association with seat-belt use and steering wheel (if driving!). Uncommon in children (because of ↑elasticity). Obtain ECG and cardiac enzymes.
- 10–12th rib fracture – suspect underlying liver, spleen, or kidney injury.

NB: carefully interpret the ossification centers (fused by adolescence).

---

[1]Antoine Louis (1723–1792) French military surgeon who was the coinventor of the guillotine!

8.3.3.3
Management

1. Analgesia – multimodal
   (a) NSAI, opiate-based regimen (including PCA)
   (b) Local infiltration at fracture site
   (c) Epidural anesthesia
2. Underlying lung contusional injury (see later)
3. Flail stabilization – (controversial but ranges from simple "strapping," to operative fixation)

8.3.4
Parenchymal Injury

There is a wide range of pathology from simple contusion through laceration, and segmental vessel injury to major hilar injury involving bronchus, tracheal, and pulmonary vessels.
   The effect of injury is manifest in three interrelated ways

- *Contusion –* $\downarrow$*ventilation/perfusion (i.e.,* $\downarrow pO_2$ $\uparrow pCO_2$*)*
- *Air leak (i.e., pneumothorax)*
   — Open – penetrating
   — Closed
   — Tension – valve effect leading to accumulation under pressure.
- *Bleeding (i.e., hemothorax)*

8.3.4.1
Clinical Features

8.3.4.1.1
Lung Contusion

This is the commonest type of thoracic injury in children and results from blunt force trauma. The injury evolves from simple blood and edema inside alveoli to a widespread inflammatory reaction (ARDS) over about 24 h. Secondary bacterial pneumonia is possible after 3–5 days.

8.3.4.2
Investigation

1. CXR – usually underestimates the degree of injury. Serial CXR will show the development of ARDS (usually with lag period).
2. Arterial blood gas – $\downarrow O_2$ saturation (<90%), $\downarrow pO_2$ $\uparrow pCO_2$ (late).
3. Chest CT scan – sensitive.

8.3.4.3
Treatment

- Supportive – supplemental O_2, CPAP, IPPV
- Avoidance of fluid overload, caution with blood products (exacerbates ARDS)

8.3.5
Pneumothorax

A "sucking" wound may be obvious, but a *tension pneumothorax* needs to be looked for. The key signs are hyperresonance, mediastinal shift (trachea, cardiac impulse) and ↓breath sounds. If untreated, this will cause impairment of venous return, caval kinking, hypotension, and death.

Surgical emphysema and crepitus implies that air is leaking from the pleural space into the subcutaneous tissues via fascial planes.

8.3.5.1
Investigation

1. CXR (in expiration if possible) confirms the diagnosis, but if there are clinical signs, then ACT.

8.3.5.2
Treatment

- *Urgent needle thoracostomy* (followed by formal tube thoracostomy).
  — Second IC space, midclavicular line.
- *Tube thoracostomy*.
  — "Large-bore" but *compatible with rib-space* (~32 Fg in adolescent).
  — 4/5th IC space – anterior/midaxillary line.
  — Incise skin, blunt dissection through rib-space with artery forceps. Enter pleural cavity. NB "Finger sweep" usually impossible in child.
  — Insert tube (apex for air, base for blood).
- Open pneumothorax – implies single-lung ventilation only. Close/occlude defect and insert chest tube (at a different site).

8.3.6
Hemothorax

The chest cavity is large, albeit usually occupied by air-filled lung, but can hide a significant quantity of blood. Key signs are dullness to percussion, ↓breath sounds, mediastinal shift (rarely), together with evidence of shock and impaired ventilation.

8.3.6.1
Investigation

1. CXR – may show fluid in pleural space (interpret supine and erect films differently), air/fluid level or a "white-out."

8.3.6.2
Treatment

- Tube thoracostomy (large-bore) (as above)
- *Thoracotomy* is indicated if there is
  - Initial loss of >1 L (adult).
  - Evidence of on-going losses (200 mL/h for 4 h – adult).
  - Possible intervention includes oversew of lacerations, repair of central bronchovascular injury etc.

8.3.7
Great Vessel Injury

Only rarely seen in pediatric practice, and rarely in isolation ......but still possible. Usually seen in MVAs with sudden deceleration injury. Possible signs include evidence of aortic dissection (e.g., impalpable distal limb pulses). CT angiography is indicated if injury is thought possible, looking for evidence of mediastinal or cervical inlet hematoma. Intervention remains the province of the cardiothoracic surgeon.

8.3.8
Cardiac Injury

This is seen either with penetrating injuries (right > left ventricle), or as a result of severe central blunt force trauma (± sternal fracture). There are a whole gamut of possible injuries ranging from contusion, pericardial effusion and tamponade to laceration, septal defects, and acute valve dysfunction. Pericardial tamponade causes muffling of the heart sounds, impaired venous return (distended neck veins), and diminished cardiac output ($\downarrow$BP).

8.3.8.1
Investigations

1. ECG (looking for arrhythmia, ST elevation, etc.)
2. Cardiac enzymes
3. Echocardiography

Specific treatment is outside the remit of this book, but aspiration of a tamponade is an achievable object (ECG controlled, subxiphoid approach – aiming for tip of left scapula).

8.3.9
Diaphragm Injury

These usually arise as a result of penetrating injury and are frequently missed during the first 24 h. Severe blunt trauma (from MVA etc.) to the abdomen can cause a blow-out injury (left » right) causing postero-lateral tearing. Right-sided injuries are almost inevitably associated with severe liver injury (often caval) and frequently fatal. In adults at least, there is also a specific association of thoracic aortic injury and left diaphragm rupture.

Delayed presentation is possible as visceral herniation is a secondary phenomenon, and may lead to small bowel obstruction, presenting some weeks after the initial trauma.

8.3.9.1
Investigation

1. CXR and AXR – blurring of the hemidiaphragm is the first clue, but ~50% appear "normal."
2. US and CT scan – should identify visceral herniation, or lack of muscular integrity.

8.3.9.2
Treatment

- Diaphragm repair – abdominal approach, in the absence of other injury, usually straight-forward primary apposition.

Further Reading

1. American College of Surgeons (2009) Advanced trauma life support for doctors 7th edn. American College of Surgeons, IL
2. Bliss D, Silen M (2002) Pediatric thoracic trauma. Crit Care Med 30(11 suppl):S409–S415
3. Feliciano DV, Rozycki GS (1999) Advances in the diagnosis and treatment of thoracic trauma. Surg Clin North Am 79:1417–1429
4. Miller PR, Croce MA, Bee TK et al (2001) ARDS after pulmonary contusion: accurate measurement of contusion volume identifies high-risk patients. J Trauma 51:223–228
5. TRAUMA.org http://www.trauma.org/archive/thoracic/index.html

Basic Brain Injury

8.4

Mark Davenport

Single commonest cause of death in trauma.
Of patients with a GCS ≤8 at 6 h postinjury, ~50% will die.

8.4.1

- Common
- Mechanisms – MVA, falls from a height, penetrating, sports-related, horse-related, assaults
- M > F 2:1

8.4.2

- *Primary injury* – the motor vehicle, the horse, etc.
  (a) Damage done
- *Secondary injury* – consequent on hypoxia, hypoperfusion, ↑ICP (*intracranial pressure*). This is the only injury that can be influenced by active treatment.
  (a) Damage waiting to be done

8.4.3
Classification: Morphological

- Skull fractures
  — Linear, stellate
  — Depressed

M. Davenport
Paediatric Surgery Department, Kings College Hospital, London, UK

C. K. Sinha and M. Davenport (eds.), *Handbook of Pediatric Surgery*,
DOI: 10.1007/978-1-84882-132-3_8.4, © Springer-Verlag London Limited 2010

— Base of skull ± CSF leak (otorhea, rhinorhea) ± seventh nerve palsy
  ○ Periorbital hematoma – Battle's sign[1]
  ○ Retroauricular hematoma
● Intracranial hematomas
  — Extradural – (arterial, "talk and die"), temporal (middle meningeal artery), lenticular[2] hematoma
  — Subdural – (venous, slower onset), hematoma covers entire hemisphere, ↑ mortality
  — Intracerebral
● Diffuse brain injury
  — Mild concussion – confusion ± amnesia
  — Classic concussion – LOC (reversible), amnesia
  — Diffuse axonal injury – LOC, coma, autonomic dysfunction (e.g., ↑BP)

Monro–Kellie[3] Doctrine – volume of intracranial content is fixed in a rigid box. Therefore, an expansile mass can only move out of the liquid components (i.e., CSF and venous blood).
● Compensated – ICP → (if CSF/venous blood = mass volume)
● Uncompensated – ICP↑↑ (when compensation mechanism exhausted)

ICP (~10 mmHg, 13.6 cm H_2O adult).
Cerebral perfusion pressure = Arterial blood pressure (mean) – ICP.

8.4.4
Clinical Features

See Table 8.4.1

8.4.4.1
Evidence of Raised Intracranial Pressure

1. Cushing[4] reflex (↑ systolic pressure, ↓ pulse, ↓ respiratory rate).
2. Herniation of brain (cerebrum and cerebellum) outside fossa.
   (a) Transtentorial temporal lobe herniation
     ○ Third nerve compression
     ○ Brainstem compression

[1]William Henry Battle (1855–1936) English surgeon at St Thomas' Hospital, London. First man to describe laparotomy for postoperative adhesions.
[2]*Lenticular* (latin) – lens-shaped (bi-convex obviously).
[3]Alexander Monro (1733–1817); George Kellie (1758–1829). Both Scottish physicians. Clearly prempted the *other* Monroe Doctrine, best expressed as (to European states), Keep Off my Land! [President James Monroe, 1823].
[4]Harvey Williams Cushing (1869–1939) – Eminent American neurosurgeon and founder of the specialty.

Table 8.4.1 Quantification of degree of coma and LOC – Glasgow Coma Scale (GCS)

	Pediatric[1]	Adult	Score
Best eye opening	Spontaneously		4
	To speech		3
	To pain		2
	No response		1
Best verbal response	Coos/babbles "normal"	Orientated	5
	Irritable/cries continuously	Confused conversation	4
	Cries to pain	Inappropriate words	3
	Moans to pain	Incomprehensible sounds	2
	No response		1
Best motor response	Spontaneous/purposeful movements	Obeys command	6
	Withdraws from touch	Localizes pain	5
	Withdraws from pain	Normal flexion	4
	Abnormal flexion	Abnormal flexion	3
	Abnormal extension	Extension – decerebrate	2
	No response		1

[1]Pediatric GCS (3–15) – use if <2 years (i.e., preverbal)

(b) Tonsilar herniation "Coning" – cerebellar tonsils through foramen magnum
(c) Midline shift

- *Ipsilateral dilated, fixed pupil* – pupil size is governed by balance of sympathetic (dilating) and parasympathetic (constricting) action. Third (oculomotor) nerve carries parasympathetic fibers. False-positive in direct ocular trauma, some drugs, previous eye surgery, etc. Not affected by neuromuscular paralysis.
- *Contracoup injury* – movement of soft brain against the opposite side of the skull (e.g., occipital lobe trauma from frontal blunt force trauma).

8.4.5
Investigations

1. *Skull X-ray and C-spine* – fracture (400-fold risk of underlying hematoma in conscious patient). Ten percent of severe brain injury will have cervical injury.
2. CT head (indications vary).
   (a) GCS <13 at any point since the injury or GCS 13 or 14 (at 2 h post injury).
   (b) Open or depressed skull fracture.? Basal skull fracture.
   (c) Post-traumatic seizure.
   (d) Focal neurological deficit.
   (e) >1 episode of vomiting.
   (f) Amnesia for >30 min of events before impact.

8.4.6
Management

Up to 8% of children with a GCS of 15 following head injury will show radiographic injury on brain CT, of which ~50% may need intervention (surgeon/anticonvulsants).

Complex, but principles are:

1. Maintain oxygenation
    (a) Intubation and ventilation – GCS < 8, absence of protective (laryngeal) reflexes. Evidence of hypoxia (pO$_2$ < 8 KPa), maxillo-facial injury
2. Maintain cerebral perfusion
    (a) Avoid hypotension (usually extracranial)
3. Reduce ICP
    (a) Mannitol (20% solution) (1–2 mg/kg) (causes ↓ brain volume)
    (b) Barbiturates (e.g., phenobarbitone) by ↓ cerebral metabolism
    (c) Hyperventilation (↓pCO$_2$ causes reflex ↓ cerebral blood flow)
    (d) Neuromuscular paralysis – avoids coughing, straining, etc.
    (e) steroids, progesterone, dexamethasone
4. Evacuate hematoma

N.B. Posttraumatic epilepsy – up to 5% of closed brain injuries (requiring hospital admission)

Further Reading

1. Brain Trauma Foundation, American Association of Neurological Surgeons, Joint Section on Neurotrauma and Critical Care (1996) Guidelines for the management of severe head injury. J Neurotrauma 13:641–734
2. Teasdale G, Jennett B (1974) Assessment of coma and impaired con-sciousness. A practical scale. Lancet 2:81–84
3. Schouten JW (2007) Neuroprotection in traumatic brain injury: a complex struggle against the biology of nature. Curr Opin Crit Care 13:134–142

Part IX

Spina Bifida and Hydrocephalus

Spina Bifida

9.1

Ajay N. Gangopadhyay, Vijai D. Upadhyaya, and Anand Pandey

Spina bifida is a major and common cause of life-long disability, which can largely be prevented by increased dietary or supplemental folate.

Neural tube defects (NTD), a group of complex congenital anomalies of the central nervous system (CNS), are the second most common birth defects.

- 2–3/1,000 births
- Female predominance (most marked in anencephaly)
- Geographical variation – incidence ↑ Ireland, Scotland; ↓ Japan
- White > black

9.1.1
Etiology

1. Genetic – the recurrence risk for NTD in siblings is 2–5%.
2. Environmental.
   (a) X-irradiation.
   (b) Hyperthermia.
   (c) Drugs, e.g., thalidomide, folate antagonists, androgenic hormones, antiepileptics (valproate and carbamazepine), and hypervitaminosis A; substance abuse (e.g., alcohol); chemical agents (e.g., organic mercury, lead).
   (d) Maternal infections, e.g., rubella, cytomegalovirus, *Toxoplasma gondii*, syphilis.
   (e) Maternal metabolic conditions (e.g., phenylketonuria, diabetes mellitus, endemic cretinism).
3. Nutritional, e.g., folate deficiency, possibly due to polymorphisms in folate metabolizing enzymes and enhanced likelihood of meiotic nondisjunctions.

[Periconceptual dietary supplementation of folate can reduce incidence of NTD by 50%.]

A. N. Gangopadhyay (✉)
Department of Pediatric Surgery, Institute of Medical Sciences, BHU, Varanasi, India

C. K. Sinha and M. Davenport (eds.), *Handbook of Pediatric Surgery*,
DOI: 10.1007/978-1-84882-132-3_9.1, © Springer-Verlag London Limited 2010

9.1.2
Embryology

The human embryo passes through 23 stages of development after conception, each occupying approximately 2–3 days (Carnegie Stages[1]). Two different processes form the CNS.

Primary neurulation – formation of neural structures into a tube, thereby forming the brain and spinal cord.

1. Thickening of the ectoderm (from primitive node of Hensen[2] caudally to the prochordal plate rostrally).
2. Formation of neural plate is formed at stage 8 (days 17–19).
3. Neural folding occurs at stage 9 (days 19–21).
4. Fusion of the neural folds (days 22–23).
    (a) Closure of anterior neuropore (days 24–26).
    (b) Closure of posterior neuropore (days 26–28).

Secondary neurulation – formation of the lower spinal cord and future lumbar and sacral elements.

- Open NTDs are due to failure of primary neurulation.
- Closed NTDs result from a defect in secondary neurulation (Table 9.1.1).

9.1.3
Spina Bifida Occulta (SBO)

- Up to 20% of otherwise normal population

Table 9.1.1 Possible NTD malformations

Cranial	
Anencephaly	Failure of closure of anterior neuropore – incompatible with life. F ≫ M
Encephalocele	Failure of closure of anterior neuropore – ranges from occiput (visual impairment) to frontal bones
Craniorachischisis totalis	Exposure of entire neural plate. Incompatible with life
Spinal	
Spina bifida occulta	See below
Spina bifida cystica (or aperta)	See below

---

[1]CA Victor Hensen (1835–1924) German zoologist who also coined the term "plankton".

---

[2]Andrew Carnegie (1835-1919) Scottish-born industrialist, donated fortune to various scientific institutes and foundations. Original embryos classified at Carnegie Institute, Washington DC.

Bony defect but no herniation of meninges. Skin covered, although there may be a hairy patch, dermal sinus tract, dimple, hemangioma, or lipoma. *Occult spinal dysraphism* is the term used for uncommon (~2%) association with neurological abnormality or symptoms. MR scans may be indicated.

9.1.4
Spina Bifida Cystica

- *Myelomeningocele* (75%) – spinal cord and nerve roots herniate into a meningeal sac. The spinal cord often ends in this sac and is splayed open, exposing the central canal. Orthopedic and neurological effects common (Fig. 9.1.1).
- *Meningocele* (10%) – herniation of the meninges only through the bony defect. Neurological effects are not common.
- *Lipomeningocele or lipomyelomeningocele* (5%)–skin-covered lipomatous mass that herniates through the bony defect and attaches to the spinal cord, causing tethering of the cord and nerve roots (Fig. 9.1.2).
- *Myelocystocele* (rare) – the spinal cord has a large terminal cystic dilatation resulting from hydromyelia. It is associated with other major defects (e.g., cloacal extrophy, exomphalos).
- *Myelocele* (rare) – most severe form with complete failure of closure of the neural tube. It is usually fatal.

9.1.5
Diagnosis & Treatment

9.1.5.1
Prenatal

Open NTDs can be detected by measuring alpha-fetoprotein (α-FP) in the amniotic fluid and maternal serum. The latter one is commonly used as the basis for screening from 15th to 20th

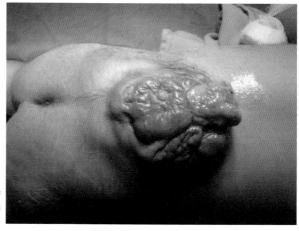

Fig. 9.1.1 Meningomyelocele (open neural tube defect) with patulous anus

Fig. 9.1.2 Lipomeningocele

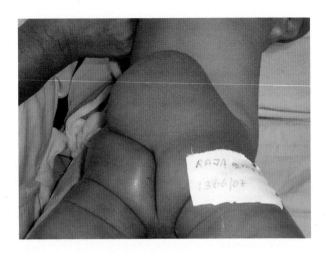

week. Fetal US (other causes include gastroschisis, etc.) and amniocentesis together with prenatal counseling are then used to complete the diagnosis and plan the next step. Options include termination (if society allows) or planned cesarean section delivery at appropriate tertiary care center.

The randomized *Management of Myelomeningocele Study* (MOMS) in the USA is currently recruiting affected fetuses to in utero skin coverage of the lesion (vs. conventional postnatal closure), with the aim of preserving neurology.

9.1.5.2
Postnatal

Treatment of spina bifida in neonates has evolved over the past half century from a period of nihilism and allowing nature to take its course through a period of aggressive early (almost emergency) back closure and unrestricted surgery in the 1960s and 1970s to a more selective policy based on the prediction of likely ("acceptable") outcome.

9.1.6
Surgery

Back closure is indicated to protect the compromised neural tissue. It should be sufficiently elective to avoid hypovolemia, hypothermia, and airway compromise but ideally within 36–48 h, to avoid infective complications.

9.1.6.1
Closure of Myelomeningocele

1. Circumferential skin incision.
2. Identification and dissection of the dura. Cover the neural placode by watertight closure of the dura. If the dura is absent, muscle fascia should be reflected off adjacent

muscle groups and again used to create a watertight tube to enclose the neural placode.

3. Skin closure is achieved by mobilizing the skin from the underlying paraspinal fascia in an avascular plane. Care is taken to avoid necrosis or ischemia.

9.1.6.2
Lipomeningocele

- The surgical goal in treating these lesions is to detach the lipoma of the buttocks from the lipoma that emerges through the dura, fascia, and bony defect.
- Identify normal anatomy and locate where the lipoma pierces the dura and enters the spinal cord. The lipoma is disconnected from the spinal cord (microsurgical technique or a carbon dioxide laser). Care should be taken to leave some lipoma on the cord to avoid injuring the underlying neural substrate. The filum terminale also is divided to further untether the cord.

9.1.6.3
Postnatal: Late

There is a spectrum of disability and deformity in spina bifida because of the varying degree of neurological involvement. It can be difficult to describe the typical child with SB. However, the three main areas that cause most problems are:

- *Central neurological* – typically related to the development of hydrocephalus (usually following back closure) and due to impaired CSF drainage (associated Arnold-Chiari malformation) (see chapter 9.2).
- *Orthopedic and peripheral neurological* – again the degree is related to the level of neural involvement.
- *Urology* – related to the level of neural involvement with a potential to develop life-threatening renal failure.

9.1.6.4
Central Neurology

Approximately 20% of all infants with myelomeningoceles will have significant hydro-cephalus at birth and a further 70% develop it after the back is closed. In some infants, shunt placement may be performed at the same time as back closure.

Management of hydrocephalus and its complication is considered in chapter 9.2.

9.1.7
Orthopedic/Peripheral Neurology

At birth, there is a flaccid paralyis of the muscle groups affected; however, thereafter various lower limb deformities have the potential to occur depending on level. Usually, this is due to unapposed muscle action across a joint. e.g. fixed flexion deformity of hip occurs with functioning hip flexors (L1) and absent extension (S2). Pressure sores are the principle complication of anesthetic skin.

Spinal radiography, CT, and MRI spine will detect relevant bony pathology and evaluate the risk of scoliosis and propensity to secondary neurological pathology (e.g., *tethered cord, diastematomelia,* intraspinal division of cord due to bony spur) and *syringomelia* (i.e., expansion of central canal, usually in cervical or thoracic parts, often associated with A–C malformation) (see chapter 9.2).

Management is complex (and outside limit of this chapter), but may include operations to centralize joints (tenotomies and casting), and correct scoliosis; together with braces and devices to aid development of walking, standing, etc.

9.1.8
Urological

Principle problem is the development of a *neuropathic bladder* (small volume, hypercontractile, ↑ intravesical pressure). This may lead to dilatation of upper tracts, hydronephrosis, and ultimately chronic renal failure. Serial US and urodynamics will direct the management strategy with the aim of preserved renal cortical function, an uninfected urinary tract, and a dry child.

Management

- Crede maneuver – emptying bladder by suprapubic pressure.
- Clean intermittent catheterization (from ~6 months) – urethral (usually anesthetic), or via Mitrofanoff[3] conduit (appendix) or Monti[4] (tubularized ileum).
- Bladder augmentation (stomach, ileum, colon) – ↑ capacity, ↓ upper tract pressure.
- Bladder neck reconstruction/closure.

9.1.9
Constipation and Incontinence

Sphincter control is often disturbed in SB, leading to incontinence, whereas poor colon motility and reduced activity lead to constipation. Regular laxatives may help timed defecation and a clear colon so aiding sphincter control. This principle can be taken a step further by the creation of an ACE (antegrade continent enema) stoma or cecostomy device to allow daily colon lavage.

9.1.10
Outcome

1. Intellect – in most series, 60–70% of the children with myelomeningocele have IQs > 80; others will have IQs in the delayed or severely delayed range.

---

[3]Paul Mitrofanoff – French urologist, technique first described in 1980.
[4]Paolo Ricardo Monti – Brazilian urologist, technique described in 1997.

   (a) IQ~102 – without hydrocephalus

   (b) IQ~95 – with hydrocephalus

   (c) IQ~73 – hydrocephalus + CNS infection

2. Bowel and bladder continence.

   (a) Only 10–15% of all children with myelomeningoceles are continent of urine

3. Ambulation – some children can ambulate in the community, some only in the home, others can only stand but not walk and the rest are wheelchair bound.

   (a) Many children with NTDs lose their ability to ambulate as they get older

Further Reading

1. Danzer E, Gerdes M, Bebbington MW et al (2009) Lower extremity neuromotor function and short-term ambulatory potential following in utero myelomeningocele surgery. Fetal Diagn Ther 25:47–53

2. Northrup H, Volcik KA (2000) Spina bifida and other neural tube defects. Curr Probl Pediatr 30:313–332

3. Thompson DN (2009) Postnatal management and outcome for neural tube defects including spina bifida and encephalocoeles. Prenat Diagn 29(4):412–419

Hydrocephalus

9.2

Ajay N. Gangopadhyay, Vijai D. Upadhyaya, and Anand Pandey

Hydrocephalus, obvious to the Ancients, is still seen in up to 1 in 500 births today.

Hydrocephalus[1] is an excessive accumulation of cerebrospinal fluid (CSF) within brain cavities (ventricles). Acute hydrocephalus occurs over days, subacute over weeks, and chronic over months or years. It is broadly classified into two groups:

- *Communicating* – full communication exists between the ventricles and subarachnoid space.
- *Noncommunicating* – CSF flow is obstructed within the ventricular system or in its outlets to the arachnoid space.

9.2.1
Physiology

- Normal CSF production ranges from 12 to 36 mL/h – mostly produced by the choroid plexus, which is located within the ventricular system (lateral and fourth ventricles 50–80%) but also from ventricular ependyma and brain parenchyma (20–50%).
- Total volume of CSF is 120 mL.
- Normal intracranial pressure is ~7 cm of H_2O ($\equiv$5 mmHg).
- CSF formation is energy-dependent.

---

[1]*Hydrocephalus* – Greek "water" and "of the head."

A. N. Gangopadhyay (✉)
Department of Pediatric Surgery, Institute of Medical Sciences, BHU, Varanasi, India

C. K. Sinha and M. Davenport (eds.), *Handbook of Pediatric Surgery*,
DOI: 10.1007/978-1-84882-132-3_9.2, © Springer-Verlag London Limited 2010

9.2.2
Anatomy (Fig. 9.2.1)

CSF (produced in the choroid plexus) flows from the lateral ventricles, through the inter-ventricular Foramina of Monro,[2] third ventricle, Aqueduct of Sylvius,[3] fourth ventricle, two lateral Foramina of Luschka[4] and one median Foramen of Magendie[5], and into the subarachnoid space. It is absorbed by arachnoid granulations into the dural sinus, and finally into the venous system.

Hydrocephalus can also be divided into congenital or acquired

9.2.2.1
Congenital

- Stenoses of the aqueduct of Sylvius (10% neonatal) – ↑ lateral and third with normal fourth ventricle
- Dandy[6]–Walker[7] malformation (2–4% neonatal) – F >> M, posterior fossa cyst and ↑ fourth ventricle

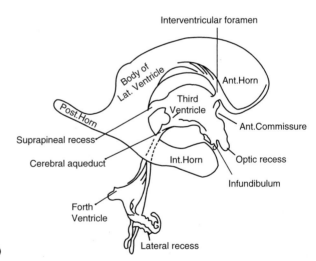

Fig. 9.2.1 Cast of ventricular system (from Gray's anatomy)

[2]Alexander Monro (1733–1817) Scottish physician.

[3]Franciscus Sylvius (1614–1762) German-born Dutch physician and scientist also credited with invention of gin!

[4]Hubert von Luschka (1820–1875) German anatomist.

[5]Francois Magendie (1783–1855) French physiologist, controversial in his day for practising live vivisection of animals.

[6]Walter E. Dandy (1886–1946) Pioneer American neurosurgeon, working at Johns Hopkins Hospital, Baltimore, USA.

- Arnold[8]–Chiari[9] malformation
  - Type 1 – cerebellar tonsillar ectopia
  - Type 2 – cerebellar vermis displacement associated with spina bifida (90%)
- Agenesis of the Foramen of Monro
- Congenital toxoplasmosis
- Bickers–Adams syndrome (X-linked recessive, severe mental retardation)

9.2.2.2
Acquired

- Intraventricular hemorrhage: It is usually due to prematurity, head injury, etc. [50% of infants < 1,500 g will develop an IVH]
- Mass lesions: tumor, cyst, abscess, or hematoma
- Meningitis
- ↑ Sinus venous pressure
- Iatrogenic – hypervitaminosis A
- Idiopathic

9.2.3
Clinical Features

These are variables depending on the rapidity of onset and age, but include poor feeding, irritability, vomiting, sleepiness, and reduced activity in infants together with headache, diminishing mental capacity, neck pain, blurred vision (papilledema), double vision (sixth cranial nerve), occasionally stunted growth, and sexual precocity in children.

Key signs in infants include progressive head enlargement (in those with unfused sutures), bulging eyes, failure to look upward, wide open fontanelles, "setting-sun" sign (visible sclera above downturned eyes), hypertonicity (due to stretching of periventricular pyramidal tract fibers). In children with a constrained cranial capacity, the signs are somewhat different but include papilledema (and later optic atrophy), failure of upward gaze (due to pressure on tectal plate), MacEwen's sign[10] ("cracked pot" feeling on skull percussion), unsteady gait, and a sixth cranial nerve palsy. Increasing head circumference is possible in children because of abnormal head growth (Fig. 9.2.2).

---

[7]Earl Walker (1907–1995) Canadian neurosurgeon, described second case (after Dandy's) in 1942.

[8]Julius Arnold (1835–1915) German pathologist – described after but independently from Chiari's description.

[9]Hans Chiari (1851–1916) Austrian pathologist.

[10]Sir William MacEwen (1848–1924) Scottish surgeon.

Fig. 9.2.2 This figure shows
enlarged head with dilated
veins and "setting-sun" sign

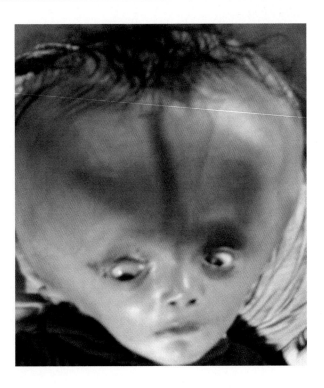

Hydrocephalus may be diagnosed prenatally, but does not develop until the third trimester and may be missed on early US.

- CSF protein content (esp. postthemorrhagic and postmeningitic).
- Genetic testing and counseling (if family history, when X-linked hydrocephalus is suspected).

9.2.4
Imaging

- Skull radiographs – erosion of sella turcica or "beaten copper cranium" (called by some authors "beaten silver cranium"). The latter can also be seen in craniosynostosis.
- US (in infants) evaluation of subependymal and intraventricular hemorrhage.
- *CT/MRI criteria for acute hydrocephalus* include the following:
  1. Temporal horns >2 mm; sylvian and interhemispheric fissures are not visible.
  2. Ratio between the largest width of the frontal horns and the internal diameter from inner table to inner table at this level should be >0.5.
  3. Ratio of the largest width of the frontal horns to maximal biparietal diameter (Evans ratio) is >30%.
  4. Transependymal absorption is translated on images as periventricular low density.

5. Ballooning of frontal horns of lateral ventricles and third ventricle ("Mickey Mouse[11]" ventricles) indicates aqueductal obstruction.
6. Upward bowing of the corpus callosum on sagittal MRI indicates acute hydrocephalus.

- *Radionuclide cisternography* can be done in normal pressure hydrocephalus (NPH) to evaluate the prognosis with regard to possible shunting. If a late scan (48–72 h) shows persistence of ventricular activity, the patient is more likely to benefit from shunting (75% chance).

9.2.5
Management

9.2.5.1
Medical

Medical treatment is used to delay surgical intervention but may induce metabolic consequences.

1. Acetazolamide (carbonic anhydrase inhibitor) and furosemide – ↓ CSF secretion by choroid plexus.
2. Isosorbide – ↑ CSF reabsorption (effectiveness).
3. Cyproheptadine or propranol – some children patients with neurological deterioration after functioning shunt surgery may benefit.

9.2.5.2
Surgery

Resectional surgery is indicated if the cause is removable (e.g., adenoma of choroid plexus, papilloma, cyst, or tumor). However, the majority of cases require a shunt procedure to alleviate the hydrocephalus rather than treat the underlying cause. The principle is to establish a communication between the CSF (ventricular or lumbar) and a drainage cavity (peritoneum, right atrium, pleura).

The modern era begins in the 1950s with Eugene Spitz inserting a totally implantable one-way pressure-regulated valve, allowing the ventricle to drain into the right atrium via the jugular vein (Spitz–Holter valve).

- Ventriculoperitoneal (VP) shunt (commonest)
  - Has intrinsic growth factor with long peritoneal catheter.
- Ventriculoatrial (VA) shunt
  - Uses jugular vein and SVC/right atrium.
  - Used when abdomen is contraindicated (e.g., peritonitis, morbid obesity, or after extensive abdominal surgery).

---

[11]Mickey Mouse – Walt Disney creation, this feature refers to the appearance of his ears!

- Lumboperitoneal shunt
  - for communicating hydrocephalus, CSF fistula, or pseudotumor cerebri.
- *Torkildsen shunt* (rare)
  - Shunts the ventricle to cisternal space and is effective only in acquired obstructive hydrocephalus.

9.2.5.3
Shunt Complications

Only about 50% of shunts inserted will be normally functional at 2 years postoperatively. Most cases of shunt malfunction are due to *occlusion of the proximal ventricular catheter*. In these instances, pumping of the shunt will show a valve that is slow to refill, or does not refill at all.

- *Proximal catheter obstruction* – ↑ risk in the first months following placement, usually due to choroid plexus or blood clot generated from the initial insult.
- *Distal shunt malfunction* – Most are related to bacterial colonizaton of the shunt, rather than length problems. Abdominal pseudocyst formation (detected on abdominal US or CT scan) is presumptive of shunt infection.
- *Shunt infections* (10–15%) – Most of them occurring in the first 5 days after surgery. Signs include fever, neck stiffness, light sensitivity, and headaches (Commonest coagulase negative *Staphyloccocal spp.*). Treatment is by externalization or removal and replacements of shunt components + appropriate antibiotics.
- *Shunt fracture* – Common cause of shunt failure is disconnection or fracture of tubing. Incidence has been lessened by the use of one-piece shunts.
- *Over-drainage* – This may cause headaches, lethargy, and nausea. Change to a higher pressure valve or insertion of an "anti-syphon device" may help but not invariably. This may lead to:
- *Slit ventricle syndrome* – It occurs after several years and is characterized by chronic or recurring headaches and slit-like ventricles on CT scan.
- *Extrusion of shunt* – It may occur through the umbilicus, abdominal wall, anus, vagina, and scrotum.
- *Under-drainage* – This may occur due to inability to keep up with CSF production and recurrence of hydrocephalus due to blockage or disconnection. Pressure may sometimes build up rapidly, resulting in loss of consciousness and necessitating urgent treatment.

9.2.5.4
Alternatives to Shunting

- Choroid plexectomy or choroid plexus coagulation.
- *Opening of a stenosed aqueduct* (↑ morbidity rate and a ↓ success rate than shunting).
- *Endoscopic fenestration* of the floor of the third ventricle establishes an alternative route for CSF toward the subarachnoid space. It is contraindicated in communicating hydrocephalus.

9.2.6
Outcome

If untreated, the prognosis is poor (~50% mortality within 3 years) and ~25% survive until adulthood with below average intelligence.

With shunt surgery, ~50% will achieve a normal IQ – this is reduced if there is history of convulsions, shunt complications, and with certain underlying causes (e.g., intraventricular hemorrhage and prematurity).

Further Reading

1. Czosnyka M, Pickard JD (2004) Monitoring and interpretation of intracranial pressure. J Neurol Neurosurg Psychiatr 75:813–821
2. Libenson MH, Kaye EM, Rosman NP (1999) Acetazolamide and furosemide for posthemorrhagic hydrocephalus of the newborn. Pediatr Neurol 20:185–191
3. Lima MM, Pereira CU, Silva AM (2007) Ventriculoperitoneal shunt infections in children and adolescents with hydrocephalus. Arq Neuropsiquiatr 65:118–123
4. Sansone JM, Iskandar BJ (2005) Endoscopic cerebral aqueductoplasty: a trans-fourth ventricle approach. J Neurosurg 103:388–392

Part X

Appendices

Reference Weights and Heights

10.1

Mark Davenport

10.1.1
Conversion Factors

Depending on origin and country, parents tend to talk in traditional units when discussing their offspring's measurements. Some conversion factors may be appropriate (Tables 10.1.1 and 10.1.2).

Table 10.1.1 Anglocentric (Imperial & USA) measurements

Weight	
1 kg≡2.2 lb (pounds)	1 lb≡0.45 kg
	14 lbs=1 stone
1 kg≡34 oz (ounces)	1 oz≡28 g
1 g≡0.035 oz	
Length	
1 m≡3.3 ft (feet)	1 yd≡0.91 m
	1 ft≡0.30 m
1 cm≡0.4 in. (inches)	1 in.≡2.5 cm
Liquid	
1 L≡1.76 pt (pints) (UK)	1 pt≡570 mL (UK)
1 L≡2.11 pt (US)	1 pt (UK)=20 fl oz
	1 pt (US)=16 fl oz
	1 fl oz≡28 mL (UK)≡29 mL (US)
Energy	
1 kJ≡0.24 kcal	1 kcal≡4.2 kJ
Pressure	
1 kPa≡7.5 mmHg	1 mmHg≡133 Pa (Pascal)

M. Davenport
Paediatric Surgery Department, Kings College Hospital, London, UK

C. K. Sinha and M. Davenport (eds.), *Handbook of Pediatric Surgery*,
DOI: 10.1007/978-1-84882-132-3_10.1, © Springer-Verlag London Limited 2010

Table 10.1.2 Average and normal

Age	Weight (kg)	Height (cm)	Body surface area (m^2)
Neonate (term)	3.5	50	0.23
1 month	4.2	55	0.27
3 month	5.6	59	0.33
6 month	7.7	67	0.41
1 year	10	76	0.49
3 year	15	94	0.65
5 year	18	108	0.74
10 year	30	132	1.1
14 year	50	163	1.5
Adult (male)	70	173	1.8
Adult (female)	56	163	1.6

Anatomical Reference

10.2

Mark Davenport

10.2.1
Cranial Nerves

See Table 10.2.1

10.2.2
Dermatomes and Myotomes

See Fig. 10.2.1

10.2.3
Segmental Liver Anatomy

- The liver is the largest organ within the body. It has a dual blood supply (flow – portal vein 75%, hepatic artery 25%) and venous drainage to the IVC.
- The segments of the liver (I–VIII) are potentially independent units with limited cross-over.

Basic division into Right and Left along the *"principal plane" of Cantlie,*[1] each being supplied by right and left portal vein, respectively. The plane runs from gallbladder bed along line of middle hepatic vein toward its confluence. The *obvious falciform ligament* separates segments II and III from IV.

---

[1]Sir James Cantlie (1851–1926) – Scottish surgeon.

M. Davenport
Paediatric Surgery Department, Kings College Hospital, London, UK

C. K. Sinha and M. Davenport (eds.), *Handbook of Pediatric Surgery*,
DOI: 10.1007/978-1-84882-132-3_10.2, © Springer-Verlag London Limited 2010

- Right – V, VI, VII, VIII
- Left – II, III, IV (quadrate lobe)
  — Segment I – caudate lobe. Surrounds cava, and has separate drainage through 4–8 small direct veins (Fig. 10.2.2)

Table 10.2.1 Cranial nerves

Cranial nerve	Role	Course	Notes
I (olfactory)	S – smell	Multiple through olfactory plate	
II (optic)	S – vision	Optic canal	part of CNS
III (oculomotor)	M – all but two eye muscles	Sup. Orb. fissure	
IV (trochlear)	M – sup.obl.	Sup. Orb. fissure	Smallest, longest, exits back of brainstem
V (trigeminal)	V1 S – opthalmic V2 S – maxillary V3 S – mandibular	V1 Sup. Orb. fissure V2 F. rotundum V3 F. ovale	M – mastication
VI (abducens)	M – abducens	Sup. Orb. fissure	
VII (facial)	M/S (taste) T – temporal Z – zygomatic B – buccal M – mandibular C – cervical	Int. acoustic canal→ Facial canal (→chorda tympani) → Stylomastoid foramen	M – facial expression, platysma. Stapedius Secretory – submandibular/ lingual
VIII (vestibulocochlear)	S – hearing and balance	Int. acoustic canal	
IX (glossopharyngeal)	M/S – (taste)	Jugular foramen	M – stylopharyngeus, secretory – parotid
X (vagus)	M/S	Jugular foramen	M – larynx, pharynx, GI tract
XI (accessory)	M – neck	Jugular foramen	M – trapezius and sternomastoid
XII (hypoglossal)	M – tongue	Hypoglossal canal	

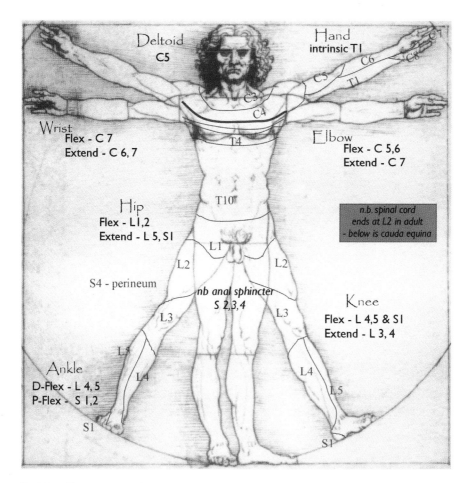

Fig. 10.2.1   Dermatomes and myotomes

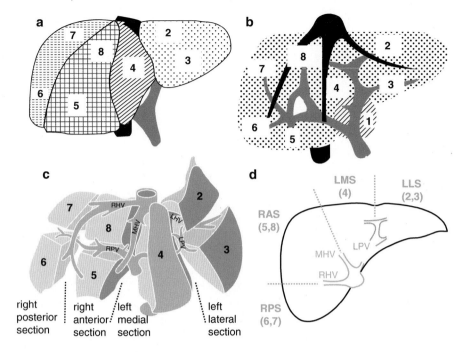

Fig. 10.2.2 Segmental anatomy of liver

Mark Davenport

10.3.1
Prenatal Development

40 weeks (280 days) gestation measured from the first day of the last period – so, fertilization should actually occur at +2 weeks.

Three trimesters[1]
First trimester – week 1 – week 13
Second trimester – week 14 – week 27
Third trimester = week 28 – week 40

- "Egg" phase
  (a) fertilization (zygote) to morula,[2] to blastocyst (58 cells+) and implantation into the wall of the uterus
  (b) 1–4 Days
- Embryonic
  (a) Controversial definition of beginning
  (b) Ends at eighth week

    1. Gastrulation and formation of trilaminar disc (16 days)
    2. Morphogenesis begins
    3. Yolk sac and amnion formation
    4. "Tube within a tube"
    5. Fusion of neural folds (22 days)

---

[1]Trimester – i.e.,3 months.
[2]*Morula* (Latin) – mulberry.

M. Davenport
Paediatric Surgery Department, Kings College Hospital, London, UK

C. K. Sinha and M. Davenport (eds.), *Handbook of Pediatric Surgery*,
DOI: 10.1007/978-1-84882-132-3_10.3, © Springer-Verlag London Limited 2010

6. Formation of urorectal septum, dorsal pancreatic bud, rupture of oro-pharyngeal membrane (26 days)
7. Formation of primary intestinal loop (32 days)
8. Ascent of the kidneys (37 days)
9. Limb buds show distinct fingers (41 days)
10. Closure of pericardio-pleural-peritoneal canals (51 days)
11. SVC formed, patency of entire GI tract (56 days)

- Fetal
  (a) Eighth week till birth

10.3.2
Ultrasound Scans in Pregnancy

1. Viability scan (6–10 weeks)
    (a) Carried out usually transvaginally. To determine number of fetuses & viability.
2. 11–13 week scan
    (a) Carried out transabdominally. To determine accurate dating, assess the risks of chromosomal anomaly (nuchal translucency etc). Some major anomalies visible.
3. Anomaly scan (18–22 weeks)
    (a) Transabdominal. Assessment of facial appearance and determines whether thoracic and abdominal organ anomalies exist.
4. Cardiac scan (20 weeks onwards)
    (a) To assess the risk of cardiac anomalies.
5. Wellbeing scan (32 weeks onwards)
    (a) To prepare for birth, and assess fetal growth and placental function.

10.3.3
Developmental Milestones

Developmental delay occurs in up to 15% of children under 5 years of age, and about half with developmental problems are detected before they begin school (Table 10.3.1).

Table 10.3.1   Developmental milestones

Age	Behavior
1–2 Months	
	Smiles, responds to bell, lifts head, regards face
6 Months	
Gross	Rises, rolls over, sits with support, raises head
Fine	Whole hand grasp, object to mouth
Verbal	Babbles
Social	"Peek-a-boo"
12 Months	
	Walks
	Pincer grasp
	Understands simple instructions, knows name
	"Wants…," plays ball
18 Months	
	Walks up stairs
	Builds 3 cube tower, drinks from cup
	Says 5–20 words, combines
	Helps in house, uses spoon
2 Years	
	Runs, kicks ball, jumps
	Tower of 8 cubes. Copies circle
	Says up to 50 words. Two-word phrases. Intelligible
	Scribbles, turns pages, puts on clothes

NB – Based on Denver Developmental Screening Test, devised in 1969 and revised in 1992.[3]

---

[3]http://developmentalscreening.org/screening_tools/denverii.htm.

Index

Printed by Printforce, the Netherlands